Molecular Pathology Library

Series Editor

Philip T. Cagle
Houston, TX, USA

Creating a diagnostic, prognostic, and therapeutic treatment strategy precisely tailored to each patient's requirements is the fundamental idea behind precision medicine. The Molecular Pathology Library series integrates molecular biology with clinical data for treatment designed for the patient's individual genetic makeup. This approach is widely recognized as the future of medicine and it is vital for practicing pathologists to know the molecular biology, diagnostics and predictive biomarkers for specific forms of cancer or other diseases and their implications for treatment. Each volume focuses on a specific type of cancer or disease and provides concise essential information in a readily accessible, user friendly, convenient format. Each volume is oriented towards the pathologist who needs this information for daily practice, tumor boards, and conferences or for preparation for certification boards or other tests. Written by experts focusing on patient care, these books are indispensible aids to pathologists' participation in precision medicine in the 21st century.

More information about this series at http://www.springer.com/series/7723

José Javier Otero • Aline Paixao Becker

Editors

Precision Molecular Pathology of Glioblastoma

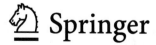

Editors
José Javier Otero
Neuropathology
The Ohio State University
Columbus, OH
USA

Aline Paixao Becker
Radiation Oncology
The Ohio State University
Columbus, OH
USA

ISSN 1935-987X   ISSN 1935-9888   (electronic)
Molecular Pathology Library
ISBN 978-3-030-69172-1   ISBN 978-3-030-69170-7   (eBook)
https://doi.org/10.1007/978-3-030-69170-7

This Springer imprint is published by the registered company Springer Nature Switzerland AG
The registered company address is: Gewerbestrasse 11, 6330 Cham, Switzerland

*To our patients, who selflessly permitted
tissue procurement for research and
contributed to all of the knowledge in
this book.
To our families, who provide us the support
to carry on in happy and in difficult times.*

J.J.O. and A.P.B.

Foreword

The modern practice of neuropathology is both stimulating and overwhelming. Making a diagnosis can be difficult enough, but the standard of care has gone far beyond simply providing a diagnosis. Over the last decade, the practice of diagnostic medicine has become increasingly complex. This was reflected in the restructuring of the 2016 WHO Classification of Tumours of the Central Nervous System to include an integrated diagnosis format combining histologic and molecular genetic data. As such, pathologists and treating physicians are necessarily becoming more familiar with the molecular pathogenesis of brain tumors and how it relates to diagnosis, prognosis, and treatment. Nowhere is this more relevant than in the study of the most common primary malignant brain tumor, glioblastoma.

Precision Molecular Pathology of Glioblastoma focuses on various aspects of cancer neuroscience, tumor pathology, epidemiology, molecular genetics, and cutting-edge treatment of this deadly disease. This book provides a deep dive into the current understanding of the neurobiology of glioblastoma and the clinical applicability of its molecular underpinnings. The authors address current obstacles in diagnosis and the barriers to implementing molecular diagnostic techniques in pathology laboratories, particularly in developing countries. Other timely topics include machine learning and learning-based automated methods for brain tumor classification and stem cell-based modeling of glioblastoma. The editors and contributing authors are a renowned group of neuroscientists, pathologists, and physicians who are experts in their fields, across many different institutions, states, and even countries.

While great strides have been made in the fields of molecular biology and neuroscience, there are still many challenges facing clinicians and pathologists in the pursuit of more accurate and prognostically relevant diagnoses. Drs. Jose Otero and

Aline Becker, both outstanding physician-scientists and neuropathologists, have edited a state-of-the-art book to aid us in the quest for precision medicine. I know you will find it informative and useful in your practice.

Michelle Madden Felicella, MD
Associate Professor of Pathology/Neuropathology,
University of Texas Medical Branch
Galveston, TX, USA

Preface

Very few human diseases require as much of an integrated approach to patient management than primary brain cancers. Primary brain tumors are the first solid tissue cancer for which widely accepted diagnostic guidelines require molecular pathology for diagnosis. The information obtained from the genomic testing is important for both prognostication and treatment planning, as well as to assist in making decisions to enroll a patient into a clinical trial that may involve targeted therapy. Implementing these diagnostic workflows creates several problems for patient care. First, in the USA, the number of pathologists per 100,000 people has declined, with now only 439 formally trained neuropathologists reported in the USA per recent reports. Formal training in neuropathology is needed to provide optimal patient care at the point of neurosurgical intraoperative consultations as well as integration of histopathological and molecular pathological testing. Exacerbating this challenge is the fact that current reimbursement rates for neuropathological intraoperative consultation is only \$63.17 per consult (CPT code = 88331)[1], rendering it financially unfeasible to staff neuropathologists to be on-call in most community clinical settings, ultimately leading to non-neuropathologists commonly fielding neurosurgical intraoperative consultations throughout the USA; neuropathology staffing problems are even worse worldwide. Furthermore, treatment planning by neuro-oncologists and radiation oncologists requires integrated histopathological/molecular pathological reports by trained neuropathologists. As primary brain cancers are rare, glioma-specific biomarkers are not commonly stocked in community and academic pathology laboratories. This even includes basic diagnostic and prognostic neuro-oncologic biomarker tests such as ATRX, H3^{K27M}, or even IDH1^{R132H} assays, all of which can be implemented on routine immunohistochemistry platforms which are widely deployed globally. A third challenge includes the US regulatory and financial landscape of molecular pathology testing. In contrast to most immunohistochemical assays which may obtain reimbursement from the same CPT code

---

[1] Current Procedural Terminology (CPT) codes, also known as service codes, are a universal system that identifies medical procedures in the USA. Reimbursement is in US Dollars as of December 28, 2020.

regardless of biomarker detected, each molecular pathology test in the USA requires a unique CPT code for each new biomarker in order to obtain reimbursement. This generates a high bar for individual molecular pathology laboratories in cancer centers to bring on new, "home-brewed" molecular assays. Also, modern technologies such as chromosomal microarray to date have not been, and will likely never be, reimbursed by most Medicare and private insurance providers. In addition, next generation sequencing (NGS) platforms have poor history of reimbursement and is therefore rarely performed outside major cancer centers in the USA. Furthermore, insurance companies in most US states that cover molecular testing will only reimburse FDA-approved NGS tests once per patient per cancer. This is problematic given the natural evolution of gliomas and the tendency to develop different molecular subclones later in the disease course.

These challenges have led to some entrepreneurial data monetization strategies, where NGS testing is cost-subsidized by private companies so that their data scientists may access patient data. Although such innovative approaches may represent positive short-term solution, instituting such an approach globally that is self-sustainable has several challenges. Furthermore, single-gene molecular pathology assays and NGS technologies benefit from economies of scale, resulting in the need to perform "batch testing." All of these factors result in excessive turnaround times (TATs) in neuropathology. At our own institution, our average TAT for neuropathology exceeds 6 business days to "result" a patient diagnosis, with molecular pathology information "resulted" typically over 12 business days following surgery. In the case of community pathologists, the TAT is even longer, as these cases would be sent out to expert neuropathologists for consultation. The net result of these challenges is delayed treatment plan generation by the neuro-oncologists and radiation oncologists.

It is with these issues in mind that we began to work on the design of this book. Although molecular sub-typing of primary brain cancers has been extremely important in providing accurate information regarding the patient diagnosis and prognosis, its implementation has not been fully equitable throughout the world. For these reasons, we attempted to provide a balanced and realistic approach review of the current state of glioblastoma understanding, ranging from traditional histological review, molecular pathology of glioma, modern radiomics, neurosurgical focus, and integration of treatment plans by neuro-oncologists. We also include chapters focused on implementing molecular pathology programs in developing countries and immunohistochemical surrogates for molecular pathology. This book is therefore aimed for a wide audience ranging from medical students and residents to practicing neuro-oncologists, radiologists, pathologists, and neurosurgeons. We hope that after reading this book, you will be inspired to work towards improving the lives of patients with high-grade glioma.

Columbus, OH, USA   José Javier Otero, MD, PhD

Contents

Part III   Key Molecular Pathways in Glioblastoma Development and Progression

Contributors

Samirkumar B. Amin The Jackson Laboratory for Genomic Medicine, Farmington, CT, USA

Sasha Beyer Department of Radiation Oncology, Arthur G. James Hospital/The Ohio State University Comprehensive Cancer Center, Columbus, OH, USA

Carlos Gilberto Carlotti Jr Division of Neurosurgery, Department of Surgery and Anatomy, Ribeirão Preto, SP, Brazil

Clinics Hospital, Ribeirão Preto School of Medicine, University of São Paulo, São Paulo, SP, Brazil

School of Medicine of Ribeirao Preto University of Sao Paulo, São Paulo, SP, Brazil

Arnab Chakravarti Department of Radiation Oncology, Arthur G. James Hospital/The Ohio State University Comprehensive Cancer Center, Columbus, OH, USA

Benedicto Oscar Colli Division of Neurosurgery, Department of Surgery and Anatomy, Ribeirão Preto, SP, Brazil

Clinics Hospital, Ribeirão Preto School of Medicine, University of São Paulo, São Paulo, SP, Brazil

School of Medicine of Ribeirao Preto University of Sao Paulo, São Paulo, SP, Brazil

David J. Cote, PhD Channing Division of Network Medicine, Brigham and Women's Hospital, Harvard Medical School, Boston, MA, USA

Computational Neuroscience Outcomes Center, Department of Neurosurgery, Brigham and Women's Hospital, Harvard Medical School, Boston, MA, USA

Huifang Dai Department of Pathology, Duke University School of Medicine, Durham, NC, USA

Ayca Ersen Danyeli, MD Acibadem MAA University, Faculty of Medicine, Pathology Department, Istanbul, Turkey

Ricardo Santos de Oliveira Division of Neurosurgery, Department of Surgery and Anatomy, Ribeirão Preto, SP, Brazil

Clinics Hospital, Ribeirão Preto School of Medicine, University of São Paulo, São Paulo, SP, Brazil

School of Medicine of Ribeirao Preto University of Sao Paulo, São Paulo, SP, Brazil

Macarena Ines de La Fuente, MD Department of Neurology and Sylvester Comprehensive Cancer Center, University of Miami, Miami, FL, USA

Maria del Pilar Guillermo Prieto, MD Department of Neurology and Sylvester Comprehensive Cancer Center, University of Miami, Miami, FL, USA

Khan M. Iftekharuddin, PhD Vision Lab, Electrical & Computer Engineering, Old Dominion University, Norfolk, VA, USA

Balveen Kaur, PhD The Department of Neurosurgery, McGovern Medical School, The University of Texas Health Science Center at Houston, Houston, TX, USA

Peter J. Kobalka, MD The Ohio State University Medical Center, Department of Pathology and Laboratory Medicine, Columbus, OH, USA

Giselle Y. López, MD, PhD Department of Pathology, Duke University School of Medicine, Durham, NC, USA

The Preston Robert Tisch Brain Tumor Center, Duke University School of Medicine, Durham, NC, USA

Duke Cancer Institute, Duke University School of Medicine, Durham, NC, USA

Marcus M. Matsushita, MD, PhD Department of Pathology, Barretos Cancer Hospital, São Paulo, Brazil

Ryan McCormack The Department of Neurosurgery, McGovern Medical School, The University of Texas Health Science Center at Houston, Houston, TX, USA

Quinn T. Ostrom, PhD Central Brain Tumor Registry of the United States, Hinsdale, IL, USA

Section of Epidemiology and Population Sciences, Department of Medicine, Dan L. Duncan Comprehensive Cancer Center, Baylor College of Medicine, Houston, TX, USA

Yoshihiro Otani The Department of Neurosurgery, McGovern Medical School, The University of Texas Health Science Center at Houston, Houston, TX, USA

Linmin Pei Department of Radiology, University of Pittsburgh, Pittsburgh, PA, USA

Hillman Cancer Center, University of Pittsburgh Medical Center, Pittsburgh, PA, USA

Vision Lab, Electrical & Computer Engineering, Old Dominion University, Norfolk, VA, USA

Christopher R. Pierson, MD, PhD Department of Pathology, Nationwide Children's Hospital, Columbus, OH, USA

Guilherme Gozzoli Podolsky-Gondim Division of Neurosurgery, Department of Surgery and Anatomy, Ribeirão Preto, SP, Brazil

Clinics Hospital, Ribeirão Preto School of Medicine, University of São Paulo, São Paulo, SP, Brazil

School of Medicine of Ribeirao Preto University of Sao Paulo, São Paulo, SP, Brazil

Appaji Rayi, MD The Ohio State University Medical Center, Department of Neurology/Neuro-oncology, Columbus, OH, USA

Charleston Area Medical Center, Department of Neurology, Charleston, WV, USA

Miranda M. Tallman Department of Radiation Oncology, James Cancer Hospital and Comprehensive Cancer Center, The Ohio State University College of Medicine, Columbus, OH, USA

Biomedical Graduate Program, The Ohio State University, Columbus, OH, USA

Diana L. Thomas, MD, PhD Department of Pathology, The Ohio State University and Nationwide Children's Hospital, Columbus, OH, USA

Monica Venere Department of Radiation Oncology, James Cancer Hospital and Comprehensive Cancer Center, The Ohio State University College of Medicine, Columbus, OH, USA

Yuanfan Yang Department of Pathology, Duke University School of Medicine, Durham, NC, USA

The Preston Robert Tisch Brain Tumor Center, Duke University School of Medicine, Durham, NC, USA

Kwanha Yu, PhD Center for Cell and Gene Therapy, Department of Neurosurgery, Baylor College of Medicine, Houston, TX, USA

Abigail A. Zalenski Department of Radiation Oncology, James Cancer Hospital and Comprehensive Cancer Center, The Ohio State University College of Medicine, Columbus, OH, USA

Neuroscience Graduate Program, The Ohio State University, Columbus, OH, USA

Part I
General Principles

Chapter 1
Epidemiology and Etiology of Glioblastoma

David J. Cote and Quinn T. Ostrom

Introduction

Glioblastoma (GB) is the most common primary brain malignancy, comprising more than half of all malignant brain and CNS tumors (Fig. 1.1) [1]. GB encompasses all gliomas categorized as grade IV in the World Health Organization classification system, which defines grades by increasing levels of aggressiveness and histological features. As a group, GB are highly aggressive and diffusely invasive of the healthy brain parenchyma, with dismal survival rates despite ongoing research into more effective therapies.

As a relatively rare disease, the epidemiology of GB has been assembled from a variety of contexts, including large prospective cohort, retrospective cohort, and case-control studies. Several randomized controlled trials have evaluated treatment efficacy for GB patients, but the vast majority of high-quality data for GB epidemiology derives from population based registries [1]. More recently, high-quality Mendelian randomization (MR) and genome-wide association (GWAS) studies have provided new evidence for behavioral and genetic risk factors, respectively [2, 3].

D. J. Cote (✉)
Channing Division of Network Medicine, Brigham and Women's Hospital, Harvard Medical School, Boston, MA, USA

Computational Neuroscience Outcomes Center, Department of Neurosurgery, Brigham and Women's Hospital, Harvard Medical School, Boston, MA, USA
e-mail: david_cote@hms.harvard.edu

Q. T. Ostrom
Central Brain Tumor Registry of the United States, Hinsdale, IL, USA

Section of Epidemiology and Population Sciences, Department of Medicine, Dan L. Duncan Comprehensive Cancer Center, Baylor College of Medicine, Houston, TX, USA

J. J. Otero, A. P. Becker (eds.), *Precision Molecular Pathology of Glioblastoma*, Molecular Pathology Library, https://doi.org/10.1007/978-3-030-69170-7_1

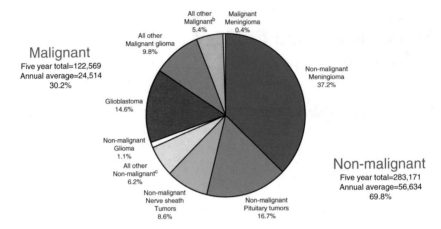

Fig. 1.1 Distribution of primary brain and other CNS tumors in the United States, 2012–2016. (From: Ostrom et al. [1])

Recent developments in GB epidemiology include an increasing emphasis on molecular markers, which play an important prognostic role for GB patients and in basic and clinical research on these tumors [4, 5]. In addition, progress has been made in the investigation of risk factors for these tumors, given the accumulation of sufficient cases in high quality cohort and case-control studies [2, 6, 7].

In this chapter, we briefly review the epidemiology of GB, with the aim of providing context to epidemiological, basic, and clinical research on these tumors. In particular, we describe the overall epidemiology of GB, the molecular factors that are relevant to prognosis, and etiologic risk factors that may play a role in incidence.

Epidemiological Features of GB

The epidemiology of GB has been described thoroughly in prior publications [1, 8, 9]. To briefly review, GB is overall a rare malignancy. Glioma, of which GB is the high-grade form, has an annual age-adjusted incidence rate of only 6.0 per 100,000 in the United States; roughly half of these are GB [1]. In general, GB occurs among older adults, particularly in the sixth and seventh decade of life, and is more common among men than women, with a male:female incidence ratio around 1.4 [1, 8].

Previous studies have demonstrated substantial differences in incidence of GB by race and ethnicity, with incidence rates of GB among White Americans roughly doubling those among Black Americans [10]. These results have been extended to other countries, with consistent findings that incidence of GB is highest among White individuals, but no underlying mechanisms for this disparity have been identified. Due to its rarity, most patients presenting with GB do not have a family history, but a family history of GB has been shown to increase risk roughly two-fold [9]. Other factors that are purported to affect risk are discussed later in the chapter.

Despite intensive research, survival rates for GB have remained relatively unchanged since the introduction of the Stupp protocol in 2005 [11]. This treatment protocol, consisting of administration of oral temozolomide with radiotherapy and an adjuvant course of temozolomide, was shown to increase median survival from 12 to 15 months compared with radiotherapy only [8]. In addition to maximum safe neurosurgical resection, temozolomide and radiotherapy are the mainstay of modern treatment for GB. Despite these interventions, current survival rates for GB remain dismal, with a 1 year relative survival of around 40% and a 5 year relative survival around 5% [10]. Roughly 1% of patients with GB will develop drop metastases to the spinal cord, but otherwise GB almost never metastasizes. Short survival in the context of GB is often attributable to expansion of the primary lesion, with diffuse invasion of the brain and mass effect and disruption of healthy brain architecture.

Survival rates have also been shown to vary by demographic features, with recent evidence that survival rates are worst among White patients compared to other racial and ethnic groups (Fig. 1.2). In addition to receipt of standard therapy, extent of surgical resection plays an important role in prognosis, with maximal resection providing the greatest survival benefit compared to subtotal resection or biopsy alone [4].

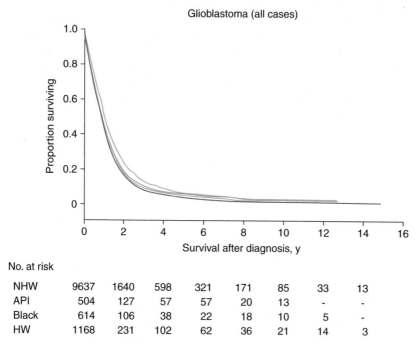

Glioblastoma (all cases)

No. at risk

NHW	9637	1640	598	321	171	85	33	13
API	504	127	57	57	20	13	-	-
Black	614	106	38	22	18	10	5	-
HW	1168	231	102	62	36	21	14	3

Fig. 1.2 Survival for GB patients by race/ethnicity, adjusted for age and extent of resection, 2000–2014. (From: Ostrom et al. [10])

Molecularly, GB is a highly heterogeneous group of tumors, with recent publications highlighting that classical categorization of GB by histologic features alone is insufficient. In particular, molecular classification of GB is paramount to generate groups of tumors that behave in a more homogenous fashion. In 2016, the WHO modified classification of GB according to the presence or absence of isocitrate dehydrogenase 1 or 2 (*IDH1/2*) gene mutation. The prognostic significance of *IDH1/2* mutation is substantial. Among the roughly 90% of GB patients with wild-type *IDH1/2* mutations, median survival is around 1 year; among the remainder with *IDH1/2* mutant tumors, median survival is greater than 3 years [4]. Additionally, methylation status of the promoter region of the enzyme O6-methylguanine-DNA methyltransferase (*MGMT*) has an important prognostic role in the natural history of GB. Patients with MGMT-methylated tumors have substantially longer survival than those with unmethylated tumors, in part because *MGMT* methylated tumors appears to be more responsive to the Stupp treatment protocol [12].

Etiology of Glioblastoma

Many potential risk factors have been examined as potential contributors to individual risk of developing GB, but few have been validated in repeat studies. Identification of risk factors has proven challenging given the rarity of GB, its rapid clinical course, and cognitive changes due to the effects of tumor that may affect the accuracy of patient recall. The most consistent associations that have been demonstrated are for increased risk after ionizing radiation exposure to the head, and decreased risk with a history of allergies or atopic disease [13, 14]. The potential influence of other factors has been examined extensively but consistent associations have not been identified, and although some studies have studied GB specifically, many have used more heterogeneous categories of all gliomas or all brain tumors in an effort to improve power. As such, many of the results reviewed below are not specific to GB alone, as indicated when relevant.

Ionizing Radiation

Moderate-to-high doses of radiation (e.g., therapeutic radiation) is the strongest and most consistently documented environmental risk factor for brain tumors in general, having been independently observed in atomic bomb survivor cohort and among individuals receiving therapeutic radiation, for example, for childhood cancers. The carcinogenic effect is stronger in children, who are more radiosensitive and have more years of potential life to express risk. Estimated latency between irradiation and incidence has been estimated at 7–9 years [15, 16].

Allergies and Atopic Disease

Both case-control and cohort studies have consistently shown that a history of atopic conditions (including asthma, hay fever, eczema, and allergies) is associated with reduced GB risk [17]. History of respiratory allergies has been shown to decrease risk of GB by ~30% [17], while eczema decreases risk of glioma overall (including lower grade tumors) by 30% [18]. The underlying mechanism through which allergy protects against development of GB has not been specifically identified, but the primary hypothesis is that allergic conditions may lead to a heightened state of immune-surveillance, prohibiting abnormal cell growth that would otherwise lead to development of a GB [17, 19, 20]. A potential protective association between autoimmune conditions and gliomas in general has also been studied, though results have been mixed [21, 22].

An MR analysis was conducted using glioma GWAS summary statistics to test the causal association between different allergic phenotypes (including respiratory allergy, asthma, and eczema) and glioma. These studies identified no causal relationship between asthma or respiratory allergies, and glioma, but did identify a weak causal association between eczema and reduced risk of glioma [23].

Aspirin and Other Medications

Non-steroidal anti-inflammatory drugs (NSAIDs), including aspirin, have been associated with decreased risk of multiple cancers of other sites. A recently conducted meta-analysis pooling results from observational studies and limited randomized studies found that regular use of aspirin was associated with significantly decreased risk of GB (~30%) [2]. The study reported no significant associations between use of other NSAIDs and GB risk.

Exposures with Mixed or Limited Evidence

Cellular Phone Use

Cellular phone technology was introduced in the 1980s and use of these devices has rapidly increased, with more than 90% of adults globally now using cellular phones. Cellular phones emit radiofrequency fields (RF) during normal functioning. When used against the head, the brain absorbs the largest dose of these fields compared to other organs. Due to the large-scale public health concerns any significant health risks of cellular phone use would pose, the association between risk of brain tumors and cellular phone use has been investigated extensively. In 2011, the International Agency for Research on Cancer (IARC) classified RF fields as a possible carcinogen, based largely on preliminary findings of an increased risk of glioma and vestibular schwannoma in heavy cellular phone users [24]. Since 2011, there have been at least six published epidemiological studies reporting on glioma risk in relation to cellular phone use [25–30], and multiple meta-analyses have been conducted. The majority of these have identified no significant associations between cellular phone use and glioma incidence. Furthermore, if cellular phones significantly affect risk for GB and other brain tumors, increases in incidence should ostensibly be identifiable during or soon after the period of increased use. There have been at least seven studies that have examined incidence trends for glioma since 2011, covering the period of increasing cellular phone use or the time immediately thereafter [31–39]. The majority of these studies have identified little to no change in incidence of glioma, with the exception of two analyses of data from Israel and the UK, which found increased incidence of GB [36–39]. Two studies assessing US and Australian data found that the small observed increases in incidence in those data were not compatible with the magnitude of risks reported by case-control studies, which may be biased by patient recall or inappropriate control selection [32, 33].

Overall, the sum of epidemiological evidence published since the IARC Monograph was published in 2011 does not support an association between use of cellular phones and risk of brain tumors, including GB. If such an association were to exist, the latency period for this exposure would still be unknown; therefore, monitoring of incidence trends as described above has been advised to consider the possibility of delayed effects.

Low Frequency Electromagnetic Fields

In line with studies of cellular phone use and GB risk, several studies have reported on the association between extremely low frequency magnetic fields (ELFs) and glioma risk [40–42]. Despite some observed positive associations that were mostly confined to case-control studies, the IARC in 2002 concluded that existing data was insufficient to classify ELFs as a risk factor for glioma [43]. Similarly, recent analyses carried out by the INTEROCC consortium have failed to identify any significant association between lifetime cumulative occupational exposure to ELF and glioma [41].

Hormonal Exposures

Several observational studies have investigated the association between both endogenous and exogenous sex hormones and glioma incidence [44]. The male preponderance in GB incidence has led to hypotheses that perhaps higher lifetime exposure to estrogens may play a protective role against developing GB. Although lifetime exposure to circulating hormones can be difficult to measure accurately, several analyses have examined associations between surrogate measures and glioma incidence, age at menarche, parity, age at menopause as well as use of supplemental estrogen or progesterone. While a few reports have found negative associations between glioma and estrogen exposure, results have generally been conflicting or null [45–47].

Dietary Factors

Studies of diet and GB risk are limited, due both to the rarity of GB and the limitations of case-control studies for assessing diet. A recent investigation pooling three, large prospective cohorts did not demonstrate an association between consumption of any food groups, nutrients, or dietary patterns and risk of glioma [48]. The associations between processed meats, nitrites and glioma risk have been previously examined, with largely null results [49–52]. Associations between glioma and various vitamins have been mixed [53–55]. Coffee and tea intake have been associated with lower risk of several cancers, but when examined in relation to glioma risk associations have largely been null [56–60], although some recent evidence suggests a possible link between higher tea intake and lower GB incidence [56, 60, 61].

Non-radiation Occupational Exposures

Possible associations between specific occupations and/or non-radiation occupational exposures and glioma have been studied extensively [62–64]. To date, there have been no occupational exposures consistently associated with glioma.

Smoking

Tobacco smoking remains one of the most significant and well-documented causes of cancer worldwide, but the association between malignant brain tumors, including GB, and smoking has consistently been found to be null [65–69].

Height, Weight and Metabolic Traits

Height and body mass index (BMI) have been repeatedly studied in relation to glioma risk. Taller adult height has been identified as a glioma and GB risk factor, with approximately a 20% increase in risk for every 10 cm increase in height [70–72]. There is less evidence for an association between adult BMI and risk of GB, and studies into this association have mostly been null [7, 70, 73–77]. Summary statistics from GWAS have been utilized in a variety of MR analyses to assess the possibility of causal associations between factors related to body habitus, such as height or BMI and glioma incidence. In general, these analyses have reported null associations between waist-to-hip ratio, circulating lipid levels, hyperglycemia, type II diabetes, and BMI and glioma [78].

Mendelian Cancer Syndromes and Rare Variants

The vast majority of glioma cases are diagnosed in individuals reporting no family history of glioma. In approximately 5% of cases, however, individuals will report that at least one additional member of their family has been previously diagnosed with a glioma [79]. An even smaller proportion of cases (1–2% of adult glioma) can be attributed to known Mendelian disorders (where a single gene is found to vary an oncogenic mutation) or in more complex inherited genetic syndromes [9, 80]. The mutations identified in most of these cases are loss-of-function mutations in tumor suppressor genes, which may arise *de novo* or may be inherited [81, 82]. A summary of these is included in Table 1.1.

Table 1.1 Inherited syndromes associated with brain and other CNS tumors

Gene (Chromosome location)	Disorder/ Syndrome (OMIM ID)	Mode of inheritance	Phenotypic features	Associated brain tumors
APC, MMR (5q21)	Familial adenomatous polyposis (FAP, 175100), Turcot syndrome type 2	Dominant	Development of multiple adenomatous colon polyps (>100), predisposition to colorectal cancer, and brain tumors	Medulloblastoma, glioma
ATM (11q22.3)	Ataxia-telangiectasia (208900)	Autosomal recessive trait	Progressive cerebellar ataxia, susceptibility to infections, predisposition to lymphoma and lymphocytic leukemia.	Astrocytoma and medulloblastoma
CDKN2A (9p21.3)	Melanoma-neural system tumor syndrome (155755)	Dominant	Predisposition to malignant melanoma and malignant brain tumors	Glioma
IDH1/IDH2 (2q33.3/15q26.1)	Ollier disease	Acquired post-zygotic mosaicism, dominant with reduced penetrance	Development of intraosseous benign cartilaginous tumors, cancer predisposition	Glioma

Table 1.1 (continued)

Gene (Chromosome location)	Disorder/ Syndrome (OMIM ID)	Mode of inheritance	Phenotypic features	Associated brain tumors
MLH1, PMS2	Turcot syndrome type 1	Autosomal recessive trait	Development of multiple adenomatous colon polyps (<100), predisposition to colorectal cancer, and brain tumors	Medulloblastoma, glioma,
MSH2,MLH1,MSH6,PMS2	Lynch syndrome (120435), Biallelic mismatch repair deficiency, constitutional MMR *deficiency* [101]	Dominant	Predisposition to gastrointestinal, endometrial and other cancers	GB, other gliomas
MSH2,MLH1,MSH6,PMS2	Mismatch repair deficiency syndrome (276300)	Recessive	Pediatric cancer predisposition; café-au-lait spots; colon polyps	Glioma
TP53 (17p13.1)	Li-Fraumeni syndrome (151623) [102, 103]	Dominant	Predisposition to numerous cancers, especially breast, brain, and soft-tissue sarcoma	GB, other gliomas

For more information please see:
Farrell and Plotkin [110]
Melean et al. [111]
Abbreviations used: *APC* adenomatous polyposis coli, *CDKN2A* cyclin-dependent kinase inhibitor 2A, *IDH1/2* isocitrate dehydrogenase 1/2, *GB* glioblastoma, *MLH1* MutL homolog 1, colon cancer, nonpolyposis type 2, *MSH2* MutS protein homolog 2, *MSH6* MutS protein homolog 6, *PMS2* PMS1 homolog 2, mismatch repair system component, *TP53* tumor protein p53

Common Genetic Variants in Adult GB

Since the development of rapid whole genome genotyping, eight GWAS of glioma have been conducted [83–90]. Together, these studies identified 11 common genetic variants affecting risk for GB in European adults (Table 1.2). The proportion in incidence variance of GB attributable to genetic factors is estimated to be 26%. Of this, ~27% is explained by currently identified variants, with 73% of the genetic risk currently unexplained [87, 91].

Table 1.2 Previously reported GB risk loci identified by genome-wide association studies including allele frequencies, p-values, odds ratios (OR), and 95% confidence intervals (95% CI)

SNP RSID[a] (Locus)	Associated gene	Population	RAF in studied population[b]	P value	Odds ratio (95% CI)
rs4977756 (9p21.3)	CDKN2B-AS1	European	0.400	2.28×10^{-14}	1.20 (1.15–1.26) [87]
rs2252586 (7p11.2)	EGFR	European	0.281	7.89×10^{-15}	1.20 (1.15–1.26) [87]
rs11979158 (7p11.2)	EGFR	European	0.831	1.94×10^{-19}	1.31 (1.24–1.39) [87]
rs730437 (7p11.2)	EGFR	East Asian	--	0.0160	1.32 (1.05–1.66) [104]
rs1468727 (7p11.2)	EGFR	East Asian	--	0.0080	1.31 (1.04–1.65) [104]
rs10852606 (16q12.1)	HEATR3	European	0.713	1.29×10^{-11}	1.18 (1.13–1.24) [87]
rs11233250 (11q14.1)	Intergenic	European	0.868	9.95×10^{-10}	1.24 (1.16–1.33) [87]
rs17748 (11q23.2)	PHLDB1	East Asian	0.227	$2.36 \times 10^{-5*}$	1.36 (1.17–1.59) [105]*
rs4774756 (15q21.3)	RAB27A	East Asian	0.297	6.12×10^{-8}	1.24 (1.15–1.33) [83]
rs12752552 (1p31.3)	RAVER2	European	0.870	2.04×10^{-9}	1.22 (1.15–1.31) [87]
rs2562152 (16p13.3)	RHBDF1	European	0.850	1.93×10^{-8}	1.21 (1.13–1.29) [87]
rs6010620 (20q13.33)	RTEL1	European/ East Asian	Eur: 0.794 EA: 0.293	Eur: 5.49×10^{-4} EA: 0.021	Eur: 1.46 (1.38–1.54) [87] EA: 1.28 (1.04–1.57) [106]
rs2235573 (22q13.1)	SLC16A8	European	0.507	1.76×10^{-10}	1.15 (1.10–1.20) [87]
rs10842893 (12p11.23)	STK38L	East Asian	0.035	2.33×10^{-12}	2.07 (1.71–2.50) [83]*
rs1920116 (3q26.2)	TERC	European/ East Asian	Eur: 0.720 EA: 0.389	Eur: 2.68×10^{-5} EA: 0.016	Eur: 1.11 (1.06–1.17) [87] EA: 1.21 (1.04–1.42) [107]*

Table 1.2 (continued)

SNP RSID[a] (Locus)	Associated gene	Population	RAF in studied population[b]	P value	Odds ratio (95% CI)
rs10069690 (5p15.33)	*TERT*	European	0.276	8.33×10^{-74}	1.61 (1.53–1.69) [87]
rs2853676 (5p15.33)	*TERT*	European/ East Asian	Eur: 0.290 EA: 0.611	Eur: 4.0×10^{-14} EA: 0.0001	Eur: 1.26 (1.20–1.32) [87] EA: 1.53 (1.21–1.94) [106]
rs78378222 (17p13.1)	*TP53*	European	0.013	4.82×10^{-29}	2.63 (2.22–3.11) [87]

Abbreviations: *95%CI* 95% confidence interval, *CDKN2B-AS1* cyclin dependent kinase inhibitor 2B antisense RNA 1, *EGFR* epidermal growth factor receptor, *HEATR* HEAT repeat containing 3, *IRF4* interferon regulatory factor 4, *PHLDB1* Pleckstrin homology like domain family B member 1, *RAF* risk allele frequency, *RAVER2* ribonucleoprotein, PTB binding 2, *RHBDF1* rhomboid 5 homolog 1, *RTEL* regulator of telomere elongation helicase 1, *SLC16A8* solute carrier family 16 member 8, *SNP* single nucleotide polymorphism, *TERT* telomerase reverse transcriptase, *TP53* tumor protein p53
*P value and odds ratio for pooled glioma sample, includes lower grade gliomas
[a]Included SNPs are those identified within cited publications, and generally represent the strongest independent association within a linkage block
[b]Allele frequencies from: 1000 genomes project phase 3 [108] and gnomAD [109]

Gliomas are a heterogeneous disease, but most analyses focused on identifying germline risk variants have been conducted on pooled histologies (all glioma together), or with classifications that are derived from histologically assigned type and WHO grade. GB case cohorts are usually ascertained at multiple centers over extended periods of time due to their rarity, and as a result, molecular classification data may not be available on all cases. Many centers that have participated in these genetic studies are attempting to molecularly classify these cases now, as this testing is now part of standard of care for GB diagnosis as well as essential to current histological classification standards. One analysis using a subset of glioma cases previously included in GWAS that underwent molecular classification estimated ORs for 25 previously-identified risk loci by molecular subtypes [5]. While some SNPs were significantly associated with all molecular subtypes, most varied in their association. SNPs previously found to have strong association with GB, such as those at 5p15.33/*TERT* (telomerase reverse transcriptase) and 20q13.33/*RTEL1* (regulator of telomere elongation helicase 1), showed the strongest association with *TERT*-mutant tumors. Due to sample size limitations, further research is necessary as more cases are molecularly classified in order to characterize the association between glioma risk SNPs and somatic variation.

Telomere Length

Many of the common variants associated with GB through GWAS are located near genes associated with telomere maintenance functions, such as *TERT* and *RTEL1* [92]. SNPs found to be associated with leukocyte telomere length (LTL) have been used to build a polygenic risk score (PRS) to estimate individual telomere length [93]. Using this PRS, it has been found that longer genetically estimated LTL is associated with increased risk of glioma [92, 94]. This association between longer relative LTL and glioma has also been confirmed using measurements generated by qPCR [95].

Genetic Ancestry

GB incidence is highest in countries with primarily European-ancestry populations, such as northern European countries, the Unites States, and Australia. Most glioma GWAS to date have been conducted in European-ancestry populations [96]. Many candidate SNP studies, which focus on SNPs within genes that are thought to be relevant due to association with other diseases or known cancer predisposing function, have been conducted in East Asian populations. These have found several novel associations as well as replicated associations previously discovered in European-ancestry populations, including loci in telomerase RNA component (*TERC*), *TERT*, epidermal growth factor receptor (*EGFR*), and pleckstrin homology like domain family b member 1 (*PHLDB1*) [97, 98]. One recent glioma GWAS to date has been conducted in a Chinese population and this also confirmed associations near *TERT*, *PHLDB1* and *RTEL1*, and identified two new variants (Table 1.2). Due to the strong signal apparently in the human leukocyte antigen (HLA) region, this analysis may be biased by lack of adjustment for population stratification [83]. Previous analyses have also attempted to compare allele frequencies of previous GWAS hits identified in Europeans within reference data sets, such as the HapMap project, stratified by continental groups, but these have not identified new risk variants [99]. One prior analysis of patterns of continental genetic ancestry in African-Americans and Hispanics identified increased overall European-ancestry in Hispanic glioma cases as compared to controls, and also several normally significant loci in African Americans where probability of European ancestry varied between cases and controls [100].

Conclusion

GB is a relatively rare illness associated with significant morbidity and short survival. Recent research has identified substantial heterogeneity in the epidemiology and clinical behavior of GB by molecular subtypes, and future studies should carefully identify GB by these subtypes. Although few risk factors have been identified for GB, recent research has identified significant differences in risk by both sociodemographic and behavioral characteristics.

Disclosures The authors have nothing to disclose.
FundingNational Institutes of Health F30 CA235791 (DJC). QTO is supported by a Research Training Grant from the Cancer Prevention and Research Institute of Texas (CPRIT; RP160097T).

References

1. Ostrom QT, Cioffi G, Gittleman H, et al. CBTRUS statistical report: primary brain and other central nervous system tumors diagnosed in the United States in 2012–2016. Neuro-Oncology. 2019;21(Suppl 5):v1–v100.
2. Amirian ES, Ostrom QT, Armstrong GN, et al. Aspirin, non-steroidal anti-inflammatory drugs (NSAIDs), and glioma risk: original data from the glioma international case-control study and a meta-analysis. Cancer Epidemiol Biomarkers Prev. 2019 Mar;28(3):555–62
3. Amirian ES, Armstrong GN, Zhou R, et al. The glioma international case-control study: a report from the genetic epidemiology of Glioma International Consortium. Am J Epidemiol. 2016;183(2):85–91.
4. Molinaro AM, Hervey-Jumper S, Morshed RA, et al. Association of maximal extent of resection of contrast-enhanced and non-contrast-enhanced tumor with survival within molecular subgroups of patients with newly diagnosed glioblastoma. JAMA Oncol. 2020;6(4):495–503.
5. Labreche K, Kinnersley B, Berzero G, et al. Diffuse gliomas classified by 1p/19q co-deletion, TERT promoter and IDH mutation status are associated with specific genetic risk loci. Acta Neuropathol. 2018;135(5):743–55.
6. Cote DJ, Rosner BA, Smith-Warner SA, Egan KM, Stampfer MJ. Statin use, hyperlipidemia, and risk of glioma. Eur J Epidemiol. 2019;34(11):997–1011.
7. Kitahara CM, Gamborg M, Rajaraman P, Sorensen TI, Baker JL. A prospective study of height and body mass index in childhood, birth weight, and risk of adult glioma over 40 years of follow-up. Am J Epidemiol. 2014;180(8):821–9.
8. Omuro A, DeAngelis LM. Glioblastoma and other malignant gliomas: a clinical review. JAMA. 2013;310(17):1842–50.
9. Ostrom QT, Bauchet L, Davis F, et al. The epidemiology of glioma in adults: a "state of the science" review. Neuro-Oncology. 2014;16(7):896–913.
10. Ostrom QT, Cote DJ, Ascha M, Kruchko C, Barnholtz-Sloan JS. Adult glioma incidence and survival by race or ethnicity in the United States from 2000 to 2014. JAMA Oncol. 2018;4(9):1254–62.
11. Stupp R, Mason WP, van den Bent MJ, et al. Radiotherapy plus concomitant and adjuvant temozolomide for glioblastoma. N Engl J Med. 2005;352(10):987–96.
12. Hegi ME, Diserens AC, Gorlia T, et al. MGMT gene silencing and benefit from temozolomide in glioblastoma. N Engl J Med. 2005;352(10):997–1003.
13. Ostrom QT, Fahmideh MA, Cote DJ, et al. Risk factors for childhood and adult primary brain tumors. Neuro-Oncology. 2019;21:1357–75.
14. Thakkar JP, Dolecek TA, Horbinski C, et al. Epidemiologic and molecular prognostic review of glioblastoma. Cancer Epidemiol Biomark Prev. 2014;23(10):1985–96.
15. Ohgaki H, Kleihues P. Epidemiology and etiology of gliomas. Acta Neuropathol. 2005;109(1):93–108.
16. Braganza MZ, Kitahara CM, Berrington de Gonzalez A, Inskip PD, Johnson KJ, Rajaraman P. Ionizing radiation and the risk of brain and central nervous system tumors: a systematic review. Neuro-Oncology. 2012;14(11):1316–24.
17. Amirian ES, Zhou R, Wrensch MR, et al. Approaching a scientific consensus on the association between allergies and glioma risk: a report from the glioma international case-control study. Cancer Epidemiol Biomarkers Prev. 2016;25(2):282–90.
18. Wang G, Xu S, Cao C, et al. Evidence from a large-scale meta-analysis indicates eczema reduces the incidence of glioma. Oncotarget. 2016;7(38):62598–606.
19. Turner MC. Epidemiology: allergy history, IgE, and cancer. Cancer Immunol Immunother. 2012;61(9):1493–510.
20. Cui Y, Hill AW. Atopy and specific cancer sites: a review of epidemiological studies. Clin Rev Allergy Immunol. 2016;51(3):338–52.
21. Anssar TM, Leitzmann MF, Linker RA, et al. Autoimmune diseases and immunosuppressive therapy in relation to the risk of glioma. Cancer Med. 2020;9(3):1263–75.
22. Schwartzbaum J, Jonsson F, Ahlbom A, et al. Cohort studies of association between self-reported allergic conditions, immune-related diagnoses and glioma and meningioma risk. Int J Cancer. 2003;106(3):423–8.

23. Disney-Hogg L, Cornish AJ, Sud A, et al. Impact of atopy on risk of glioma: a Mendelian randomisation study. BMC Med. 2018;16(1):42.
24. Baan R, Grosse Y, Lauby-Secretan B, et al. Carcinogenicity of radiofrequency electromagnetic fields. Lancet Oncol. 2011;12(7):624–6.
25. Benson VS, Pirie K, Schuz J, et al. Mobile phone use and risk of brain neoplasms and other cancers: prospective study. Int J Epidemiol. 2013;42(3):792–802.
26. Cardis E, Armstrong BK, Bowman JD, et al. Risk of brain tumours in relation to estimated RF dose from mobile phones: results from five interphone countries. Occup Environ Med. 2011;68(9):631–40.
27. Momoli F, Siemiatycki J, McBride ML, et al. Probabilistic multiple-bias modeling applied to the Canadian data from the interphone study of mobile phone use and risk of glioma, meningioma, acoustic neuroma, and parotid gland tumors. Am J Epidemiol. 2017;186(7):885–93.
28. Aydin D, Feychting M, Schuz J, et al. Mobile phone use and brain tumors in children and adolescents: a multicenter case-control study. J Natl Cancer Inst. 2011;103(16):1264–76.
29. Hardell L, Carlberg M, Soderqvist F, Mild KH. Case-control study of the association between malignant brain tumours diagnosed between 2007 and 2009 and mobile and cordless phone use. Int J Oncol. 2013;43(6):1833–45.
30. Interphone Study Group. Brain tumour risk in relation to mobile telephone use: results of the INTERPHONE international case-control study. Int J Epidemiol. 2010;39(3):675–94.
31. Nilsson J, Järås J, Henriksson R, et al. No evidence for increased brain tumour incidence in the Swedish national cancer register between years 1980–2012. Anticancer Res. 2019;39(2):791–6.
32. Chapman S, Azizi L, Luo Q, Sitas F. Has the incidence of brain cancer risen in Australia since the introduction of mobile phones 29 years ago? Cancer Epidemiol. 2016;42:199–205.
33. Little MP, Rajaraman P, Curtis RE, et al. Mobile phone use and glioma risk: comparison of epidemiological study results with incidence trends in the United States. BMJ. 2012;344:e1147.
34. Davis FG, Smith TR, Gittleman HR, Ostrom QT, Kruchko C, Barnholtz-Sloan JS. Glioblastoma incidence rate trends in Canada and the United States compared with England, 1995–2015. Neuro-Oncology. 2020;22(2):301–2.
35. Deltour I, Auvinen A, Feychting M, et al. Mobile phone use and incidence of glioma in the Nordic countries 1979–2008: consistency check. Epidemiology. 2012;23(2):301–7.
36. Barchana M, Margaliot M, Liphshitz I. Changes in brain glioma incidence and laterality correlates with use of mobile phones--a nationwide population based study in Israel. Asian Pac J Cancer Prev. 2012;13(11):5857–63.
37. Philips A, Henshaw DL, Lamburn G, O'Carroll MJ. Brain tumours: rise in glioblastoma multiforme incidence in England 1995–2015 suggests an adverse environmental or lifestyle factor. J Environ Public Health. 2018;2018:7910754.
38. Philips A, Henshaw DL, Lamburn G, O'Carroll MJ. Authors' comment on "brain tumours: rise in glioblastoma multiforme incidence in England 1995–2015 suggests an adverse environmental or lifestyle factor". J Environ Public Health. 2018;2018:2170208.
39. de Vocht F. Analyses of temporal and spatial patterns of glioblastoma multiforme and other brain cancer subtypes in relation to mobile phones using synthetic counterfactuals. Environ Res. 2019;168:329–35.
40. Vila J, Turner MC, Gracia-Lavedan E, et al. Occupational exposure to high-frequency electromagnetic fields and brain tumor risk in the INTEROCC study: an individualized assessment approach. Environ Int. 2018;119:353–65.
41. Turner MC, Benke G, Bowman JD, et al. Occupational exposure to extremely low-frequency magnetic fields and brain tumor risks in the INTEROCC study. Cancer Epidemiol Biomarkers Prev. 2014;23(9):1863–72.
42. Carlberg M, Koppel T, Ahonen M, Hardell L. Case-control study on occupational exposure to extremely low-frequency electromagnetic fields and glioma risk. Am J Ind Med. 2017;60(5):494–503.
43. IARC Working Group on the evaluation of carcinogenic risks to humans. Non-ionizing radiation, part 1: static and extremely low-frequency (ELF) electric and magnetic fields. Lyon, France; IARC. 2002.

44. Cowppli-Bony A, Bouvier G, Rue M, et al. Brain tumors and hormonal factors: review of the epidemiological literature. Cancer Causes Control. 2011;22(5):697–714.
45. Zong H, Xu H, Geng Z, et al. Reproductive factors in relation to risk of brain tumors in women: an updated meta-analysis of 27 independent studies. Tumour Biol. 2014;35(11):11579–86.
46. Qi ZY, Shao C, Zhang X, Hui GZ, Wang Z. Exogenous and endogenous hormones in relation to glioma in women: a meta-analysis of 11 case-control studies. PLoS One. 2013;8(7):e68695.
47. Benson VS, Kirichek O, Beral V, Green J. Menopausal hormone therapy and central nervous system tumor risk: large UK prospective study and meta-analysis. Int J Cancer. 2015;136(10):2369–77.
48. Kuan AS, Green J, Kitahara CM, et al. Diet and risk of glioma: combined analysis of three large prospective studies in the UK and USA. Neuro-Oncology. 2019;21(7):944–52.
49. Ward HA, Gayle A, Jakszyn P, et al. Meat and haem iron intake in relation to glioma in the European Prospective Investigation into Cancer and Nutrition study. Eur J Cancer Prev. 2018;27(4):379–83.
50. Michaud DS, Holick CN, Batchelor TT, Giovannucci E, Hunter DJ. Prospective study of meat intake and dietary nitrates, nitrites, and nitrosamines and risk of adult glioma. Am J Clin Nutr. 2009;90(3):570–7.
51. Li Y. Association between fruit and vegetable intake and risk for glioma: a meta-analysis. Nutrition. 2014;30(11–12):1272–8.
52. Alles B, Pouchieu C, Gruber A, et al. Dietary and alcohol intake and central nervous system tumors in adults: results of the CERENAT multicenter case-control study. Neuroepidemiology. 2016;47(3–4):145–54.
53. Zhou Q, Luo ML, Li H, Li M, Zhou JG. Coffee consumption and risk of endometrial cancer: a dose-response meta-analysis of prospective cohort studies. Sci Rep. 2015;5:13410.
54. Lv W, Zhong X, Xu L, Han W. Association between dietary vitamin A intake and the risk of glioma: evidence from a meta-analysis. Nutrients. 2015;7(11):8897–904.
55. Takahashi H, Cornish AJ, Sud A, et al. Mendelian randomisation study of the relationship between vitamin D and risk of glioma. Sci Rep. 2018;8(1):2339.
56. Malmir H, Shayanfar M, Mohammad-Shirazi M, Tabibi H, Sharifi G, Esmaillzadeh A. Tea and coffee consumption in relation to glioma: a case-control study. Eur J Nutr. 2019;58(1):103–11.
57. Malerba S, Galeone C, Pelucchi C, et al. A meta-analysis of coffee and tea consumption and the risk of glioma in adults. Cancer Causes Control. 2013;24(2):267–76.
58. Dubrow R, Darefsky AS, Freedman ND, Hollenbeck AR, Sinha R. Coffee, tea, soda, and caffeine intake in relation to risk of adult glioma in the NIH-AARP Diet and Health Study. Cancer Causes Control. 2012;23(5):757–68.
59. Holick CN, Smith SG, Giovannucci E, Michaud DS. Coffee, tea, caffeine intake, and risk of adult glioma in three prospective cohort studies. Cancer Epidemiol Biomarkers Prev. 2010;19(1):39–47.
60. Ogawa T, Sawada N, Iwasaki M, et al. Coffee and green tea consumption in relation to brain tumor risk in a Japanese population. Int J Cancer. 2016;139(12):2714–21.
61. Cote DJ, Bever AM, Wilson KM, Smith TR, Smith-Warner SA, Stampfer MJ. A prospective study of tea and coffee intake and risk of glioma. Int J Cancer. 2020;146(9):2442–9.
62. Lacourt A, Cardis E, Pintos J, et al. INTEROCC case-control study: lack of association between glioma tumors and occupational exposure to selected combustion products, dusts and other chemical agents. BMC Public Health. 2013;13:340.
63. Ruder AM, Yiin JH, Waters MA, et al. The Upper Midwest health study: gliomas and occupational exposure to chlorinated solvents. Occup Environ Med. 2013;70(2):73–80.
64. Parent ME, Turner MC, Lavoue J, et al. Lifetime occupational exposure to metals and welding fumes, and risk of glioma: a 7-country population-based case-control study. Environ Health. 2017;16(1):90.
65. Shao C, Zhao W, Qi Z, He J. Smoking and glioma risk: evidence from a meta-analysis of 25 observational studies. Medicine. 2016;95(2):e2447.
66. Braganza MZ, Rajaraman P, Park Y, et al. Cigarette smoking, alcohol intake, and risk of glioma in the NIH-AARP diet and health study. Br J Cancer. 2014;110(1):242–8.

67. Zheng T, Cantor KP, Zhang Y, Chiu BC, Lynch CF. Risk of brain glioma not associated with cigarette smoking or use of other tobacco products in Iowa. Cancer Epidemiol Biomarkers Prev. 2001;10(4):413–4.

68. Efird JT, Friedman GD, Sidney S, et al. The risk for malignant primary adult-onset glioma in a large, multiethnic, managed-care cohort: cigarette smoking and other lifestyle behaviors. J Neuro-Oncol. 2004;68(1):57–69.

69. Holick CN, Giovannucci EL, Rosner B, Stampfer MJ, Michaud DS. Prospective study of cigarette smoking and adult glioma: dosage, duration, and latency. Neuro-Oncology. 2007;9(3):326–34.

70. Wiedmann MKH, Brunborg C, Di Ieva A, et al. The impact of body mass index and height on the risk for glioblastoma and other glioma subgroups: a large prospective cohort study. Neuro-Oncology. 2017;19(7):976–85.

71. Benson VS, Pirie K, Green J, Casabonne D, Beral V. Lifestyle factors and primary glioma and meningioma tumours in the Million Women Study cohort. Br J Cancer. 2008;99(1):185–90.

72. Moore SC, Rajaraman P, Dubrow R, et al. Height, body mass index, and physical activity in relation to glioma risk. Cancer Res. 2009;69(21):8349–55.

73. Sergentanis TN, Tsivgoulis G, Perlepe C, et al. Obesity and risk for brain/CNS tumors, gliomas and meningiomas: a meta-analysis. PLoS One. 2015;10(9):e0136974.

74. Niedermaier T, Behrens G, Schmid D, Schlecht I, Fischer B, Leitzmann MF. Body mass index, physical activity, and risk of adult meningioma and glioma: a meta-analysis. Neurology. 2015;85(15):1342–50.

75. Cote DJ, Downer MK, Smith TR, Smith-Warner SA, Egan KM, Stampfer MJ. Height, waist circumference, body mass index, and body somatotype across the life course and risk of glioma. Cancer Causes Control. 2018;29(8):707–19.

76. Michaud DS, Bove G, Gallo V, et al. Anthropometric measures, physical activity, and risk of glioma and meningioma in a large prospective cohort study. Cancer Prev Res (Phila). 2011;4(9):1385–92.

77. Little RB, Madden MH, Thompson RC, et al. Anthropometric factors in relation to risk of glioma. Cancer Causes Control. 2013;24(5):1025–31.

78. Disney-Hogg L, Sud A, Law PJ, et al. Influence of obesity-related risk factors in the aetiology of glioma. Br J Cancer. 2018;118(7):1020–7.

79. Wrensch M, Lee M, Miike R, et al. Familial and personal medical history of cancer and nervous system conditions among adults with glioma and controls. Am J Epidemiol. 1997;145(7):581–93.

80. Johnson KJ, Cullen J, Barnholtz-Sloan JS, et al. Childhood brain tumor epidemiology: a brain tumor epidemiology consortium review. Cancer Epidemiol Biomarkers Prev. 2014;23(12):2716–36.

81. Ranger AM, Patel YK, Chaudhary N, Anantha RV. Familial syndromes associated with intracranial tumours: a review. Childs Nerv Syst. 2014;30(1):47–64.

82. Vijapura C, Saad Aldin E, Capizzano AA, Policeni B, Sato Y, Moritani T. Genetic syndromes associated with central nervous system tumors. Radiographics. 2017;37(1):258–80.

83. Chen H, Chen G, Li G, et al. Two novel genetic variants in the STK38L and RAB27A genes are associated with glioma susceptibility. Int J Cancer. 2019;145(9):2372–82.

84. Rajaraman P, Melin BS, Wang Z, et al. Genome-wide association study of glioma and meta-analysis. Hum Genet. 2012;131(12):1877–88.

85. Shete S, Hosking FJ, Robertson LB, et al. Genome-wide association study identifies five susceptibility loci for glioma. Nat Genet. 2009;41(8):899–904.

86. Enciso-Mora V, Hosking FJ, Kinnersley B, et al. Deciphering the 8q24.21 association for glioma. Hum Mol Genet. 2013;22(11):2293–302.

87. Melin BS, Barnholtz-Sloan JS, Wrensch MR, et al. Genome-wide association study of glioma subtypes identifies specific differences in genetic susceptibility to glioblastoma and non-glioblastoma tumors. Nat Genet. 2017;49(5):789–94.

88. Wrensch M, Jenkins RB, Chang JS, et al. Variants in the CDKN2B and RTEL1 regions are associated with high-grade glioma susceptibility. Nat Genet. 2009;41(8):905–8.

89. Walsh KM, Codd V, Smirnov IV, et al. Variants near TERT and TERC influencing telomere length are associated with high-grade glioma risk. Nat Genet. 2014;46(7):731–5.
90. Kinnersley B, Labussiere M, Holroyd A, et al. Genome-wide association study identifies multiple susceptibility loci for glioma. Nat Commun. 2015;6:8559.
91. Kinnersley B, Mitchell JS, Gousias K, et al. Quantifying the heritability of glioma using genome-wide complex trait analysis. Sci Rep. 2015;5:17267.
92. Walsh KM, Codd V, Rice T, et al. Longer genotypically-estimated leukocyte telomere length is associated with increased adult glioma risk. Oncotarget. 2015;6(40):42468–77.
93. Codd V, Nelson CP, Albrecht E, et al. Identification of seven loci affecting mean telomere length and their association with disease. Nat Genet. 2013;45(4):422–7, 427e421–422.
94. Walsh KM, Wiencke JK, Lachance DH, et al. Telomere maintenance and the etiology of adult glioma. Neuro-Oncology. 2015;17(11):1445–52.
95. Andersson U, Degerman S, Dahlin AM, et al. The association between longer relative leukocyte telomere length and risk of glioma is independent of the potentially confounding factors allergy, BMI, and smoking. Cancer Causes Control. 2019;30(2):177–85.
96. Leece R, Xu J, Ostrom QT, Chen Y, Kruchko C, Barnholtz-Sloan JS. Global incidence of malignant brain and other central nervous system tumors by histology, 2003–2007. Neuro-Oncology. 2017;19(11):1553–64.
97. Li G, Jin T, Liang H, et al. RTEL1 tagging SNPs and haplotypes were associated with glioma development. Diagn Pathol. 2013;8:83.
98. Liu HB, Peng YP, Dou CW, et al. Comprehensive study on associations between nine SNPs and glioma risk. Asian Pac J Cancer Prev. 2012;13(10):4905–8.
99. Jacobs DI, Walsh KM, Wrensch M, et al. Leveraging ethnic group incidence variation to investigate genetic susceptibility to glioma: a novel candidate SNP approach. Front Genet. 2012;3:203.
100. Ostrom QT, Egan KM, Nabors LB, et al. Glioma risk associated with extent of estimated European genetic ancestry in African-Americans and Hispanics. Int J Cancer. 2020;146(3):739–48.
101. Bouffet E, Larouche V, Campbell BB, et al. Immune checkpoint inhibition for hypermutant glioblastoma multiforme resulting from germline biallelic mismatch repair deficiency. J Clin Oncol. 2016;34(19):2206–11.
102. Bougeard G, Renaux-Petel M, Flaman JM, et al. Revisiting Li-Fraumeni syndrome from TP53 mutation carriers. J Clin Oncol. 2015;33(21):2345–52.
103. Li FP, Fraumeni JF Jr, Mulvihill JJ, et al. A cancer family syndrome in twenty-four kindreds. Cancer Res. 1988;48(18):5358–62.
104. Hou WG, Ai WB, Bai XG, et al. Genetic variation in the EGFR gene and the risk of glioma in a Chinese Han population. PLoS One. 2012;7(5):e37531.
105. Chen H, Sun B, Zhao Y, et al. Fine mapping of a region of chromosome 11q23.3 reveals independent locus associated with risk of glioma. PLoS One. 2012;7(12):e52864.
106. Jin TB, Zhang JY, Li G, et al. RTEL1 and TERT polymorphisms are associated with astrocytoma risk in the Chinese Han population. Tumour Biol. 2013;34(6):3659–66.
107. Wang D, Hu E, Wu P, et al. Genetic variant near TERC influencing the risk of gliomas with older age at diagnosis in a Chinese population. J Neuro-Oncol. 2015;124(1):57–64.
108. Genomes Project C, Auton A, Brooks LD, et al. A global reference for human genetic variation. Nature. 2015;526(7571):68–74.
109. Lek M, Karczewski KJ, Minikel EV, et al. Analysis of protein-coding genetic variation in 60,706 humans. Nature. 2016;536(7616):285–91.
110. Farrell CJ, Plotkin SR. Genetic causes of brain tumors: neurofibromatosis, tuberous sclerosis, von Hippel-Lindau, and other syndromes. Neurol Clin. 2007;25(4):925–46, viii.
111. Melean G, et al. Genetic insights into familial tumors of the nervous system. Am J Med Genet C Semin Med Genet. 2004;129C(1):74–84.

Chapter 2
The Role of Molecular Genetics of Glioblastoma in the Clinical Setting

Maria del Pilar Guillermo Prieto and Macarena Ines de La Fuente

Introduction

Neuro-oncology clinical practice has evolved at a rapid pace over the last decade, especially in the most recent years. The World Health Organization (WHO) 2016 classification of central nervous system (CNS) tumors became a pivotal point in the diagnosis and management of brain tumors. The incorporation of molecular biomarkers in addition to histology has importantly impacted the clinical management of gliomas, leading to more accurate diagnosis, better prognostication of tumor behavior, and overall survival (OS) and, at the same time, it has opened new horizons in term of therapeutic approaches [1–3].

The Consortium to Inform Molecular and Practical Approaches to CNS Tumor Taxonomy (cIMPACT-NOW) was announced in December 2016 as a response to the accelerated expansion of advances on novel molecular markers and their clinical implication in the management of CNS tumors, providing regular and timely updates in between WHO CNS tumor classification editions and proposing future changes to future CNS tumor classifications [4, 5]. In April 2020, cIMPACT-NOW published their 6th update and their recommendations will be further discussed [2].

In this chapter, we will review the molecular markers that are relevant in clinical practice for glioblastoma (GBM) along with emerging novel biomarkers with a potential diagnostic or therapeutic role (Table 2.1).

M. del Pilar Guillermo Prieto · M. I. de La Fuente (✉)
Department of Neurology and Sylvester Comprehensive Cancer Center, University of Miami, Miami, FL, USA
e-mail: pilar.prieto@med.miami.edu; mdelafuente@med.miami.edu

J. J. Otero, A. P. Becker (eds.), *Precision Molecular Pathology of Glioblastoma*,
Molecular Pathology Library, https://doi.org/10.1007/978-3-030-69170-7_2

Table 2.1 Clinically relevant and emergent biomarkers in Glioblastoma

Biomarker	Diagnostic role	Prognostic role	Prospective treatment target
IDH 1/2 mutations	Defining feature of the majority of WHO grade II–IV gliomas.	*IDH* mutations are correlated with better OS in astrocytic tumors WHO grade II–IV	Yes
MGMT hypermethylation status	No diagnostic role	Predict benefit from alkylating chemotherapy in patients with *IDH* wild-type gliomas. Associated with increased incidence of pseudo-progression Key component in treatment decision in elderly population	No
EGFR amplification	Supports GBM diagnosis in *IDH*-wildtype WHO grade II and III astrocytomas	Associated with poor prognosis	Yes
EGFRvIII expression	Supports diagnosis of GBM	May be associated with poor prognosis, controversial	Yes
PTEN deletion	Supports diagnosis of GBM	May be associated with poor prognosis, controversial	Yes
BRAF V600E	Not diagnostic for GBM. Associated with epithelioid variant of GBM, pleomorphic xanthoastrocytoma and ganglioglioma.	Associated with poor prognosis in epithelioid variant of GBM. On specific cases, the use of BRAF and MEK inhibitors can dramatically improve PFS.	Yes
FGFR-TACC gene fusions	No diagnostic role	Not defined	Yes
PDGFRA	Associated with proneural subtype and secondary GBM	Poor prognosis on *IDH*-mutant WHO grade III and III astrocytomas and very poor prognosis on GBM with H3K27M mutation	Yes
CDKN2A/B homozygous deletion	Supports GBM diagnosis in *IDH*-mutant WHO grade II and III astrocytomas	Poor prognosis	No
TERTp mutation	Supports GBM diagnosis in IDH-wildtype WHO grade II and III astrocytomas	Poor prognosis	No

Table 2.1 (continued)

Biomarker	Diagnostic role	Prognostic role	Prospective treatment target
Chromosome 7 gains and chromosome 10 losses (+7/−10) -not reviewed in this chapter	Supports GBM diagnosis in IDH-wildtype WHO grade II and III astrocytomas	Poor prognosis	No

IDH isocitrate dehydrogenase, *MGMT* O6-methylguanine-DNA methyl- transferase, *EGFR* epidermal growth factor receptor, *PTEN* phosphatase and tensin homolog, *FGFR-TACC* fibroblast growth factor receptor-transforming acidic coiled-coil, *PDGFRA* platelet derived growth factor receptor alpha, *CDKN* cyclin dependent finase inhibitor, *TERT* telomerase reverse transcriptase promoter mutation

Isocitrate Dehydrogenase (*IDH*)

Isocitrate dehydrogenases (IDH1, IDH2, IDH3) are metabolic enzymes that participate in the Krebs cycle by catalyzing the oxidative carboxylation of isocitrate to α-ketoglutarate and carbon dioxide, resulting in the production of nicotinamide adenine dinucleotide phosphate hydrogen (NADPH) or nicotinamide adenine dinucleotide hydrogen in the case of IDH3 [6–11].

Mutations in the *IDH1* and *IDH2* genes result in a single amino acid substitution and are considered to be mutually exclusive [8, 11]. The most common mutation of *IDH1* in glioma is found at the arginine codon 132 (R132) with the most frequent substitution is of arginine by histidine (R132H), which occurs in more than 90%. On the *IDH2* gene, the most common mutation is at codon 172 (R172) and (R140) which is analogous for *IDH1* [8, 9]. Mutations in *IDH1* and *IDH2* have been identified in other malignancies such as chondrosarcoma, intrahepatic cholangiocarcinoma, acute myeloid leukemia and myelodysplastic syndromes [10, 12, 13].

Mutations in *IDH* result in the production of the oncometabolite R(−)-2-hydroxyglutarate (2HG). 2HG competitively inhibits α-ketoglutarate-dependent enzymes affecting histone and DNA demethylation, and adaption to hypoxia, leading to abnormalities of epigenetic regulation, genetic instability, T cell differentiation, and tumor immunity. 2HG also impairs cellular differentiation in a variety of cell lineages promoting oncogenic transformation in association with other cancer genes [6, 9, 10, 14, 15].

IDH1 mutations are present in up to 7% of GBM and in over 70% of grade II and grade III gliomas. Mutations have been also identified in the *IDH2* gene in approximately 4–8% of gliomas [13, 15, 16]. *IDH* mutation has been recognized as an early event in gliomagenesis. It has become a fundamental element for diagnosis, treatment decision and prognostication of tumor behavior.

The presence of *IDH1/2* mutation in gliomas has been associated with younger age and better prognosis [11, 17]. The mean age at diagnosis for *IDH*-mutant GBM is 40 years and median overall survival (mOS) 27–31 months. For *IDH*-wildtype GBM the mean age at diagnosis is 64 years and mOS 15–18 months [17–19].

Recent research advances suggest that *IDH*-wildtype and *IDH*-mutant GBM are two separate diseases, with a completely different age of presentation, molecular profile, and overall survival. This has been translated to the clinical research setting where most clinical trial studies designed for newly diagnosed or recurrent GBM are focused on *IDH*-wildtype GBM and exclude *IDH*-mutant tumors. In the recent years, *IDH* mutation has been explored as a potential therapeutic target in glioma [20–22], with clinical trials designed for *IDH*-mutant solid tumors including dedicated arms for *IDH*-mutant gliomas [23, 24].

The third update of cIMPACT-NOW recognized WHO grade II diffuse astrocytic glioma, *IDH*-wildtype, with molecular features of GBM as an equivalent to a WHO grade IV tumor. This new concept applies to lower grade astrocytic tumors by histology, that contain the presence of *TERT* promoter mutation, *EGFR* gene amplification, and/or the combination of gain of entire chromosome 7 and loss of entire chromosome 10 (+7/−10); given that their behavior is similar than classic *IDH*-wildtype GBM [25, 26]. This was further reviewed in the sixth update from cIMPACT-NOW. On an effort to simplify nomenclature, and clinical trial eligibility, it was proposed that *IDH*-wildtype diffuse astrocytic gliomas can be classified as GBM, *IDH*-wildtype WHO grade 4 (now suggesting the use of Arabic numerals) in the presence of one or more of the aforementioned mutations. For *IDH*-mutant astrocytomas with microvascular proliferation or necrosis or *CDKN2/B* homozygous deletion, or any combination of any of these features will be designated astrocytoma, *IDH*-mutant, WHO grade 4 [2].

These guidelines from C-IMPACT-NOW are giving the clinician timely updates based on recent validated findings for more accurate diagnosis and prognostication that may change clinical management in daily practice, allowing the physician to provide a more tailored treatment recommendation and the possibility to offer a clinical trial that better suit the molecular profile for each patient's tumor.

O^6-Methylguanine-DNA Methyl- Transferase (*MGMT*)

Despite the fact it was not incorporated to the 2016 WHO classification of CNS tumors, *MGMT* promoter methylation status is one of the most relevant biomarkers used in the management of GBM as its presence predicts benefit from alkylating chemotherapy in patients with glioblastoma [27, 28]. The *MGMT* gene is located on chromosome 10 (10q26). It encodes the repair protein MGMT that reverses the damage created by alkylating agents by repairing damaged guanine nucleotides by transferring the methyl at O^6 site of guanine to its cysteine residues. Epigenetic modification of the cytosine-phosphate-guanine (CpG) island at specific CpG sites within the *MGMT* promoter silences the gene, causing defective repair of DNA alkylation, promoting gene mutation and cell death [29, 30].

MGMT promoter methylation has been associated with better OS in glioma [28, 31–33]. *MGMT* promoter methylation status has been defined according to the percentage or level of methylation detected. Different testing methods have been studied, however, there is no agreement on the best test modality. Among the testing with the most reliability are methylation specific PCR (qMSP) and pyrosequencing [32, 34, 35]. Thresholds on the level of methylation have been studied in GBM: Unmethylated ≤9%, indeterminate or "gray zone" 10–29% and methylated >30%. Methylation levels above 30% have been correlated with better PFS and OS than below 30% (25.2 vs 15.2 months) [32]. Additional studies demonstrated that patients in the indeterminate methylation status also benefit of radiation and temozolomide therapy reflecting an OS of 10–17 months for truly unmethylated, 15.4–20 months for indeterminate and 19.7–34.1 months in methylated patients [35, 36]. It is important to underline that these studies did not correlate consistently with *IDH* status of the tumor samples studied.

Reliable and consistent assessment of *MGMT* methylation status at the first clinic visit is of utmost importance in the evaluation of patients with GBM due to its role in patient counseling and clinical trials eligibility. *MGMT* status has become relevant in the design of clinical trials for newly diagnosed GBM with some trials excluding patients with *MGMT* promoter hypermethylated tumors, other trials include it as a parameter for randomization.

A special population in which the value of *MGMT* has been particularly important for consideration of treatment decision, is the elderly. Multiple trials have demonstrated that concomitant treatment with temozolomide and hypofractionated radiotherapy increased OS regardless of the *MGMT* promoter methylation status [37–41]. However, for older patients who are not candidates for a combined-modality approach because of poor functional status or significant comorbidity, *MGMT* promoter methylation has a particularly important role. Emerging data support the use of temozolomide chemotherapy as an alternative to radiation therapy, in those patients with *MGMT* methylated tumors. Radiation therapy alone is an effective alternative for patients with *MGMT* unmethylated tumors.

Pseudoprogression is defined as a new or expanding area(s) of contrast enhancement that occur early after the end of radiation therapy, within the first 6 months (typically between 3 and 4 months), in the absence of true tumor growth, and that tends to stabilize or resolve without a change in therapy. In GBM, *MGMT* promoter methylation was associated with a 3.5-fold greater risk of developing pseudoprogression in up to 30% of patients treated with chemoradiation with concomitant temozolomide and has been linked to a better outcome. Pseudoprogression can also occur in unmethylated tumors, but to a lesser frequency. The response assessment in neuro-oncology (RANO) criteria recommended that patients should be excluded from clinical trials for recurrent disease within the first 12 weeks after radiation therapy, unless progression is clearly outside the radiation field or there is histologic documentation of progression [42–46]. In the clinical setting, magnetic resonance perfusion and spectroscopy and 18-FDG brain PET may aid in the differentiation between pseudoprogression versus progressive disease although histopathological analysis continues to be the gold standard.

Epidermal Growth Factor Receptor (*EGFR*)

Epidermal growth factor receptor (EGFR) is a member of the ErbB family of receptor tyrosine kinase (RTK). Its structure includes an N-terminal extracellular domain, a transmembrane domain, an extracellular kinase domain, and a cytoplasmic C-terminal tail containing several phosphorylation sites that serve as signal transduction modules. Binding of one of several ligands to the extracellular ligand-binding domain induces receptor homo-dimerization or hetero-dimerization and results in kinase activation. In normal cells, this leads to DNA synthesis, cell proliferation, migration, and adhesion. *EGFR* mutations lead to production of mitogenic RTKs that inhibit the activity of p53 [47, 48].

EGFR is one of the first oncogenes identified in GBM. *EGFR* gene amplification is presented in about 40% of GBM [47, 49–51]. *EGFRvIII* mutation is found in 20% of GBM and it is particularly interesting as it is constitutively active and a potential neoantigen. The presence of *EGFR* amplification supports a GBM diagnosis and differentiates from other gliomas [47, 48, 50, 52–54]. *EGFRvIII* mutation alone is not predictive of outcome, however, the downstream altered molecular pathways associated as a result of its deletion may have a clinical impact [50, 52, 55]. *EGFR* has become one of the hallmark alterations that, if present in *IDH*-wildtype anaplastic astrocytoma, it supports the diagnosis of WHO grade IV astrocytoma [25].

EGFR has been extensively studied as therapeutic target. However, the results of multiple clinical trials evaluating *EGFR* tyrosine kinase inhibitors (TKI) and peptide treatment/vaccine, such as rindopepimut, in recurrent and/or newly diagnosed GBM patients have been disappointing [56, 57]. Clinical trials with newer generation *EGFR* TKI, *EGFRvIII* CAR-T cells alone and in combination with PD-1 inhibitors are currently ongoing and may elucidate the precise role of *EGFR* as a therapeutic target in GBM [50].

Phosphatase and Tensin Homolog (*PTEN*) Deletion

PTEN plays a major role regulating multiple biological functions at the level of the membrane and nucleus. It regulates genomic stability, cellular proliferation, migration and survival, tumor microenvironment among other functions. It has been implicated in multiple malignancies including gliomas. The loss of *PTEN* expression has been associated with glioma cells proliferation. This alteration is present in approximately 40% of primary GBM, and its relevance in OS has been under debate. However, it is considered an additional biomarker in the diagnosis of GBM [58–60]. Recent clinical trials have focused on the PI3K/Akt pathway, with targeted therapies such as buparlisib, sonolisib, pilaralisib, dactolisib, alone or in combination with mTOR inhibitors, are ongoing or have demonstrated no clinical benefit [61, 62].

BRAF V600E Mutation

The BRAF protein is an intermediary in the RAS-RAF pathway. After a ligand-mediated receptor tyrosine kinase is triggered by extracellular growth factors, it activates *RAS*, which initiates BRAF-mediated activation of MEK and ERK, causing transcription of factors for cell proliferation. The *BRAF* V600E mutation results in constitutive activation of the MEK-ERK pathway and uncontrolled cell division [63, 64]. *BRAF* mutations are drivers of oncogenesis in approximately 6% of human malignancies including melanoma, thyroid, colorectal and non-small cell lung cancer [65]. *BRAF* V600E mutations have been identified in a variety of primary brain tumors such as pleomorphic xanthoastrocytoma (up to 60%) [66, 67] and 47–58% ganglioglioma [68, 69], but they are uncommon in GBM (1–2%), except for the epithelioid variant in which is present in about 56% [65, 70, 71]. Epithelioid GBM is a rare and aggressive variant that is more common in children and young adults. It carries a dismal prognosis of about 6 months OS and frequently has leptomeningeal dissemination [72–74].

Even though *BRAF* mutations are rare in GBM, it is important to consider testing for it, especially in the younger population, as the use of BRAF and MEK inhibitors have shown a dramatic response on imaging and prolonged PFS [65, 74].

FGFR-TACC Gene Fusions

Fibroblast growth factor receptor-transforming acidic coiled-coil (*FGFR-TACC*) gene fusions are present in 3% of GBM. In astrocytes, fusions between *FGFR3* and *TACC3* genes can lead to malignant transformation and GBM progression due to the activation of mitogenic, antiapoptotic and migratory functions. Preliminary data of a Phase 2 trial with infigratinib showed PFS6 of 16% with a mOS of 6.7 months, demonstrating a partial response or stable disease in approximately one-third of patients with recurrent GBM and other glioma subtypes [75]. Futibatinib, another *FGFR* inhibitor, has shown to be well tolerated, however, efficacy results have not been published yet [76].

Platelet Derived Growth Factor Receptor Alpha (*PDGFRA*)

PDGFRA amplification is found in approximately 15–20% of adult GBM, especially in cerebellar variant. *PDGFRA* amplification increases with grade and is associated with a less favorable prognosis in WHO grade II and III *IDH1*-mutant astrocytoma comparable to WHO grade IV [49, 52]. In GBM harboring *H3F3A*-K27M mutation, positive *PDGFRA* expression was linked to even worse prognosis [77]. *PDGFRA* has been studied as a potential target in the treatment for GBM using dasatinib and other multikinase inhibitors alone or in combination with bevacizumab with no significant results [78, 79].

CDKN2A/B Homozygous Deletion

Cyclin Dependent Kinase Inhibitor 2A (*CDKN2A*) encodes Ink4a and Arf proteins, which play an important role in activating Rb and p53, respectively. *CDKN2B* encodes the tumor suppressor p15INK4b. Ink4a and p15INK4b inhibit *CDK4* and *CDK6* and maintain the growth-suppressive function of the Rb gene. When dysregulated, uncontrolled cell growth occurs [52, 80].

The prevalence of homozygous deletion of *CDKN2A/B* has been reported in 22–35% of all gliomas (16–47% *IDH*-mutant GBM and up to 58% of *IDH*-wildtype GBM) [54]. The presence of *CDKN2A* homozygous deletion in LGG and *IDH*-mutant GBM was associated with lower PFS and OS when compared to *CDKN2A* intact tumors [81]. The fifth and sixth updates of C-IMPACT-NOW have incorporated *CDKN2A/B* homozygous deletion as a marker for malignant behavior *IDH*-mutant WHO grade 2 and 3 astrocytomas, upgrading them to WHO grade 4 astrocytoma [2, 82].

These recent changes are quite impactful to daily clinical practice, as the presence of this mutation in astrocytic tumors dramatically changes the prognosis. *CDKN2A/B* deletion should be obtained routinely in the pathological analysis of *IDH*-mutant astrocytoma of any grade [83]. This marker could become a landmark parameter for clinical trial inclusion criteria in the near future [82, 84–86].

Telomerase Reverse Transcriptase Promoter Mutation (*TERTp*)

Telomerase reverse transcriptase (TERT) is a rate-limiting catalytic subunit of telomerase, an RNA-dependent DNA polymerase that lengthens telomeric DNA to maintain shorter telomeres in human cells function to prevent uncontrolled cellular proliferation. *TERT* promoter mutations result in the upregulation of *TERT* transcription, have been identified in over 50 different types of cancer, including several CNS neoplasms [87, 88]. Somatic hot spot mutations in *TERTp* occur in

IDH-wildtype GBM and in *1p/19q* co-deleted *IDH*-mutant oligodendroglioma. *ATRX* mutations are found to be mutually exclusive with *TERT*p mutations in adult GBM [89–91]. *TERT*p mutation has been linked to worse prognosis if found on *IDH*-wildtype astrocytoma WHO grade II or III as their clinical course resembles to the one of a WHO grade IV GBM [25, 90, 92]. Although *TERT* promoter mutation has not become a major pharmacological target for cancer therapy yet, it has significant role in glioma diagnosis and prognosis.

Conclusion

Advances in tumor molecular profiling technologies have allowed molecular characterization of GBM as never before. The addition of molecular biomarkers and histology to the 2016 WHO Classification of CNS Tumors has deeply impacted the clinical management of gliomas providing not only a more accurate diagnosis and prognostication, but also the opportunity to develop innovative clinical trials tailored to the genetic and epigenetic alterations of each tumor. The inclusion of next generation sequence-based assays and other molecular methods in the evaluation of newly diagnosed and recurrent GBM is becoming essential, as it may dramatically impact the diagnosis and management of our patients.

As more discoveries rapidly arise, and the pathogenesis of GBM continues to be better understood, it is likely that more markers will become part of additional classifications of this complex and heterogeneous tumor.

References

1. van den Bent MJ, et al. A clinical perspective on the 2016 WHO brain tumor classification and routine molecular diagnostics. Neuro-Oncology. 2017;19(5):614–24.
2. Louis DN, et al. cIMPACT-NOW update 6: new entity and diagnostic principle recommendations of the cIMPACT-Utrecht meeting on future CNS tumor classification and grading. Brain Pathol. 2020;30(4):844–56.
3. Louis DN, et al. The 2016 World Health Organization classification of tumors of the central nervous system: a summary. Acta Neuropathol. 2016;131(6):803–20.
4. Louis DN, et al. Announcing cIMPACT-NOW: the consortium to inform molecular and practical approaches to CNS tumor taxonomy. Acta Neuropathol. 2017;133(1):1–3.
5. Louis DN, et al. cIMPACT-NOW (the consortium to inform molecular and practical approaches to CNS tumor taxonomy): a new initiative in advancing nervous system tumor classification. Brain Pathol. 2017;27(6):851–2.
6. Zhang C, et al. IDH1/2 mutations target a key hallmark of cancer by deregulating cellular metabolism in glioma. Neuro-Oncology. 2013;15(9):1114–26.
7. Parsons DW, et al. An integrated genomic analysis of human glioblastoma multiforme. Science. 2008;321(5897):1807–12.
8. Romanidou O, Kotoula V, Fountzilas G. Bridging cancer biology with the clinic: comprehending and exploiting IDH gene mutations in gliomas. Cancer Genomics Proteomics. 2018;15(5):421–36.

 9. Miyata S, et al. Comprehensive metabolomic analysis of IDH1R132H clinical glioma samples reveals suppression of β-oxidation due to carnitine deficiency. Sci Rep. 2019;9(1):9787.
10. Clark O, Yen K, Mellinghoff IK. Molecular pathways: isocitrate dehydrogenase mutations in cancer. Clin Cancer Res. 2016;22(8):1837–42.
11. Hartmann C, et al. Type and frequency of IDH1 and IDH2 mutations are related to astrocytic and oligodendroglial differentiation and age: a study of 1,010 diffuse gliomas. Acta Neuropathol. 2009;118(4):469–74.
12. Dang L, Yen K, Attar EC. IDH mutations in cancer and progress toward development of targeted therapeutics. Ann Oncol. 2016;27(4):599–608.
13. Ohgaki H, Kleihues P. The definition of primary and secondary glioblastoma. Clin Cancer Res. 2013;19(4):764.
14. Waitkus MS, Diplas BH, Yan H. Isocitrate dehydrogenase mutations in gliomas. Neuro-Oncology. 2016;18(1):16–26.
15. Jalbert LE, et al. Metabolic profiling of IDH mutation and malignant progression in infiltrating glioma. Sci Rep. 2017;7:44792.
16. Ostrom QT, et al. CBTRUS statistical report: primary brain and other central nervous system tumors diagnosed in the United States in 2012–2016. Neuro-Oncology. 2019;21(Suppl_5):v1–v100.
17. Yan H, et al. IDH1 and IDH2 mutations in gliomas. N Engl J Med. 2009;360(8):765–73.
18. Molinaro AM, et al. Genetic and molecular epidemiology of adult diffuse glioma. Nat Rev Neurol. 2019;15(7):405–17.
19. Christians A, et al. The prognostic role of IDH mutations in homogeneously treated patients with anaplastic astrocytomas and glioblastomas. Acta Neuropathol Commun. 2019;7(1):156.
20. Tejera D, et al. Ivosidenib, an IDH1 inhibitor, in a patient with recurrent, IDH1-mutant glioblastoma: a case report from a phase I study. CNS Oncol. 2020;9:Cns62.
21. Mellinghoff, I. K., et al. Ivosidenib in Isocitrate Dehydrogenase 1-Mutated Advanced Glioma. J Clin Oncol 2020;38(29):3398–406.
22. De La Fuente MI, et al. A phase Ib/II study of olutasidenib in patients with relapsed/refractory IDH1 mutant gliomas: safety and efficacy as single agent and in combination with azacitidine. J Clin Oncol. 2020;38(15_Suppl):2505.
23. Galanis E, et al. Integrating genomics into neuro-oncology clinical trials and practice. Am Soc Clin Oncol Educ Book. 2018;38:148–57.
24. Popovici-Muller J, et al. Discovery of AG-120 (Ivosidenib): a first-in-class mutant IDH1 inhibitor for the treatment of IDH1 mutant cancers. ACS Med Chem Lett. 2018;9(4):300–5.
25. Brat DJ, et al. cIMPACT-NOW update 3: recommended diagnostic criteria for "diffuse astrocytic glioma, IDH-wildtype, with molecular features of glioblastoma, WHO grade IV". Acta Neuropathol. 2018;136(5):805–10.
26. Tesileanu CMS, et al. Survival of diffuse astrocytic glioma, IDH1/2 wildtype, with molecular features of glioblastoma, WHO grade IV: a confirmation of the cIMPACT-NOW criteria. Neuro-Oncology. 2019;22(4):515–23.
27. Stupp R, et al. Effects of radiotherapy with concomitant and adjuvant temozolomide versus radiotherapy alone on survival in glioblastoma in a randomised phase III study: 5-year analysis of the EORTC-NCIC trial. Lancet Oncol. 2009;10(5):459–66.
28. Binabaj MM, et al. The prognostic value of MGMT promoter methylation in glioblastoma: a meta-analysis of clinical trials. J Cell Physiol. 2018;233(1):378–86.
29. Yu W, et al. O(6)-methylguanine-DNA methyltransferase (MGMT): challenges and new opportunities in glioma chemotherapy. Front Oncol. 2020;9:1547.
30. Mansouri A, et al. MGMT promoter methylation status testing to guide therapy for glioblastoma: refining the approach based on emerging evidence and current challenges. Neuro-Oncology. 2019;21(2):167–78.
31. Dahlrot RH, et al. Posttreatment effect of MGMT methylation level on glioblastoma survival. J Neuropathol Exp Neurol. 2019;78(7):633–40.

32. Brigliadori G, et al. Defining the cutoff value of MGMT gene promoter methylation and its predictive capacity in glioblastoma. J Neuro-Oncol. 2016;128(2):333–9.
33. Hegi ME, et al. MGMT gene silencing and benefit from temozolomide in glioblastoma. N Engl J Med. 2005;352(10):997–1003.
34. Estival A, et al. Pyrosequencing versus methylation-specific PCR for assessment of MGMT methylation in tumor and blood samples of glioblastoma patients. Sci Rep. 2019;9(1):11125.
35. Hsu C-Y, et al. Prognosis of glioblastoma with faint MGMT methylation-specific PCR product. J Neuro-Oncol. 2015;122(1):179–88.
36. Pinson H, et al. Weak MGMT gene promoter methylation confers a clinically significant survival benefit in patients with newly diagnosed glioblastoma: a retrospective cohort study. J Neuro-Oncol. 2020;146(1):55–62.
37. Malmström A, et al. Temozolomide versus standard 6-week radiotherapy versus hypofractionated radiotherapy in patients older than 60 years with glioblastoma: the Nordic randomised, phase 3 trial. Lancet Oncol. 2012;13(9):916–26.
38. Kalra B, Kannan S, Gupta T. Optimal adjuvant therapy in elderly glioblastoma: results from a systematic review and network meta-analysis. J Neuro-Oncol. 2020;146(2):311–20.
39. Wee CW, et al. Chemoradiation in elderly patients with glioblastoma from the multi-institutional GBM-molRPA cohort: is short-course radiotherapy enough or is it a matter of selection? J Neuro-Oncol. 2020;148(1):57–65.
40. Hanna C, et al. Treatment of newly diagnosed glioblastoma in the elderly: a network meta-analysis. Cochrane Database Syst Rev. 2020;3(3):Cd013261.
41. Perry JR, et al. Short-course radiation plus temozolomide in elderly patients with glioblastoma. N Engl J Med. 2017;376(11):1027–37.
42. Zhou M, et al. The value of MGMT promote methylation and IDH-1 mutation on diagnosis of pseudoprogression in patients with high-grade glioma: a meta-analysis. Medicine. 2019;98(50):e18194.
43. Brandes AA, et al. MGMT promoter methylation status can predict the incidence and outcome of pseudoprogression after concomitant radiochemotherapy in newly diagnosed glioblastoma patients. J Clin Oncol. 2008;26(13):2192–7.
44. Wen PY, et al. Response assessment in neuro-oncology clinical trials. J Clin Oncol Off J Am Soc Clin Oncol. 2017;35(21):2439–49.
45. Thust SC, van den Bent MJ, Smits M. Pseudoprogression of brain tumors. J Magn Reson Imaging. 2018;48(3):571–89.
46. Chukwueke UN, Wen PY. Use of the response assessment in neuro-oncology (RANO) criteria in clinical trials and clinical practice. CNS Oncol. 2019;8(1):CNS28.
47. Maire CL, Ligon KL. Molecular pathologic diagnosis of epidermal growth factor receptor. Neuro-Oncology. 2014;16 Suppl 8(Suppl 8):viii1–6.
48. Cimino PJ, et al. A wide spectrum of EGFR mutations in glioblastoma is detected by a single clinical oncology targeted next-generation sequencing panel. Exp Mol Pathol. 2015;98(3):568–73.
49. Brennan CW, et al. The somatic genomic landscape of glioblastoma. Cell. 2013;155(2):462–77.
50. An Z, et al. Epidermal growth factor receptor and EGFRvIII in glioblastoma: signaling pathways and targeted therapies. Oncogene. 2018;37(12):1561–75.
51. Mellinghoff IK, et al. Molecular determinants of the response of glioblastomas to EGFR kinase inhibitors. N Engl J Med. 2005;353(19):2012–24.
52. Aldape K, et al. Glioblastoma: pathology, molecular mechanisms and markers. Acta Neuropathol. 2015;129(6):829–48.
53. Neftel C, et al. An integrative model of cellular states, plasticity, and genetics for glioblastoma. Cell. 2019;178(4):835–849.e21.
54. Kessler T, et al. Molecular profiling-based decision for targeted therapies in IDH wild-type glioblastoma. Neurooncol Adv. 2020;2(1):vdz060.

55. Brito C, et al. Clinical insights gained by refining the 2016 WHO classification of diffuse gliomas with: EGFR amplification, TERT mutations, PTEN deletion and MGMT methylation. BMC Cancer. 2019;19(1):968.
56. Alexandru O, et al. Receptor tyrosine kinase targeting in glioblastoma: performance, limitations and future approaches. Contemp Oncol (Pozn). 2020;24(1):55–66.
57. Weller M, et al. Rindopepimut with temozolomide for patients with newly diagnosed, EGFRvIII-expressing glioblastoma (ACT IV): a randomised, double-blind, international phase 3 trial. Lancet Oncol. 2017;18(10):1373–85.
58. Milella M, et al. PTEN: multiple functions in human malignant tumors. Front Oncol. 2015;5:24.
59. Han F, et al. PTEN gene mutations correlate to poor prognosis in glioma patients: a meta-analysis. Onco Targets Ther. 2016;9:3485–92.
60. Yang J-M, et al. Characterization of PTEN mutations in brain cancer reveals that pten mono-ubiquitination promotes protein stability and nuclear localization. Oncogene. 2017;36(26):3673–85.
61. Rosenthal M, et al. Buparlisib plus carboplatin or lomustine in patients with recurrent glioblastoma: a phase Ib/II, open-label, multicentre, randomised study. ESMO Open. 2020;5(4):e000672.
62. Wen PY, et al. Phase I, open-label, multicentre study of buparlisib in combination with temozolomide or with concomitant radiation therapy and temozolomide in patients with newly diagnosed glioblastoma. ESMO Open. 2020;5(4):e000673.
63. Maraka S, Janku F. BRAF alterations in primary brain tumors. Discov Med. 2018;26(141):51–60.
64. Bond CE, Whitehall VLJ. How the BRAF V600E mutation defines a distinct subgroup of colorectal cancer: molecular and clinical implications. Gastroenterol Res Pract. 2018;2018:9250757.
65. Kushnirsky M, et al. Prolonged complete response with combined dabrafenib and trametinib after BRAF inhibitor failure in BRAF-mutant glioblastoma. JCO Precis Oncol. 2020;4:44–50.
66. Ida CM, et al. Pleomorphic xanthoastrocytoma: natural history and long-term follow-up. Brain Pathol. 2015;25(5):575–86.
67. Dias-Santagata D, et al. BRAF V600E mutations are common in pleomorphic xanthoastrocytoma: diagnostic and therapeutic implications. PLoS One. 2011;6(3):e17948.
68. Koelsche C, et al. Mutant BRAF V600E protein in ganglioglioma is predominantly expressed by neuronal tumor cells. Acta Neuropathol. 2013;125(6):891–900.
69. Phadnis S, et al. Rare-20. BRAF mutations in pediatric gangliogliomas and the clinical significance an MD Anderson Cancer Center experience. Neuro-Oncology. 2018;20(Suppl_6):vi240.
70. Korshunov A, et al. Epithelioid glioblastomas stratify into established diagnostic subsets upon integrated molecular analysis. Brain Pathol. 2018;28(5):656–62.
71. Behling F, et al. Frequency of BRAF V600E mutations in 969 central nervous system neoplasms. Diagn Pathol. 2016;11(1):55.
72. Zeng Y, et al. Clinicopathological, immunohistochemical and molecular genetic study on epithelioid glioblastoma: a series of fifteen cases with literature review. Onco Targets Ther. 2020;13:3943–52.
73. Kanemaru Y, et al. Dramatic response of BRAF V600E-mutant epithelioid glioblastoma to combination therapy with BRAF and MEK inhibitor: establishment and xenograft of a cell line to predict clinical efficacy. Acta Neuropathol Commun. 2019;7(1):119.
74. Burger MC, et al. Dabrafenib in patients with recurrent, BRAF V600E mutated malignant glioma and leptomeningeal disease. Oncol Rep. 2017;38(6):3291–6.
75. Lassman A, et al. OS10.6 Infigratinib (BGJ398) in patients with recurrent gliomas with fibroblast growth factor receptor (FGFR) alterations: a multicenter phase II study. Neuro-Oncology. 2019;21:iii21–2.
76. Meric-Bernstam F, et al. Abstract CT238: TAS-120 in patients with advanced solid tumors bearing FGF/FGFR aberrations: a phase I study. Cancer Res. 2019;79(13 Supplement):CT238.

77. Zhang R-Q, et al. Biomarker-based prognostic stratification of young adult glioblastoma. Oncotarget. 2016;7(4):5030–41.
78. Lassman AB, et al. Phase 2 trial of dasatinib in target-selected patients with recurrent glioblastoma (RTOG 0627). Neuro-Oncology. 2015;17(7):992–8.
79. Galanis E, et al. A phase 1 and randomized, placebo-controlled phase 2 trial of bevacizumab plus dasatinib in patients with recurrent glioblastoma: Alliance/North Central Cancer Treatment Group N0872. Cancer. 2019;125(21):3790–800.
80. Jiao Y, Feng Y, Wang X. Regulation of tumor suppressor gene CDKN2A and encoded p16-INK4a protein by covalent modifications. Biochem Mosc. 2018;83(11):1289–98.
81. Lu VM, et al. The prognostic significance of CDKN2A homozygous deletion in IDH-mutant lower-grade glioma and glioblastoma: a systematic review of the contemporary literature. J Neuro-Oncol. 2020;148(2):221–9.
82. Brat DJ, et al. cIMPACT-NOW update 5: recommended grading criteria and terminologies for IDH-mutant astrocytomas. Acta Neuropathol. 2020;139(3):603–8.
83. Yang RR, et al. IDH mutant lower grade (WHO Grades II/III) astrocytomas can be stratified for risk by CDKN2A, CDK4 and PDGFRA copy number alterations. Brain Pathol. 2020;30(3):541–53.
84. Appay R, et al. CDKN2A homozygous deletion is a strong adverse prognosis factor in diffuse malignant IDH-mutant gliomas. Neuro-Oncology. 2019;21:1519–28.
85. Mirchia K, et al. Total copy number variation as a prognostic factor in adult astrocytoma subtypes. Acta Neuropathol Commun. 2019;7(1):92.
86. Reis GF, et al. CDKN2A loss is associated with shortened overall survival in lower-grade (World Health Organization Grades II–III) astrocytomas. J Neuropathol Exp Neurol. 2015;74(5):442–52.
87. Patel B, et al. TERT, a promoter of CNS malignancies. Neurooncol Adv. 2020;2(1):vdaa025.
88. Yuan X, Larsson C, Xu D. Mechanisms underlying the activation of TERT transcription and telomerase activity in human cancer: old actors and new players. Oncogene. 2019;38(34):6172–83.
89. Killela PJ, et al. Mutations in IDH1, IDH2, and in the TERT promoter define clinically distinct subgroups of adult malignant gliomas. Oncotarget. 2014;5(6):1515–25.
90. Bollam SR, Berens ME, Dhruv HD. When the ends are really the beginnings: targeting telomerase for treatment of GBM. Curr Neurol Neurosci Rep. 2018;18(4):15.
91. Lee Y, et al. The frequency and prognostic effect of TERT promoter mutation in diffuse gliomas. Acta Neuropathol Commun. 2017;5(1):62.
92. Reifenberger G, et al. Advances in the molecular genetics of gliomas — implications for classification and therapy. Nat Rev Clin Oncol. 2017;14(7):434–52.

Chapter 3
Neurosurgical Approach to the Patient with Glioblastoma

Guilherme Gozzoli Podolsky-Gondim, Ricardo Santos de Oliveira, Carlos Gilberto Carlotti Jr, and Benedicto Oscar Colli

Introduction

Epidemiology and Survival

Glioblastoma is the most common primary malignant brain tumor in adults, corresponding to approximately 15% of all intracranial neoplasms and 48% of all primary malignant tumors of the central nervous system (CNS) [1–3]. The incidence varies according to the country and region pooled and in the United States (US) when considering all malignant brain tumors, the highest incidence was for glioblastoma with 3.22 per 100,000 [3]. Although patients of any age may be diagnosed with glioblastoma, there is a higher incidence in older adults, with the highest rates in the 74–84 years range [3]. In a population-based study from Zurich, Switzerland, the mean age of patients with primary (*de novo*) glioblastoma was 62 years and for secondary glioblastoma (those arisen from a previous lower grade glioma) was 45 years [1]. The male-to-female ratio is 1.6 in the US [3] and 1.28 in Switzerland [1]. Prognosis is poor and median survival of secondary glioblastoma patients was 7.8 months and for primary glioblastoma patients was 4.7 months in a Swiss study [1]. In the paramount clinical trial by *Stupp* et al. [4] median overall survival increased to 14.6 months for patients with newly diagnosed glioblastoma that received both radiotherapy plus chemotherapy with temozolomide, following surgery.

G. G. Podolsky-Gondim · R. S. de Oliveira (✉) · C. G. Carlotti Jr · B. O. Colli
Division of Neurosurgery, Department of Surgery and Anatomy, Ribeirão Preto, SP, Brazil

Clinics Hospital, Ribeirão Preto School of Medicine, University of São Paulo, São Paulo, SP, Brazil

School of Medicine of Ribeirao Preto University of Sao Paulo, São Paulo, SP, Brazil
e-mail: podolsky@usp.br; rsoliveira@hcrp.usp.br; carlotti@fmrp.usp.br; bocolli@fmrp.usp.br

© The Author(s), under exclusive license to Springer Nature Switzerland AG 2021
J. J. Otero, A. P. Becker (eds.), *Precision Molecular Pathology of Glioblastoma*, Molecular Pathology Library, https://doi.org/10.1007/978-3-030-69170-7_3

Clinical Presentation

The clinical presentation of glioblastoma is highly variable, and the signs/symp-toms will depend upon the tumor location and its extension. According to two ret-rospective studies conducted at emergency medicine departments, patients that were further diagnosed with brain tumors presented with focal neurological signs – such as hemiparesis – mental status alterations, headache, seizures, trauma, visual changes, speech deficit, sensory abnormalities, nausea, vomiting or dizziness [5–8]. Seizures may affect up to half of patients with glioblastoma at some point during the course of the disease. Although the widespread adoption of antiepileptic drugs for this population is controversial, the use is recommended when a first seizure is pres-ent [9]. Also, recent evidence suggest that patients with a mutated *IDH* status had a higher chance of presenting seizures [10, 11]. Additionally, due to glioblastoma rapid growth rate, it is not unusual for the patient to first present with signs of increased intracranial pressure (ICP) – such as new onset headache associated with vomiting, nausea and consciousness compromise – due to mass effect by the lesion and associated surrounding edema. In this case, corticosteroids are usually promptly initiated, a treatment supported by data from landmark studies published in the 1960s, and patients with signs of increased ICP or consciousness compromise will be frequently treated with dexamethasone 10 mg intravenously and 4 mg orally four times a day, with a good initial response expected following the effects over the sur-rounding vasogenic edema [12, 13]. Due to the side effects expected with cortico-steroids, concomitant prescription of proton-pump inhibitors, such as omeprazole, is required.

Operative Candidate Selection

Diagnostic Workup

As previously mentioned, it is common for the patient with glioblastoma to be ini-tially admitted to the emergency department following new onset neurological defi-cit, seizures or clinical signs of increased ICP. Thus, often the first radiological imaging to investigate those symptoms is a head computed tomography (CT) with or without contrast enhancement (Fig. 3.1). A gadolinium-enhanced magnetic reso-nance imaging (MRI) is ordered following the CT, or as standard-of-care if the patient was first evaluated in an outpatient consultation. MRI allows for detailed anatomical resolution, as well as, within certain degree of certainty due to the known characteristics of anatomical location of each primary brain tumor, a diagnosis (Fig. 3.2). For instance, extra-axial lesions often represent meningiomas, whereas inflammatory and infectious lesions, such as multiple sclerosis or cerebral abscess, would demonstrate distinct neuroanatomical localizations.

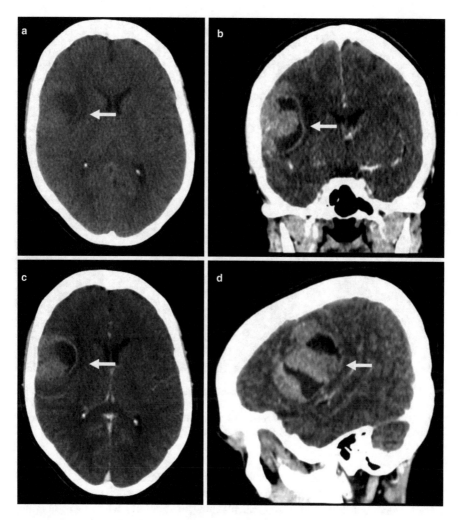

Fig. 3.1 Emergency head CT. Emergency head computed tomography (CT) of a patient with a glioblastoma initially admitted at the emergency room. (**a**) Axial reconstruction of the non-enhanced CT depicting a heterogenous lesion with surrounding edema (white arrow). (**b**) A coronal reconstruction post-contrast enhancement depicting the same lesion, with the surrounding edema and a heterogenous aspect (white arrow). (**c**) Axial contrast-enhanced view. (**d**) Sagittal contrast-enhanced reconstruction with the same features (white arrow)

Further investigation may include complementary MRI sequences. For example, MRI-spectroscopy, in which tissue metabolites are evaluated (Fig. 3.3), allowing for a higher assurance in differentiating between infection and high-grade glioma, and MRI perfusion, which allows for further resolution of areas of increased tumor cellularity and malignancy grade for gliomas [14–16] (Fig. 3.4).

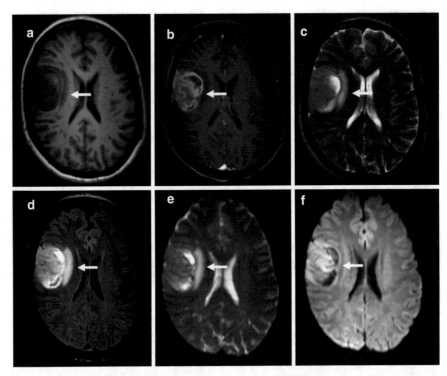

Fig. 3.2 MRI commonly used sequences. Magnetic resonance imaging of an insular glioblastoma (white arrow). Axial reconstruction in different sequences. (**a**) T1 weighted sequence. (**b**) T1 weighted gadolinium-enhanced sequence. (**c**) T2 weighted sequence. (**d**) Fluid-attenuated inversion recovery (FLAIR) sequence. (**e**) Diffusion-weighted imaging (DWI) sequence. (**f**) Iso DWI sequence

When there is involvement of eloquent brain areas, such as speech areas (eg., left inferior frontal gyrus, left temporal and parietal lobes), <u>preoperative</u> functional MRI (fMRI) may contribute to the surgical planning, particularly when there is doubt regarding lateralization of cerebral hemisphere dominance [17, 18]. Another additional preoperative imaging technique is the diffuse tensor imaging (DTI), which may contribute to the differential diagnosis between glioblastoma and brain metastases, besides helping in the surgical planning and, when coupled with a neuronavigation device, assisting in the avoidance of lesions to fibers, such as pyramidal tract when there is tumor involvement of motor pathways [16, 19–21].

Additionally, general clinical assessment is required, including but not limited to laboratorial exams (i.e., coagulation status, hemogram, renal function, serum electrolytes), chest radiography and electrocardiogram. Further clinical assessment may be needed for elderly patients, such as echocardiogram and pulmonary function. Although rare, attention to immunocompromise is needed, with a comprehensive interview regarding previous exposure to HIV and potential immunocompromise,

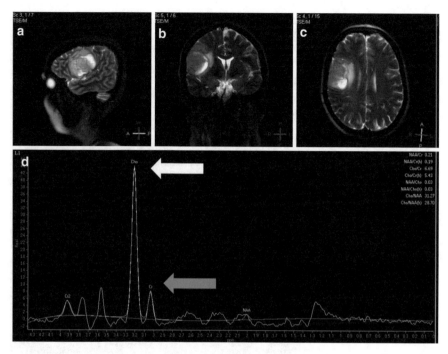

Fig. 3.3 MRI Advanced sequences – spectroscopy. Example of the MRI spectroscopy profile of an insular glioblastoma. The region of interest (red square) delimited in the sagittal (**a**), coronal (**b**) and axial (**c**) plans and the corresponding metabolic profile typical of a glioblastoma (**d**), depicting a peak of choline (white arrow) and the peak of creatine (blue arrow), among other metabolites

such as for transplanted patients, since infectious intracranial diseases may mimic clinical presentation of brain tumors.

Preoperative Performance Status

One of the mainstays of clinical assessment for patients with glioblastoma is the Karnofsky Performance Status (KPS). Published in 1949, KPS describes the patient's functional status in a comprehensive scale ranging from 100% (no evidence of disease, no symptoms) to 0% (death) (Table 3.1). Although it is not feasible to summarize and categorize the whole range of social, personal and clinical aspects of the patient with glioblastoma in one common denominator, KPS is particularly important in the attempt to determine the patient's general condition, thus showing particular utility in the setting of oncological clinical trials [22, 23]. Many clinical trials for patients with glioblastoma have considered a KPS of 70% (cares for self, unable to carry on normal activity or to do active work) or equivalent as the cutoff limit to consider major surgical resection. In the individual and personalized

Fig. 3.4 MRI Advanced sequences – MRI Perfusion. Magnetic resonance spectroscopy showing the relative cerebral blood volume (rCBV) measurement for an insular glioblastoma. Note the high rCBV (red) in parts of the lesion (white arrow)

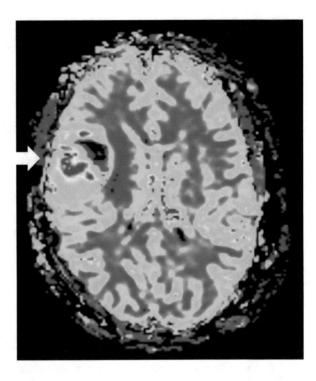

setting, other factors influence the surgical decision, however the previous assessment of the performance status help to ascertain the optimal therapeutic management strategies, in light of the relevant literature.

Surgical Strategies

Extent of Resection

One of the key factors that seems to influence overall survival and recurrence free period for patients with glioblastoma is the extent of resection. However, this is not a feasible goal for many patients – especially those with multifocal lesions, involvement of eloquent areas and poor performance status, to name some of the hindering factors. Three studies addressed the influence of the extent of resection and found evidences that favors the goal of trying to reach gross total resection in order to improve survival and recurrence free interval [24–26]. Surgical adjuncts such as 5-ALA and intraoperative imaging techniques, when available, recently held promise in assisting this goal. For the elderly population, in spite of the intrinsic clinical limitations to an aggressive resection approach, there is also evidence that tumor debulking via craniotomy also offer a survival advantage [27].

Table 3.1 Karnofsky performance status (KPS)

General status	Percentage	Criteria
Able to carry on normal activity and to work. No special care is needed	100	Normal, no complaints, no evidence of disease
	90	Able to carry on normal activity, minor signs or symptoms of disease
	80	Normal activity with effort, some signs or symptoms of disease
Unable to work. Able to live at home, care for most personal needs. A varying degree of assistance is needed	70	Cares for self, unable to carry on normal activity or to do active work
	60	Requires occasional assistance but is able to care for most of his needs
	50	Requires considerable assistance and frequent medical care
Unable to care for self. Requires equivalent of institutional or hospital care. Disease may be progressing rapidly	40	Disabled, requires special care and assistance (In bed more than 50% of the time)
	30	Severely disabled, hospitalization is indicated although death not imminent (Almost completely bedfast)
	20	Hospitalization necessary, very sick, active supportive treatment necessary (Totally bedfast and requiring extensive nursing care by professionals and/or family)
	10	Moribund, fatal processes progressing rapidly (Comatose or barely arousable)
	0	Dead

Adapted from Peus et al. [23], and Karnofsky and Burchenal [22]

We suggest a general flowchart for the decision regarding the surgical approach for newly diagnosed glioblastoma (Fig. 3.5).

Gross Total Resection

Patients with a good clinical performance status (i.e., a KPS ≥70%), no signs of involvement of eloquent areas, usually younger (<65 years) and with a suspected single lesion, are generally referred for craniotomy with a preoperative goal of gross total resection (GTR) (Fig. 3.6). Due to glioblastoma biological characteristics, the surgeon is often faced with brisk bleeding and local edema, thus challenging the goal of total macroscopic resection. Usually the planned craniotomy is large in order to alleviate the expected increased ICP for larger lesions and corticosteroids (i.e., dexamethasone) are commonly administered, alongside with mannitol or hypertonic saline in order to compensate for the high ICP, to name some of the frequently used adjuncts.

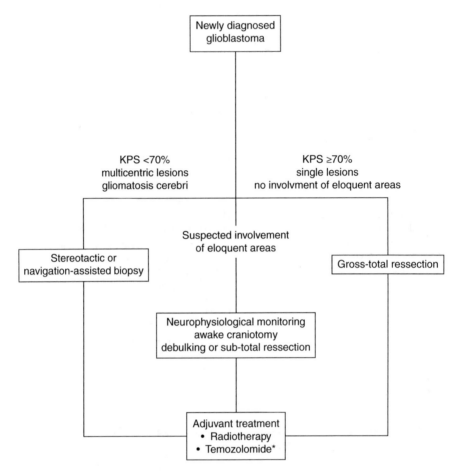

Fig. 3.5 Flowchart for newly diagnosed glioblastoma

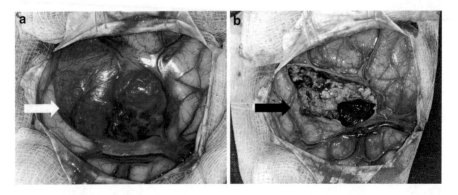

Fig. 3.6 Gross total resection. (**a**) Intraoperative photograph of an insular glioblastoma depicting the heterogenous and highly vascular aspects of the lesion (white arrow) and in (**b**). The post resection tumor bed (black arrow)

Subtotal Resection/Debulking

When gross total resection is deemed unreachable – often due to the age of the patient and/or the involvement of eloquent areas – the surgeon will try to reduce the lesion, via debulking. However, this strategy is not free of risks, since the remaining malignant tissue may lead to postoperative hemorrhage and brain edema, increasing the chance of immediate postoperative complications.

Stereotactic and Neuronavigation-Assisted Biopsy

For patients with poor preoperative clinical performance, high preoperative cardio-vascular risk, multiple lesions, and particularly for those with deep seated lesions, the surgical strategy is based in sampling the suspected area, via a single burr hole with the use of a stereotactic frame-based arch or, more recently, with the use of neuronavigation devices. This procedure may be performed under local anesthesia, thus limiting the perioperative anesthetic risks for those poor-performing patients. For frame-based stereotactic biopsy, a frame is attached to the patient's head under local anesthesia and the patient is submitted to a CT or MRI. The images of the couple head and frame are then fused in a software, and the surgeon draws a trajectory for sampling the tumor with a cannula attached to a stereotactic arch while avoiding vessels, eloquent areas and the ventricles (Fig. 3.7). The procedure is straightforward and one of the benefits is the short length of stay in hospital.

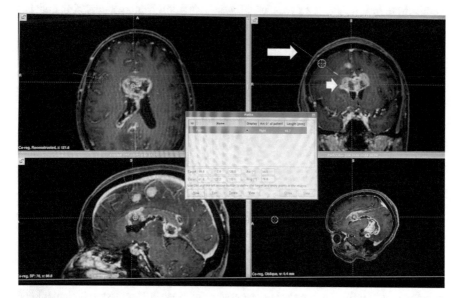

Fig. 3.7 Stereotactic biopsy. Screen capture of the planning workstation depicting a trajectory (large arrow) for stereotactic biopsy of a butterfly glioblastoma (small arrow). An optimal trajectory aims at sampling the contrast-enhanced regions of the lesion while avoiding vessels and the ventricles, in order to minimize the odds of postoperative complications

For the frameless approach, the surgeon may use a neuronavigator – a device that captures various superficial points in the patient's head, thus allowing for the representation of the anatomy in a screen promptly available for the surgical staff. The biopsy then occurs in a similar fashion to the stereotactic frame-based approach described above – burr hole and tumor sampling via a cannula.

Surgical Adjuncts and Special Techniques

Neurophysiological Monitoring and Awake Craniotomy

A special situation occurs whenever there is a suspected involvement of eloquent brain areas, such as the left-frontal opercular region or the pre-central gyrus, responsible for speech production and the primary motor cortex respectively. It may be possible to resect lesions affecting these areas, however the surgeon often relies in intraoperative brain mapping techniques, such as awake craniotomy and brain stimulation. Although the development of imaging techniques such as fMRI may assist in delimiting the speech area or the hand movement area in the motor cortex, the spatial resolution of this imaging technique is insufficient to guarantee a safe approach to lesions involving these areas [28].

Current strategies for the intraoperative brain stimulation include the detection of the areas to be preserved, such as the hand area (for lesions involving the primary motor cortex) or the speech production field (in lesions involving the dominating hemisphere inferior frontal gyrus, usually the left side). Negative-mapping consists in stablishing the safest surgical corridor to the lesion, while stimulating different areas and not incurring in any disturbance of movement or speech, when these functions may be compromised due to involvement by the tumor. High-order cortical function is better evaluated and preserved with the combination of an awake craniotomy coupled with brain stimulation (cortical and white matter) and the participation of an interdisciplinary team, usually composed of speech therapists, neurophysiologists and an experienced neuro-anesthetist [2].

Neuronavigation

Currently, neuronavigation is ubiquitous to the neurosurgical operating theater, allowing for tailored surgical approaches and smaller craniotomies, especially for neuro-oncological procedures. The general principle of this adjunct tool is to allow the spatial localization of particular intracranial structures and brain areas, playing an important role in assisting the neurosurgeon in tailoring the approaches for various intracranial pathologies. The system usually consists of an infrared camera or antenna that identifies a fixed reference near or in close contact to the patient's head (for intracranial surgeries) or bone structures in the spine (for spinal surgeries), and a touch screen that displays the preoperative CT and/or MRI images with the representation of the tip of the neuronavigation probe; or a pair of surgical instrument + camera recognizable object. One main limitation of this device is that it is based in preoperative images, thus subject to the brain-shift phenomena – in which the brain structures may be displaced following cerebral spine fluid drainage or tumor resection, hampering a reliable determination of tumor limits, for example. Recently, efforts were made in circumventing this issue, with adoption of intraoperative ultrasound imaging, allowing correction of this effect with real time intraoperative imaging, among other resources [29, 30].

Intraoperative Magnetic Resonance Imaging

In pursuing GTR, the advent of intraoperative MRI (iMRI) introduced the possibility of evaluating if the resection was satisfactory (i.e., if any residual tumor is present) or promptly detecting signs of surgical complications – while the patient is still at the operating room – allowing a higher chance of GTR. Although this would imply in increased survival and progression-free survival, to this moment no unchallenged evidence for this was published [31, 32]. One major limitation of this adjunct is the necessity of a bold institutional infrastructure, monetary resources and well-established protocols for the anesthesia, surgical and nursing teams in order to employ iMRI at the best conditions [33, 34].

Intraoperative Ultrasound Imaging (iUS)

Ubiquitous to most surgical centers worldwide, the ultrasound is an interesting adjunct for neurosurgery in general and particularly for glioblastoma surgery. Its cost-effectiveness and no need for infrastructure adaptions – such as requested for iMRI implementation – allow for real-time follow-up of brain lesions, such as glioblastoma, without suffering influence of brain-shift. Recent improvements allow for advanced iUS 3D mapping of the lesions, use of contrast-enhancement techniques and also coupling with neuronavigation devices, limiting the effects of such brain-shift [35]. Another important aspect of this surgical adjunct is the possibility of early detection of complications, such as tumor bed hemorrhage, after the dura-mater is closed and before the bone flap is fixed. One limitation for its use is its dependency on the skills of the surgeon operating the device, however the learning curve is not as steep as for other neurosurgical techniques (Fig. 3.8).

Fluorescence-Guided Surgery

Since glioblastoma is characteristically an infiltrating brain lesion, there is an underlying difficulty in differentiating the tumor from the surrounding brain tissue. One strategy for improving maximal safe tumor resection is the use of fluorescent dyes, such as the 5-aminolevulinic acid (5-ALA) – an increasingly popular substance,

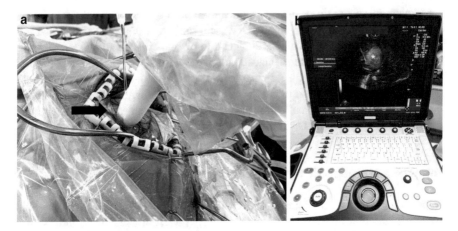

Fig. 3.8 Intraoperative Ultrasound Imaging (iUS). (**a**) Intraoperative photograph of the operative field of a large frontal glioblastoma with the ultrasound probe covered in a sterile plastic dressing (black arrow). (**b**) Ultrasonographic aspect of the tumor, depicting a hyperechogenic lesion (star)

with its use initially described in the late 1990s and administered orally [36, 37]. Although the 5-ALA is deemed safe and with minimal side effects reported, it is still not readily available worldwide and also there is the need for specific hardware (i.e., microscopes capable of fluorescent visualization), thus limiting its use.

Therapeutic Adjuncts

Brachytherapy

Following cumulative evidence of the efficacy of radiation therapy in the management of newly diagnosed and recurrent high-grade gliomas, there were reports in the late 1980s and 1990s of the use of radiotherapy via locally delivered radioactive sources, implanted into the tumor [38, 39]. This direct application delivers a high dose of radiation to the tumor, while minimizing the effects over the surrounding brain. Although many of the reports were case series, two randomized controlled trials that assessed survival following stereotactically implanted high-activity I^{125} concluded that no survival advantage was detected in the patients with newly diagnosed high-grade gliomas submitted to this approach [38–40].

In Situ Chemotherapy

Another therapeutic strategy also tested in the late 1980s and 1990s was the local administration of chemotherapy – carmustine [bis-chloroethylnitrosourea – BCNU] wafers – into the tumor bed of patients with malignant gliomas. This strategy is based in the concepts of circumventing the blood-brain barrier, avoidance of well-known side effects of systemic chemotherapy agents, and potentially deterrence of local recurrence [38]. Three randomized controlled trials were conducted and some of the results suggest a modest survival advantage for use of carmustine wafers, particularly to patients for which a near gross total resection was feasible [41–44]. Complications associated with this therapy are malignant edema, an increased frequency of wound infection, cyst formation and seizures, among others. However, more evidence is needed in order to determine the optimal combination of treatments available (i.e, systemic + carmustine wafer + radiotherapy) and the patient's characteristics that would indicate those a clear benefit of this therapy [38, 40, 45].

Reoperation

Due to the intrinsic characteristics of glioblastoma, recurrence is expected even after GTR and optimal adjuvant treatment were performed. Also, due to the high variability in presentation and patterns of recurrence, no unified consensus has been achieved regarding the decision to re-operate patients that present with glioblastoma recurrence. However, this option should be considered after careful evaluation of potential complications following surgery as well as the patient's expectations regarding the procedure, given that the patient performance status and involvement of eloquent areas may preclude further surgeries [46]. A suggested simplified flow-chart for decision is presented below (Fig. 3.9).

Also to be considered in the decision regarding reoperation is the difficult differential diagnosis between radiation necrosis – injury to the brain tissue which may span from acute (during radiation therapy), subacute (within 3 months after radiation therapy) and late (months or even years after completion of radiotherapy), – and pseudoprogression – a subacute reaction secondary to the radiation, that may be followed or not by neurological deficits [47, 48]. Although no single imaging technique consistently differentiates between these entities, novel techniques such as DWI, DTI, dynamic contrast enhancement and dynamic susceptibility contrast perfusion, magnetic resonance spectroscopy and PET/SPECT presents promise in assisting this matter, pending future studies comparing different combinations of these modalities [49].

Postoperative Care

Following surgery, the patient is usually admitted to the intensive care unit (ICU) or more recently according to specific protocols, to neurosurgical wards in which the staff is familiarized with the routines of care for neurological patients, if no risk factors requiring ICU monitoring were found [50, 51]. Attention to the level of

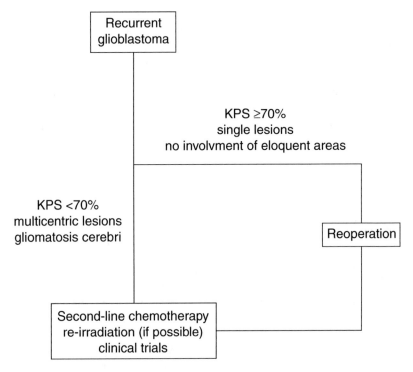

Fig. 3.9 Flowchart for recurrent glioblastoma

consciousness is brought via a neuro-check (i.e., hourly assessment of Glasgow coma scale, pupillary reaction and signs of neurological deficits, such as new-onset hemiparesis). If any new signs of neurological compromise are detected, the neurosurgery staff is notified, and an emergency non-enhanced CT of the head is performed to evaluate postoperative hemorrhage, hydrocephalus or postoperative edema. Subcutaneous drain output is measured, as well as external ventricular drain, if applicable. Continuous systemic multimodal monitoring, laboratory and imaging examinations are also warranted. Depending on the availability of resources, a postoperative gadolinium-enhanced MRI is performed in the first 72 hours after surgery, to assess the extent of tumor resection [52] – if the institution does not have iMRI. If a conventional MRI is unavailable for postoperative imaging, a contrast-enhanced head CT allows for both exclusion of postoperative complications and to roughly estimate the extent of resection. Subcutaneous drains are generally removed in the first or second postoperative day. At the authors' institution transfer to the neurosurgical ward is granted if no clinical or neurological complications were encountered and usually hospital discharge occurs 2–3 days after surgery. This of course depends on the institutional protocols and the patient general clinical condition. If the patient is bed-ridden or in need of assistance, a multidisciplinary program of rehabilitation is activated and further discussion of options for long-term care are discussed with the family (i.e., transfer for a rehabilitation or nursing facility, if no conditions for home discharge is possible).

Complications

Postoperative complications for patients with glioblastoma are highly variable, however they may be categorized as surgical field related and clinical complications. Of the former, the most common complication reported in a large retrospective series of 16,530 malignant brain tumors surgeries was iatrogenic stroke (incidence 16.3 per 1000 cases), followed by hemorrhage or hematoma (incidence of 10.3 per 1000 cases), and postoperative meningitis (incidence of 1.1 per 1000 cases). Rarely the retention of a foreign object and wrong side surgery were reported (less than 0.7 per 1000 cases) [53]. The odds of clinical complications were higher whenever a surgical complication was present and the more frequent were urinary tract infection, followed by pneumonia, deep vein thrombosis and finally – with the same incidence – pulmonary embolism, acute kidney injury, myocardial infarction and pancreatitis. As it would be expected, there was a negative impact of the presence of surgical or clinical complications and higher length of stay and mortality [53]. A literature review of adverse effects in intracranial neoplasm surgery found that complications ranged from 9% to 40%, with overall mortality rates of 1.5–16%, with a myriad of types of adverse effects. The authors reported that deep vein thrombosis was the most common complication, with an incidence ranging 0–20% – lower in a meningioma case series, and highest for eloquent area glioma surgery [54]. Thus, tackling potential causes of postoperative complications, may preclude longer length of stay periods and thus diminish the risk of mortality. However, due to the intrinsic characteristics of glioblastoma patients – such as older age of onset, intense vascularization of the tumor, early important surrounding brain edema and functional impairments, to name a few – avoiding perioperative complications poses a significant challenge for the interdisciplinary team.

Conclusions

Surgical management of glioblastoma is challenging and before surgery is considered, the patient must undergo a comprehensive preoperative assessment. The radiological and laboratory workup is a priority in order to confirm glioblastoma as the main clinical hypothesis and to predict potential risks for further functional compromise due to involvement of eloquent areas for example, as well as the need for special techniques for the resection, such as awake craniotomy or intraoperative brain stimulation. The preoperative performance status, measure by KPS, is paramount to weight the potential benefits of the surgery versus the risks of poor postoperative outcome. An interdisciplinary discussion of diagnostic and treatment goals, aligned with the patient and family interests and goals, is highly recommended.

References

1. Ohgaki H, Kleihues P. Population-based studies on incidence, survival rates, and genetic alterations in astrocytic and oligodendroglial gliomas. J Neuropathol Exp Neurol. 2005;64(6):479–89. https://doi.org/10.1093/jnen/64.6.479.
2. Louis DN, Ohgaki H, Wiestler OD, Cavenee WK, editors. WHO Classification of tumours of the central nervous system. Revised 4th ed. Lyon: IARC; 2016.
3. Ostrom QT, Cioffi G, Gittleman H, et al. CBTRUS statistical report: primary brain and other central nervous system tumors diagnosed in the United States in 2012–2016. Neuro-Oncology. 2019;21(Suppl 5):v1–v100. https://doi.org/10.1093/neuonc/noz150.
4. Stupp R, Mason WP, van den Bent MJ, et al. Radiotherapy plus concomitant and adjuvant temozolomide for glioblastoma. N Engl J Med. 2005;352(10):987–96. https://doi.org/10.1056/NEJMoa043330.
5. Snyder H, Robinson K, Shah D, Brennan R, Handrigan M. Signs and symptoms of patients with brain tumors presenting to the emergency department. J Emerg Med. 1993;11(3):253–8. https://doi.org/10.1016/0736-4679(93)90042-6.
6. Comelli I, Lippi G, Campana V, Servadei F, Cervellin G. Clinical presentation and epidemiology of brain tumors firstly diagnosed in adults in the emergency department: a 10-year, single center retrospective study. Ann Transl Med. 2017;5(13):269. https://doi.org/10.21037/atm.2017.06.12.
7. Posti JP, Bori M, Kauko T, et al. Presenting symptoms of glioma in adults. Acta Neurol Scand. 2015;131(2):88–93. https://doi.org/10.1111/ane.12285.
8. Silvani A, Gaviani P, Lamperti E, et al. Malignant gliomas: early diagnosis and clinical aspects. Neurol Sci. 2011;32(Suppl 2):S207–8. https://doi.org/10.1007/s10072-011-0788-9.
9. Julie DAR, Ahmed Z, Karceski SC, Pannullo SC, Schwartz TH, Parashar B, Wernicke AG. An overview of anti-epileptic therapy management of patients with malignant tumors of the brain undergoing radiation therapy. Seizure. 2019;70:30–7. https://doi.org/10.1016/j.seizure.2019.06.019.
10. Chen H, Judkins J, Thomas C, et al. Mutant IDH1 and seizures in patients with glioma. Neurology. 2017;88(19):1805–13. https://doi.org/10.1212/WNL.0000000000003911.
11. Lee JW. Mutating our understanding of brain tumors and seizures: Entrez IDH. Epilepsy Curr. 2017;17(6):365–7. https://doi.org/10.5698/1535-7597.17.6.365.
12. Galicich JH, French LA, Melby JC. Use of dexamethasone in treatment of cerebral oedema associated with brain tumours. J Lancet. 1961;81:46–53.
13. McLelland S, Long DM. Genesis of the use of corticosteroids in the treatment and prevention of brain oedema. Neurosurgery. 2008;62:965–8.
14. Young RM, Jamshidi A, Davis G, Sherman JH. Current trends in the surgical management and treatment of adult glioblastoma. Ann Transl Med. 2015;3(9):121. https://doi.org/10.3978/j.issn.2305-5839.2015.05.10.
15. Oberheim Bush NA, Hervey-Jumper SL, Berger MS. Management of glioblastoma, present and future. World Neurosurg. 2019;131:328–38. https://doi.org/10.1016/j.wneu.2019.07.044.
16. Shukla G, Alexander GS, Bakas S, et al. Advanced magnetic resonance imaging in glioblastoma: a review. Chin Clin Oncol. 2017;6(4):40. https://doi.org/10.21037/cco.2017.06.28.
17. Ishikawa T, Muragaki Y, Maruyama T, Abe K, Kawamata T. Roles of the Wada test and functional magnetic resonance imaging in identifying the language-dominant hemisphere among patients with gliomas located near speech areas. Neurol Med Chir (Tokyo). 2017;57(1):28–34. https://doi.org/10.2176/nmc.oa.2016-0042.
18. Gunal V, Savardekar AR, Devi BI, Bharath RD. Preoperative functional magnetic resonance imaging in patients undergoing surgery for tumors around left (dominant) inferior frontal gyrus region. Surg Neurol Int. 2018;9:126. Published 26 June 2018. https://doi.org/10.4103/sni.sni_414_17.
19. Salama GR, Heier LA, Patel P, Ramakrishna R, Magge R, Tsiouris AJ. Diffusion weighted/tensor imaging, functional MRI and perfusion weighted imaging in glioblastoma-foundations

and future. Front Neurol. 2018;8:660. https://doi.org/10.3389/fneur.2017.00660. Published 22 Jan 2018.

20. Mekkaoui C, Metellus P, Kostis WJ, et al. Diffusion tensor imaging in patients with glioblastoma multiforme using the supertoroidal model. PLoS One. 2016;11(1):e0146693. https://doi.org/10.1371/journal.pone.0146693. Published 13 Jan 2016.

21. Wang W, Steward CE, Desmond PM. Diffusion tensor imaging in glioblastoma multiforme and brain metastases: the role of p, q, L, and fractional anisotropy. AJNR Am J Neuroradiol. 2009;30(1):203–8. https://doi.org/10.3174/ajnr.A1303.

22. Karnofsky DA, Burchenal JH. The clinical evaluation of chemotherapeutic agents in cancer. In: MacLeod CM, editor. Evaluation of chemotherapeutic agents. New York: Columbia University Press; 1949. p. 191–205.

23. Péus D, Newcomb N, Hofer S. Appraisal of the Karnofsky performance status and proposal of a simple algorithmic system for its evaluation. BMC Med Inform Decis Mak. 2013;13:72. Published 19 July 2013. https://doi.org/10.1186/1472-6947-13-72.

24. Keles GE, Anderson B, Berger MS. The effect of extent of resection on time to tumor progression and survival in patients with glioblastoma multiforme of the cerebral hemisphere. Surg Neurol. 1999;52(4):371–9. https://doi.org/10.1016/s0090-3019(99)00103-2.

25. Lacroix M, Abi-Said D, Fourney DR, Gokaslan ZL, Shi W, DeMonte F, Lang FF, McCutcheon IE, Hassenbusch SJ, Holland E, Hess K, Michael C, Miller D, Sawaya R. A multivariate analysis of 416 patients with glioblastoma multiforme: prognosis, extent of resection, and survival. J Neurosurg. 2001;95:190–8.

26. Stummer W, Reulen HJ, Meinel T, Pichlmeier U, Schumacher W, Tonn JC, Rohde V, Oppel F, Turowski B, Woiciechowsky C, Franz K, Pietsch T, for the ALA-Glioma Study Group. Extent of resection and survival in glioblastoma multiforme: identification of and adjustment for bias. Lancet Oncol. 2008;7:392–401.

27. Vuorinen V, Hinkka S, Färkkilä M, Jääskeläinen J. Debulking or biopsy of malignant glioma in elderly people – a randomised study. Acta Neurochir. 2003;145(1):5–10. https://doi.org/10.1007/s00701-002-1030-6.

28. Hervey-Jumper SL, Li J, Lau D, et al. Awake craniotomy to maximize glioma resection: methods and technical nuances over a 27-year period. J Neurosurg. 2015;123(2):325–39. https://doi.org/10.3171/2014.10.JNS141520.

29. Wirtz CR, Albert FK, Schwaderer M, et al. The benefit of neuronavigation for neurosurgery analyzed by its impact on glioblastoma surgery. Neurol Res. 2000;22(4):354–60. https://doi.org/10.1080/01616412.2000.11740684.

30. Orringer DA, Golby A, Jolesz F. Neuronavigation in the surgical management of brain tumors: current and future trends. Expert Rev Med Devices. 2012;9(5):491–500. https://doi.org/10.1586/erd.12.42.

31. Senft C, Bink A, Franz K, Vatter H, Gasser T, Seifert V. Intraoperative MRI guidance and extent of resection in glioma surgery: a randomised, controlled trial. Lancet Oncol. 2011;12(11):997–1003. https://doi.org/10.1016/S1470-2045(11)70196-6.

32. Kubben PL, Scholtes F, Schijns OE, et al. Intraoperative magnetic resonance imaging versus standard neuronavigation for the neurosurgical treatment of glioblastoma: a randomized controlled trial. Surg Neurol Int. 2014;5:70. https://doi.org/10.4103/2152-7806.132572. Published 15 May 2014.

33. Pichierri A, Bradley M, Iyer V. Intraoperative magnetic resonance imaging-guided glioma resections in awake or asleep settings and feasibility in the context of a public health system. World Neurosurg X. 2019;3:100022. https://doi.org/10.1016/j.wnsx.2019.100022. Published 20 Feb 2019.

34. Napolitano M, Vaz G, Lawson TM, et al. Glioblastoma surgery with and without intraoperative MRI at 3.0T. Neurochirurgie. 2014;60(4):143–50. https://doi.org/10.1016/j.neuchi.2014.03.010.

35. Moiraghi A, Pallud J. Intraoperative ultrasound techniques for cerebral gliomas resection: usefulness and pitfalls. Ann Transl Med. 2020;8(8):523. https://doi.org/10.21037/atm.2020.03.178.

36. Stummer W, Pichlmeier U, Meinel T, Wiestler OD, Zanella F, Reulen HJ, ALA-Glioma Study Group. Fluorescence-guided surgery with 5-alaminovulinic acid for resection of malignant glioma: a randomised controlled multicentre phase III trial. Lancet Oncol. 2006;7:392–401.
37. Hadjipanayis CG, Widhalm G, Stummer W. What is the surgical benefit of utilizing 5-aminolevulinic acid for fluorescence-guided surgery of malignant gliomas? Neurosurgery. 2015;77(5):663–73. https://doi.org/10.1227/NEU.0000000000000929.
38. Johnson RD, Green AL. Landmark papers in neurosurgery. 1st ed. Oxford: Oxford University Press; 2010.
39. Laperriere NJ, Leung PM, McKenzie S, et al. Randomized study of brachytherapy in the initial management of patients with malignant astrocytoma. Int J Radiat Oncol Biol Phys. 1998;41(5):1005–11. https://doi.org/10.1016/s0360-3016(98)00159-x.
40. Selker RG, Shapiro WR, Burger P, et al. The Brain Tumor Cooperative Group NIH Trial 87-01: a randomized comparison of surgery, external radiotherapy, and carmustine versus surgery, interstitial radiotherapy boost, external radiation therapy, and carmustine. Neurosurgery. 2002;51(2):343–57.
41. Brem H, Piantadosi S, Burger PC, et al. Placebo-controlled trial of safety and efficacy of intra-operative controlled delivery by biodegradable polymers of chemotherapy for recurrent gliomas. The Polymer-Brain Tumor Treatment Group. Lancet. 1995;345(8956):1008–12. https://doi.org/10.1016/s0140-6736(95)90755-6.
42. Perry J, Chambers A, Spithoff K, Laperriere N. Gliadel wafers in the treatment of malignant glioma: a systematic review. Curr Oncol. 2007;14(5):189–94. https://doi.org/10.3747/co.2007.147.
43. Westphal M, Hilt DC, Bortey E, et al. A phase 3 trial of local chemotherapy with biodegradable carmustine (BCNU) wafers (Gliadel wafers) in patients with primary malignant glioma. Neuro-Oncology. 2003;5(2):79–88. https://doi.org/10.1093/neuonc/5.2.79.
44. Westphal M, Ram Z, Riddle V, Hilt D, Bortey E. Gliadel wafer in initial surgery for malignant glioma: long-term follow-up of a multi-center controlled trial. Acta Neurochir (Wein). 2006;148:269–75.
45. Nagpal S. The role of BCNU polymer wafers (Gliadel) in the treatment of malignant glioma. Neurosurg Clin N Am. 2012;23(2):289–ix. https://doi.org/10.1016/j.nec.2012.01.004.
46. Sughrue ME, Sheean T, Bonney PA, Maurer AJ, Teo C. Aggressive repeat surgery for focally recurrent primary glioblastoma: outcomes and theoretical framework. Neurosurg Focus. 2015;38(3):E11. https://doi.org/10.3171/2014.12.FOCUS14726.
47. Hygino da Cruz LC Jr, Rodriguez I, Domingues RC, Gasparetto EL, Sorensen AG. Pseudoprogression and pseudoresponse: imaging challenges in the assessment of posttreatment glioma. AJNR Am J Neuroradiol. 2011;32(11):1978–85. https://doi.org/10.3174/ajnr.A2397.
48. Delgado-López PD, Riñones-Mena E, Corrales-García EM. Treatment-related changes in glioblastoma: a review on the controversies in response assessment criteria and the concepts of true progression, pseudoprogression, pseudoresponse and radionecrosis. Clin Transl Oncol. 2018;20(8):939–53. https://doi.org/10.1007/s12094-017-1816-x.
49. Zikou A, Sioka C, Alexiou GA, Fotopoulos A, Voulgaris S, Argyropoulou MI. Radiation necrosis, pseudoprogression, pseudoresponse, and tumor recurrence: imaging challenges for the evaluation of treated gliomas. Contrast Media Mol Imaging. 2018;2018:6828396. https://doi.org/10.1155/2018/6828396. Published 2 Dec 2018.
50. Hecht N, Spies C, Vajkoczy P. Routine intensive care unit-level care after elective craniotomy: time to rethink. World Neurosurg. 2014;81(1):66–8. https://doi.org/10.1016/j.wneu.2013.01.119.
51. Badenes R, Prisco L, Maruenda A, Taccone FS. Criteria for intensive care admission and monitoring after elective craniotomy. Curr Opin Anaesthesiol. 2017;30(5):540–5. https://doi.org/10.1097/ACO.0000000000000503.

52. Lescher S, Schniewindt S, Jurcoane A, Senft C, Hattingen E. Time window for postoperative reactive enhancement after resection of brain tumors: less than 72 hours. Neurosurg Focus. 2014;37(6):E3. https://doi.org/10.3171/2014.9.FOCUS14479.
53. De la Garza-Ramos R, Kerezoudis P, Tamargo RJ, Brem H, Huang J, Bydon M. Surgical complications following malignant brain tumor surgery: an analysis of 2002–2011 data. Clin Neurol Neurosurg. 2016;140:6–10. https://doi.org/10.1016/j.clineuro.2015.11.005.
54. Wong JM, Panchmatia JR, Ziewacz JE, et al. Patterns in neurosurgical adverse events: intracranial neoplasm surgery. Neurosurg Focus. 2012;33(5):E16. https://doi.org/10.3171/2012.7.FOCUS12183.

Chapter 4
Machine Learning Approaches Pertinent to Glioma Classification

Samirkumar B. Amin

Prediction is very difficult, especially about the future.

– Niels Bohr

Background

Glioma classification dates back to 1920s when neurosurgeons Harvey Cushing and Percival Bailey published their seminal work on classification of gliomas into 14 types [1]. They based this classification using extensive histological and cellular characteristics of 254 surgical specimens and meticulous correlation with clinical history of respective patients. While authors' work predated discovery of DNA and genetic underpinning of cancer evolution, they justly described significance of genetics in clinically relevant glioma classification by including the keyword, "histogenetic" in their book title, *A Classification of the Tumors of the Glioma Group on a Histogenetic Basis with a Correlated Study of Prognosis.*

Current practice of glioma classification is largely based on histopathological and molecular features, and is detailed respectively in the chapters: *Histopathology of adult and pediatric gliomas, and Molecular stratification adult and pediatric gliomas.* Large-scale genomic analyses from The Cancer Genome Atlas (TCGA) and pediatric cancer genome projects have been proved valuable to refine histopathology-based classification by defining molecular subtypes [2–7]. For example, revised World Health Organization (WHO) classification [8] now defines two major glioma types: *IDH* 1/2 mutant versus wild-type gliomas. Within these two types, patients with gliomas are further classified based on specific somatic structural alterations, e.g., *IDH* wild-type class contains pediatric high-grade

S. B. Amin (✉)
The Jackson Laboratory for Genomic Medicine, Farmington, CT, USA
e-mail: sbamin@alumni.bcm.edu

© The Author(s), under exclusive license to Springer Nature
Switzerland AG 2021
J. J. Otero, A. P. Becker (eds.), *Precision Molecular Pathology of Glioblastoma*,
Molecular Pathology Library, https://doi.org/10.1007/978-3-030-69170-7_4

gliomas with a driver mutations in K27 and G34 mutations in histone gene, *H3F3A*, gliomas enriched in *TERT* promoter mutations, chromosome 7q gain and 10q loss, and also *IDH*-mutant gliomas with (Oligodendrogliomas) or without (Astrocytoma) 1p/19q co-deletion. Besides mutational subtypes, promoter methylation of O-6-methylguanine-DNA methyltransferase (*MGMT*) gene among *IDH* wild-type gliomas has been related to favorable outcome for patients getting temozolomide, a chemotherapy drug given with concurrent and adjuvant radiotherapy. *MGMT* promoter methylation is now one of the most well-studied molecular biomarkers in clinical neuro-oncology. While most of genetic alterations used in WHO classification are of potential diagnostic value, their value in treatment decision is yet debatable given several challenges [9]. First, detection of driver mutations are neither specific nor sensitive [10], and its accuracy depends on both, biological variables, e.g., intra-tumor heterogeneity and clonal dominance at primary or recurrent disease [11]; and technical variables, e.g., sequencing depth, tumor section to be sequenced, etc. [12] Second, there is lack of rigorous statistical data to support prospective prediction accuracy of these biomarkers, especially when used in combination [13, 14]. Finally, these biomarkers require invasive technique to extract tumor sample for sequencing, which may not even be feasible for certain gliomas in brainstem or those with diffuse infiltration. While overcoming these challenges is non-trivial, recent surge in applied machine learning using gene expression subtypes, methylation, and histopathological image based methods provides promising avenue towards accurate glioma classification, including for better risk stratification and personalized therapy.

Applied machine learning in cancer biology is not uncommon [15] since availability of multi-omics genomic data and increased computing power for about a decade or so, e.g., gene expression profile (GEP) based signatures have been widely published in several cancer types, including their use in clinical practice for risk stratification of patients with early-stage breast cancer and colon cancer [16, 17]. However, the machine learning field has greatly expanded since the rebirth of artificial neural network when researchers in 2012 used deep convolutional neural network (dCNN) or a deep learning model to accurately classify 1.2 million images across 1000 categories from a database, ImageNet [18]. Since then, researchers have shown potential value of deep learning based models in tumor classification, predicting underlying mutations and prognosis. In the following sections, we will review relevant machine learning approaches – both classical and deep learning – in glioma classification and clinical relevance, prevailing challenges and their potential solutions.

Classical Machine Learning Approaches

Classical methods of machine learning are classical in terms of not using deep neural networks and instead relies on commonly used statistical approaches. These approaches are mainstream in computational cancer biology and are broadly divided into two major classes: supervised versus unsupervised learning. Supervised learning requires "a supervisor" or a teacher for training in the form of known outcome label, e.g., responder versus non-responder for a feature, for example *MGMT* promoter methylation, obtained from a patient sample. Then, a machine learning algorithm, e.g., regression method(s) will learn the pattern between a feature and outcome label to classify the source (patients) with a certain value of the feature into responder versus non-responder category. Besides regression-based approaches, sample classification by support vector machine (SVM) or K-nearest neighbor (KNN) are also commonly used in supervised learning.

In contrast, unsupervised learning does not require outcome labels to learn patterns from the data, e.g., clustering approach with unsupervised hierarchical clustering and dimensionality reduction using principal component analysis are the two most common approaches used in cancer genomics to classify patient samples into molecular subtypes. Here, the training data consists of one of gene expression from bulk or single-cell profiles, copy-number, methylation, or integration of multi-omics data to derive composite molecular subtypes. These subtypes are then correlated with known patient outcomes, e.g., overall and event-free survival, mutational status, etc., to infer significant properties of each molecular subtype. In the rest of this section, we will review a few major implementations of classical machine learning approaches for glioma classification.

Gene Expression Based Subtypes

Gene expression profile (GEP) based subtypes are one of the most cited applications of machine learning in cancer genomics. GEP subtype analysis is often the most ubiquitous analysis in TCGA published articles where researchers did extensive genomic profiling of more than 30 adult cancer types [19]. Expression subtypes provide valuable gene regulatory and pathway-level context [20, 21] of underlying cancer biology and its impact on patient's risk stratification, treatment response to targeted therapies, and survival outcomes [22].

Early in 2000s, researchers using microarray based GEPs did supervised learning to correlate gene expression among known histopathological subtypes, and came up with GEP signatures to classify histology of gliomas [23, 24]. While studies did not show robust accuracy in prospective prediction of classifying tumor samples from new patients, these studies provided significant associations of gene expression profiles with clinical variables, e.g., tumor histology, grade, age cohort, and survival outcomes. These results were an impetus in the high-throughput genomic era to learn expression patterns and improve glioma classification via unsupervised machine learning approaches.

In 2006, Phillips et al. published the first major work on molecular subtypes of high-grade gliomas [25]. The authors first selected 108 genes based on their microarray profiling expression that correlate significantly with patient survival across 76 primary astrocytoma samples. Then, they used two-way agglomerative clustering – an unsupervised learning – to identify three distinct subsets of patient tumor samples that differed significantly in their expression profiles of those 108 genes (features). Subsequently, the authors selected candidate 35 genes signature based on the strongest and consistent expression of top 35 genes in each of three subtypes. Finally, authors used these 35 genes to do (semi) unsupervised KNN clustering and reported three major subtypes of high-grade gliomas, namely Proneural, Proliferative, and Mesenchymal subtypes. Authors also conducted validation of their 35 genes signatures in two independent sets to infer a few novel and clinically relevant findings: First, 35 genes signature of three subtypes represented underlying developmental cues and potential cell-of-origin of gliomas, e.g., Proneural signature had a high correlation with gene expression profiles from fetal and adult normal brain tissues while those from Mesenchymal signature had higher similarity to GEP from bone, smooth muscle, and vascular cells, i.e., a lineage dependent expression profile. Second, expression subtypes were predictive of disease progression independent of histology grade. Proneural subtype with normal-brain like GEP was shown to have better prognosis than Proliferative and Mesenchymal subtypes which were more aligned to GEPs found with cell proliferation or angiogenesis, respectively. Altogether, this work provided a strong rationale for use of GEP based subtypes to refine prevalent practice of histopathology based glioma classification and advocate use of GEP signatures as a prognostic biomarkers. Nonetheless, this work, given limited availability of next generation sequencing, required independent and robust statistical validation using the larger dataset of high-grade gliomas and importantly, integration of copy-number and mutational data to ascertain prognostic value of three subtypes.

TCGA glioblastoma (GBM) work [2] expanded earlier work on glioma classification where authors detailed the robust GEP classifier based on comprehensive expression, copy-number, and mutational data from 200 patients with GBM. Authors first included microarray GEP from three different sequencing platforms and did thorough feature selection or gene filtering to minimize potential confounding effects of sample batch, sample purity, and sample quality. Next, authors used unbiased gene filtering approach based on expression variance to select 1740 genes which were then used for an unsupervised consensus hierarchical clustering to derive four major subtypes of GBM: Classical (or proliferative), Mesenchymal, Proneural, and Neural. The resulting 840 gene signature (210 genes per subtype) was then rigorously validated using cross-validation as well as using an independent set of 260 GBM expression profiles, including 76 cases from the initial work on GBM subtypes. Unique to TCGA data was availability of copy-number and mutational profiles on core set of 170/200 GBM patients. Using this data, TCGA study provided the most granular classification of four subtypes and its relevance to underlying somatic alterations, e.g., aberrations in *EGFR*, *NF1*, and *PDGFRA/IDH1* were significantly enriched among the Classical, Mesenchymal, and Proneural subtypes, respectively. These subtypes, independent of underlying tumor histology, also reflected variable to response to chemotherapy and related survival. Notably, intensive chemotherapy significantly reduced mortality in Classical and

Mesenchymal subtypes, but it did not alter survival in Proneural subtype. Subsequent work from TCGA Glioma consortium, including for low-grade gliomas [6, 7], further validated histology-independent prognostic value of expression subtypes and their potential significance in decision making as highlighted by inclusion of mutational biomarkers in revised WHO classification.

While TCGA GBM subtypes provided robust gene signatures per subtype of prognostic value, signatures derived from the bulk tumor tissue could not address pervasive intra-tumor heterogeneity and cellular states of evolving glioma cells in tumor stroma [26, 27]. Recent studies using multi-sector tumor expression profiling from the same patient showed that TCGA subtypes can vary across these sector biopsies with around 60% of discordance among different tumor sub-specimens from the same patient's tumor or in other case, tumor margins were classified as neural subtype while core tumor tissue was classified as other three subtypes [28, 29].

Recently, a revised classification of TCGA [30] refined original subtypes in an attempt to address intra-tumoral heterogeneity and tumor microenvironment confounding glioma molecular subtypes. In this study, authors used single-cell RNA-seq profile of 596 isolated glioma cells from eight GBM patients to quantify glioma-specific gene expression. For robustness of glioma-specific gene expression, authors used glioma sphere-forming cell cultures and expression profile from additional bulk tumors with at least two sections – core tumor specimen and leading edge specimen. Authors then used resulting expressed genes (7425) for unsupervised learning using consensus non-negative matrix factorization (CNMF) method and re-classified TCGA *IDH* wild-type GBMs (n = 369) into three major subtypes. Compared to original TCGA subtypes, they did not find Neural subtype with updated gene (feature) list, suggesting Neural subtype is not reflective of glioma intrinsic subtypes, and rather it was a result of contamination from non-tumor cells. This study also revealed that Mesenchymal subtype is a composite of glioma cells and tumor-associated immune and other cells from tumor microenvironment, and significantly correlated with loss of *NF1* activity. Importantly, this study, along with parallel studies using single-cell RNA-seq (scRNAseq) profiling [28, 31–33], emphasized role of phenotypic plasticity and resulting change in GEP subtypes as growing tumor interacts with host immune and other stromal cells as well as growing tumor's response to treatments.

Finally, intra-tumoral heterogeneity is not limited to presence of tumor vs non-tumor cells but rather it is a property of intrinsic and inherent clonal heterogeneity – competing tumor cells with different sets of driver mutations – that drives adaptation of an evolving tumor [34–36]. Multiple studies in last 5 year have extensively studied tumor heterogeneity at single-cell resolution using scRNAseq and single-cell DNA sequencing. Collectively, these studies signify that tumors carry expression signatures that show their identity with respect to cell-of-origin but also the ability of cancer cells to change their expression and potentially phenotypic state as they adapt to tumor microenvironment and anti-proliferative treatments. While detailed review of these studies is beyond the scope of this chapter, readers are encouraged to review additional reading listed in the references [31, 37].

Methylation Based Subtypes

DNA methylation – methylation of cytosine to form 5-methylcytosine – is a frequent event across cancers in all age groups. DNA methylation in the context of CG dinucleotide pair (CpG) near gene promoter regions is a potent transcriptional repressor, and has been implicated in epigenetic remodeling of gene expression programs in cancers. Hence, similar to GEP based subtypes, DNA methylation signatures should dictate underlying gene expression patterns and of potential prognostic value.

Early studies in the 1990s studied the role of the DNA repair protein MGMT in protecting cancer cells from cytotoxic effects of alkylating agents [38]. This sparked research interest in studying basal MGMT activity in normal brain versus glioma samples which finally revealed prevalent MGMT promoter methylation (30% of gliomas) and thus, rationalizing use of temozolomide – an alkylating agent – in patients with promoter methylation of *MGMT* gene [39, 40]. Subsequent studies with availability of methylation-based microarrays and advent of reduced representation bisulfite sequencing (RRBS), enabled high-throughput, genome-wide screening of DNA methylation, and thus paving the way to use DNA methylation at base-pair level resolution (features) for machine learning based classification of tumors, including gliomas.

In 2010, TCGA group reported detailed methylation subtypes [41] using unsupervised KNN clustering of 272 TCGA GBM samples with methylation signal derived from two different microarray platforms. Despite having wide range of prob-set distribution between two platforms (1505 CpGs/807 genes versus 27,578 CpGs/14,473 genes), authors showed 97% concordance of three subtypes for common set of samples (61/63) that were ran on both microarray platforms. Authors designated cluster 1 as Glioma CpG Island Methylator Phenotype (G-CIMP) based on earlier study showing cancer-specific hypermethylated genes in the CIMP cluster in colorectal cancer. G-CIMP subtype represented 24/272 (8.8%) GBM samples. Importantly, G-CIMP tumors were part of 30% (21/71) of GBM Proneural expression subtype which is also enriched for *IDH1/2* mutations and have favorable prognosis with slow disease progression. Association of G-CIMP with *IDH1/2* mutation was further supported by studies showing similar pattern among low-grade gliomas, suggesting gradual progression of G-CIMP subtype over the life history of gliomas. Collectively, discovery of G-CIMP and its association with *IDH1/2* mutations led to discovery of mechanistic nature of *IDH1*-mutant G-CIMP phenotype when series of experimental studies [42, 43] showed that *IDH1* mutation produces an oncometabolite, 2-hydroxyglutarate that in turn inhibits DNA demethylating enzyme, TET1 to cause genome-wide hypermethylation phenotype or G-CIMP. Discovery of G-CIMP in adult gliomas was then followed by detailed G-CIMP correlative analyses with mutational and expression subtypes of adult gliomas [7] as well as pediatric gliomas [44], thus providing potential value of methylation-based classification in of brain tumors across all age and histological grades.

The largest and perhaps most of the direct clinical impact so far came from a study [45] in 2018 when an international group of researchers collected genome-wide methylation profiles of 2801 CNS tumors across 76 histopathological classes and took on the daunting task of classifying these tumors based on DNA methylation patterns. Authors initially developed the reference cohort by performing unsupervised clustering within each histological class and those with higher similarity to designate each tumor into one of 82 CNS tumor and 9 control tissue methylation classes. These classes included all of WHO defined classes as well as those which were undefined by WHO. Authors then used the elegant machine learning approach to first develop the classifier based on supervised learning using the random forest classifier – a decision tree based approach that combines predictive accuracy for each of 10,000 binary decision trees to improve overall prediction accuracy for one of 92 methylation classes developed above with the reference cohort. Resulting classifier was then used to predict methylation class for the test dataset (unused in the reference cohort) of 1104 tumor methylation profiles. Their results showed that for 60% of cases, machine learning classifier accurately matched diagnosis that of a pathologist while for 15.5% cases, the classifier and pathologist assigned the same tumor class but the classifier also assigned additional subclass. Of most clinical relevance was 12.6% where the classifier failed to concur with pathologist's diagnosis but upon manual examination, including genetic sequencing of known cancer drivers, 92.8% of those tumor samples switched from original histopathological diagnosis to the one originally given by the classifier. Importantly, 71% of these tumors were then reassigned to a different tumor grade, thereby potentially changing treatment decision, and thus validating clinical utility of methylation-based, next-generation neuropathology in tumor diagnosis, especially for aiding into accurate molecular subtyping and grading of gliomas prior to starting treatment. While the classifier has not yet been implemented in the consensus guidelines, authors have now made their classifier available at https://www.molecularneuropathology. org/mnp for use as a secondary validation by a neuropathologist for a prospective tumor methylation profile.

Deep Learning Based Approaches

Similar to classical machine learning approaches, deep learning can also be categorized into supervised and unsupervised learning. However, deep learning differs from classical learning in several ways: (1) While classical learning typically requires data preprocessing for selecting features which are the most relevant and the least redundant to outcome of interest, deep learning can tackle with raw data, e.g., gene expression across all of protein-coding genes or somatic mutational or methylation data at base-pair resolution. In other words, deep learning can be seen as a *black box learning* [46] where raw data passing through series of hierarchical supervised learning or *hidden layers* and learning (feature selection) from each of these layers is propagated into the final layer or output class label, e.g., treatment responder or non-responder, low-grade or high-grade tumor, assign predicted probability to all of WHO or methylation-based 92 classes discussed earlier. (2) Classical learning may not be practical given feature selection becomes computationally daunting with rapidly expanding multi-omics data and less effective ways to integrate these datasets. In contrast, deep learning is optimized for big data analytics, especially for gene regulatory [47] and image-based classification [48, 49] where pixel-level values (feature) of a high-resolution radiology images generate overwhelming input data for classical machine learning methods. It is worth noting that both classical and deep learning methods are equally vulnerable to poor prediction accuracy if raw data is of bad quality.

Deep learning based approaches leverage variants of artificial neural network, namely convolutional, recurrent, and fully connected neural networks (CNNs) for supervised learning [49]. For unsupervised learning, autoencoders and generative adversarial networks (GANs) are now being implemented in single-cell genomics datasets. In recent years, deep learnings methods have made significant strides into detecting several outcomes of clinical relevance directly from digital whole-slide images of histopathology [48], e.g., tumor versus normal tissue, degree of microsatellite instability [50], actionable driver mutations [51, 52], and immune cell infiltration [53]. Within glioma, deep CNNs (dCNNs) are recently being used to predict overall survival and predict glioma histology grade using radiology imaging of patients with brain tumors [54]. However, deep learning field is relatively new and yet to be benchmarked for clinical-grade utility. For in-depth review on deep learning approaches in cancer, readers are encouraged to review additional reading listed in the references [48, 49, 55].

Prevailing Challenges and Current Trends

Applied machine learning has become one of the cornerstones in the modern, genomic era with widespread use in molecular tumor subtyping, applicability for risk stratification at the diagnosis and guide personalized therapy per anticipated response to targeted therapies [15]. However, these utilities are predominantly marked as proof-of-concept and yet to be accepted widely in the clinical practice. The core principle in the clinical practice, *'First do no harm'* should apply to machine learning approaches such that several cancer-specific as well as method-specific limitations need to be addressed before its use in the standard of care for patients.

Classical and deep machine learning approaches are both quite sensitive to input data quality. Failure to develop data standardization and not follow the best practices for data collection and preprocessing can introduce technical batch effects and confounding biases, thus giving false sense of better prediction accuracy [56, 57].

Clinical grade machine learning models must pass through rigorous benchmarking, mainly for deep learning models where it is challenging to infer how and why the model predicts with high accuracy. Data preprocessing should also involve splitting of input data for training and cross validation while ideally using independent test or hold-out dataset from different institute/region/country to benchmark model performance [58–60]. For histopathology based machine learning models, cross-tumor and even cross-species histopathology can be of value to measure accuracy of models that predict histology grade, cell-of-origin, tumor purity, etc. Our recent work [61] found stronger support for the human methylation classifier [45] by using the same classifier to accurately classify spontaneous canine gliomas as human pediatric-like gliomas, and provide additional validation using orthogonal somatic structural variant data.

Classical machine learning models based on GEP signature alone have shown average performance at-large except for specific high-risk patient groups in breast and colon cancer [56, 59]. It is imperative that prediction of survival outcome or treatment response is a function of more than just gene expression. Gene regulatory networks are product of gene-gene interactions, DNA and histone modification, and higher level chromatin reorganization in cancer cells. With availability of multi-modal (genomics, radiology, histopathology), multi-omics (DNA, RNA, methylation, proteins) data, deep learning methods should leverage such heterogeneous data for learning and inference which otherwise demand significant human and computational effort for traditional data preprocessing [58, 62].

Finally, machine learning models should account for clonal evolution of tumors, including its adaptation to changing microenvironment and treatment types [34, 63–66]. With recent availability of the longitudinal glioma genomics data from the Glioma Longitudinal Analysis Consortium (GLASS), research efforts to improve glioma classification and importantly, predict patient-specific risk profiles based on underlying clonal heterogeneity will be of clinical relevance, e.g., predictive models that can integrate multi-omics data at primary and recurrent disease to capture predictive features of tumor progression or the classifier that can accurately predict hypermutation profile prior to starting Temozolomide therapy in patients with *MGMT* promoter methylation [11, 67].

Key Takeaways

- Machine learning approaches bridge histopathology with underlying molecular patterns, and can improve diagnostic classification of gliomas for optimal personalized therapies.
- Classical machine learning methods have been commonly used in identifying gene expression and methylation based subtypes of gliomas.
- Deep learning methods are recently being used to refine digital whole slide image based inference of histopathology as well as underlying cancer driver mutations, immune cell infiltration, and molecular subtypes.

- Standardization of multi-omics, multi-modal data with clinical records will be of critical value in the robust training of machine learning classifiers to enable accurate and safer prospective risk stratification of patients at the primary diagnosis.
- Tumor evolution and resulting intra-tumor and inter-tumor heterogeneity can be exploited for biomarker development by training the classifier using large-scale, longitudinal, multi-omics data from patients with glioma at multiple time-points.

References

1. Bailey P, Cushing H. A classification of the tumors of the glioma group on a histogenetic basis with a correlated study of prognosis. Philadelphia, London, etc.: J.B. Lippincott Company; 1926. 3 p. l., 175 p. incl. illus., tables, diagrs.
2. Verhaak RGW, et al. Integrated genomic analysis identifies clinically relevant subtypes of glioblastoma characterized by abnormalities in PDGFRA, IDH1, EGFR, and NF1. Cancer Cell. 2010;17(1):98–110.
3. Downing JR, et al. The pediatric cancer genome project. Nat Genet. 2012;44(6):619–22.
4. Wu G, et al. The genomic landscape of diffuse intrinsic pontine glioma and pediatric non-brainstem high-grade glioma. Nat Genet. 2014;46(5):444–50.
5. Huether R, et al. The landscape of somatic mutations in epigenetic regulators across 1,000 paediatric cancer genomes. Nat Commun. 2014;5:3630.
6. Cancer Genome Atlas Research, N, et al. Comprehensive, integrative genomic analysis of diffuse lower-grade gliomas. N Engl J Med. 2015;372(26):2481–98.
7. Ceccarelli M, et al. Molecular profiling reveals biologically discrete subsets and pathways of progression in diffuse glioma. Cell. 2016;164(3):550–63.
8. Louis DN, et al. The 2016 World Health Organization classification of tumors of the central nervous system: a summary. Acta Neuropathol. 2016;131(6):803–20.
9. Weller M, et al. Glioma. Nat Rev Dis Primers. 2015;1:15017.
10. Bailey MH, et al. Comprehensive characterization of cancer driver genes and mutations. Cell. 2018;173(2):371–385.e18.
11. Barthel FP, et al. Longitudinal molecular trajectories of diffuse glioma in adults. Nature. 2019;576(7785):112–20.
12. Gonzalez-Perez A, Sabarinathan R, Lopez-Bigas N. Local determinants of the mutational landscape of the human genome. Cell. 2019;177(1):101–14.
13. Amin SB, et al. Gene expression profile alone is inadequate in predicting complete response in multiple myeloma. Leukemia. 2014;28(11):2229–34.
14. Yuan Y, et al. Assessing the clinical utility of cancer genomic and proteomic data across tumor types. Nat Biotechnol. 2014;32(7):644–52.
15. Rajkomar A, Dean J, Kohane I. Machine learning in medicine. N Engl J Med. 2019;380(14):1347–58.
16. You YN, Rustin RB, Sullivan JD. Oncotype DX((R)) colon cancer assay for prediction of recurrence risk in patients with stage II and III colon cancer: a review of the evidence. Surg Oncol. 2015;24(2):61–6.
17. van't Veer LJ, et al. Gene expression profiling predicts clinical outcome of breast cancer. Nature. 2002;415(6871):530–6.
18. Krizhevsky A, Sutskever I, Hinton GE. ImageNet classification with deep convolutional neural networks. Commun ACM. 2017;60(6):84–90. https://doi.org/10.1145/3065386.
19. Weinstein JN, et al. The cancer genome atlas pan-cancer analysis project. Nat Genet. 2013;45(10):1113–20.

20. Ben-Hamo R, et al. Predicting and affecting response to cancer therapy based on pathway-level biomarkers. Nat Commun. 2020;11(1):3296.
21. Andersen JN, et al. Pathway-based identification of biomarkers for targeted therapeutics: personalized oncology with PI3K pathway inhibitors. Sci Transl Med. 2010;2(43):43ra55.
22. Barthel FP, et al. Evolving insights into the molecular neuropathology of diffuse gliomas in adults. Neurol Clin. 2018;36(3):421–37.
23. Rickman DS, et al. Distinctive molecular profiles of high-grade and low-grade gliomas based on oligonucleotide microarray analysis. Cancer Res. 2001;61(18):6885–91.
24. Godard S, et al. Classification of human astrocytic gliomas on the basis of gene expression: a correlated group of genes with angiogenic activity emerges as a strong predictor of subtypes. Cancer Res. 2003;63(20):6613–25.
25. Phillips HS, et al. Molecular subclasses of high-grade glioma predict prognosis, delineate a pattern of disease progression, and resemble stages in neurogenesis. Cancer Cell. 2006;9(3):157–73.
26. Venkatesan S, Swanton C. Tumor evolutionary principles: how intratumor heterogeneity influences cancer treatment and outcome. Am Soc Clin Oncol Educ Book. 2016;35:e141–9.
27. Mazor T, et al. Intratumoral heterogeneity of the epigenome. Cancer Cell. 2016;29(4):440–51.
28. Tirosh I, et al. Single-cell RNA-seq supports a developmental hierarchy in human oligodendroglioma. Nature. 2016;539(7628):309–13.
29. Patel AP, et al. Single-cell RNA-seq highlights intratumoral heterogeneity in primary glioblastoma. Science. 2014;344(6190):1396–401.
30. Wang Q, et al. Tumor evolution of glioma-intrinsic gene expression subtypes associates with immunological changes in the microenvironment. Cancer Cell. 2017;32(1):42–56.e6.
31. Suva ML, Tirosh I. The glioma stem cell model in the era of single-cell genomics. Cancer Cell. 2020;37(5):630–6.
32. Filbin MG, et al. Developmental and oncogenic programs in H3K27M gliomas dissected by single-cell RNA-seq. Science. 2018;360(6386):331–5.
33. Suva ML, et al. Reconstructing and reprogramming the tumor-propagating potential of glioblastoma stem-like cells. Cell. 2014;157(3):580–94.
34. Spiteri I, et al. Evolutionary dynamics of residual disease in human glioblastoma. Ann Oncol. 2019;30(3):456–63.
35. Sottoriva A, et al. Intratumor heterogeneity in human glioblastoma reflects cancer evolutionary dynamics. Proc Natl Acad Sci U S A. 2013;110(10):4009–14.
36. Kim H, et al. Whole-genome and multisector exome sequencing of primary and post-treatment glioblastoma reveals patterns of tumor evolution. Genome Res. 2015. p. gr.180612.114.
37. Filbin M, Monje M. Developmental origins and emerging therapeutic opportunities for childhood cancer. Nat Med. 2019;25(3):367–76.
38. Esteller M, et al. Inactivation of the DNA-repair gene MGMT and the clinical response of gliomas to alkylating agents. N Engl J Med. 2000;343(19):1350–4.
39. Hegi ME, et al. MGMT gene silencing and benefit from temozolomide in glioblastoma. N Engl J Med. 2005;352(10):997–1003.
40. Wick W, et al. MGMT testing – the challenges for biomarker-based glioma treatment. Nat Rev Neurol. 2014;10(7):372–85.
41. Noushmehr H, et al. Identification of a CpG island methylator phenotype that defines a distinct subgroup of glioma. Cancer Cell. 2010;17(5):510–22.
42. Lu C, et al. IDH mutation impairs histone demethylation and results in a block to cell differentiation. Nature. 2012;483(7390):474–8.
43. Turcan S, et al. IDH1 mutation is sufficient to establish the glioma hypermethylator phenotype. Nature. 2012;483(7390):479–83.
44. Sturm D, et al. Paediatric and adult glioblastoma: multiform (epi)genomic culprits emerge. Nat Rev Cancer. 2014;14(2):92–107.
45. Capper D, et al. DNA methylation-based classification of central nervous system tumours. Nature. 2018;555(7697):469–74.

46. Zou J, et al. A primer on deep learning in genomics. Nat Genet. 2019;51(1):12–8.
47. Park Y, Kellis M. Deep learning for regulatory genomics. Nat Biotechnol. 2015;33(8):825–6.
48. Komura D, Ishikawa S. Machine learning methods for histopathological image analysis. Comput Struct Biotechnol J. 2018;16:34–42.
49. Eraslan GK, et al. Deep learning: new computational modelling techniques for genomics. Nat Rev Genet. 2019;20(7):389–403.
50. Kather JN, et al. Deep learning can predict microsatellite instability directly from histology in gastrointestinal cancer. Nat Med. 2019;25:1054–56.
51. Coudray N, et al. Classification and mutation prediction from non-small cell lung cancer histopathology images using deep learning. Nat Med. 2018;24(10):1559–67.
52. Ainscough BJ, et al. A deep learning approach to automate refinement of somatic variant calling from cancer sequencing data. Nat Genet. 2018:1.
53. Saltz J, et al. Spatial organization and molecular correlation of tumor-infiltrating lymphocytes using deep learning on pathology images. Cell Rep. 2018;23(1):181–193 e7.
54. Ertosun MG, Rubin DL. Automated grading of gliomas using deep learning in digital pathology images: a modular approach with ensemble of convolutional neural networks. AMIA Annu Symp Proc. 2015;2015:1899–908.
55. LeCun Y, Bengio Y, Hinton G. Deep learning. Nature. 2015;521(7553):436–44.
56. Shah NH, Milstein A, Bagley SC. Making machine learning models clinically useful. JAMA. 2019;322(14):1351–52.
57. Schreiber J, et al. A pitfall for machine learning methods aiming to predict across cell types. bioRxiv. 2019.
58. Zitnik M, et al. Machine learning for integrating data in biology and medicine: principles, practice, and opportunities. arXiv [q-bio.QM]. 2018.
59. Ali M, Aittokallio T. Machine learning and feature selection for drug response prediction in precision oncology applications. Biophys Rev. 2019;11(1):31–9.
60. Chen JH, Asch SM. Machine learning and prediction in medicine — beyond the peak of inflated expectations. N Engl J Med. 2017;376(26):2507–9.
61. Amin SB, et al. Comparative molecular life history of spontaneous canine and human gliomas. Cancer Cell. 2020;37(2):243–257.e7.
62. Xu C, Jackson SA. Machine learning and complex biological data. Genome Biol. 2019;20(1):76.
63. Hall P, Ambati S, Phan W. Ideas on interpreting machine learning. O'Reilly Radar AI & ML (Blog). 2017. https://www.oreilly.com/radar/ideas-on-interpreting-machinelearning/. Accessed 25 March 2021.
64. Birkbak NJ, McGranahan N. Cancer genome evolutionary trajectories in metastasis. Cancer Cell. 2020;37(1):8–19.
65. Pogrebniak KL, Curtis CN. Harnessing tumor evolution to circumvent resistance. Trends Genet. 2018;34(8):639–51.
66. Marongiu F, Serra M, Laconi E. Development versus evolution in cancer biology. Trends Cancer Res. 2018;4(5):342–8.
67. Klughammer J, et al. The DNA methylation landscape of glioblastoma disease progression shows extensive heterogeneity in time and space. Nat Med. 2018;24(10):1611–24.

Chapter 5
Histopathology of Adult and Pediatric Glioblastoma

Appaji Rayi and Peter J. Kobalka

Introduction

Histopathologically, GBM consists of varying proportions of spindle cells, embedded within a fibrillary (eosinophilic, stringy) network (Fig. 5.1a). The cells are enlarged, irregular in morphology, with hyperchromasia and pleomorphism [1]. Tumor cells can also appear variably shaped, including rounded, giant, or even bizarre [2] (Fig. 5.1b). The impressive heterogeneity of these neoplasms is what led to the (now outdated) term "multiforme." It is not unusual for these cells to be mixed, or for tumors to be mixtures of varying subtypes, as described below.

In order to histologically diagnose GBM, the shape of the cells alone is insufficient. In addition to pleomorphism (WHO grade II criteria) and significant mitotic activity (WHO grade III criteria), one of two additional criteria must be met: microvascular proliferation (Fig. 5.1c, d), and/or necrosis (WHO grade IV criteria) (Fig. 5.1e, f).

With the modern push for integrated diagnoses, an astrocytic glioma with less than grade IV histological features can meet GBM criteria, provided certain molecular features are present; these include TERT promoter mutation, and/or EGFR amplification, and/or gain of chromosome 7 with loss of chromosome 10 [3]. The scope of this chapter focuses on histopathology, and the molecular abnormalities will be discussed separately in other chapters.

A. Rayi
The Ohio State University Medical Center, Department of Neurology/Neuro-oncology, Columbus, OH, USA

Charleston Area Medical Center, Department of Neurology, Charleston, WV, USA

P. J. Kobalka (✉)
The Ohio State University Medical Center, Department of Pathology and Laboratory Medicine, Columbus, OH, USA
e-mail: Peter.Kobalka@osumc.edu

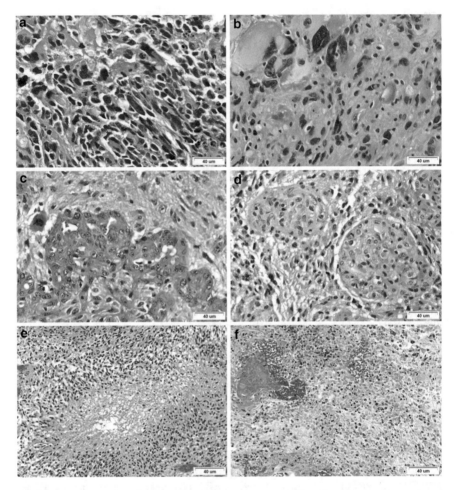

Fig. 5.1 General histology features of GBM. (**a**) Malignant spindle cells with hyperchromasia and pleomorphism. Note the frequent mitotic activity (**b**) A GBM displaying a mixture of variably-shaped cell types, some of which appear rather bizarre. Microvascular proliferation, (**c**) glomeruloid type and (**d**) endothelial proliferation within a single vessel. Ischemic necrosis of (**e**) pseudopallisading type and (**f**) geographic type

Under physiological conditions, the CNS vessels are lined by a single layer of endothelial cells. However, as the GBM mass increases to a critical level, a hypoxic state reached within the tumor mass causes the tumor cells to release angiotrophic factors (including VEGFA) that ultimately lead to increased angiogenesis [4–6]. These nascent vessels usually emerge as glomeruloid tufts consisting of numerous, juxtaposed small vessels lined by multiple layers of endothelial cells [7–10]. The term is said to have arisen due to the resemblance to glomeruli of the kidney. Often, vascular thrombosis is present, known to the surgeon as "black veins" [1, 2]. In the less common form, proliferation of endothelial cells within a single vessel is seen

[1]. Unsurprisingly, these proliferating vessels are most common in close proximity to areas of necrosis [2], which is another hallmark of GBMs. In the archetypical form, serpiginous, slit-like areas of non-viable tumor cell debris are lined perpendicularly by crowded, more viable neoplastic cells [1, 2]. Sometimes, this takes the appearance of longitudinal, long palisades. Necrosis can also take on an infarct-like appearance, with large swaths of coagulative necrosis containing dead blood vessels [1, 2].

Although not a grading criterion, GBMs have histological features of infiltration (i.e. secondary structures), wherein normal brain tissue is invaded and overrun by neoplastic cells [2]. Infiltration is present in all diffuse gliomas, although the rate of spread is typically more rapid in GBMs [11]. Histopathologically, secondary structures seen include perineuronal satellitosis (tumor cells cluster around neurons), perivascular congregations (numerous tumor cells crowd around vessels), or subpial spread (the molecular layer of the cortex, the most superficial layer, is invaded by neoplastic cells) [12]. These tumor cells are present even well-beyond where imaging or gross assessment can detect them, and are therefore, the most likely source of tumor recurrences [2].

By immunohistochemistry (IHC), most cases of GBM stain, in varying proportions, with the typical glial markers GFAP and Olig-2, [1, 2] S-100, a less specific marker, is also generally positive. Secondary GBM frequently express *IDH*1 R132H positivity that can also be seen in lower grade infiltrating astrocytic tumors and oligodendrogliomas. However, these tumors can be clearly differentiated from GBMs due to their different histological features and molecular phenotypes. Ki-67 is positive, with high percentages of positive nuclei, though expression levels have not been shown to correlate well with prognosis [13]. Frustratingly, cytokeratins may be positive, especially AE1/3, [2] potentially causing diagnostic confusion for metastatic carcinoma in certain GBM subtypes (i.e. Epithelioid GBM) [2].

Small Cell GBM

A quite common architectural pattern, small cell GBM is seen in perhaps 10% or more of glioblastomas, mostly in adults [14, 15]. Histopathology reveals highly cellular sheets of quite uniform small cells, rounded to slightly oblong in appearance [1, 2, 14] (Fig. 5.2a). Both microvascular proliferation and pseudopallisading necrosis are generally present [14, 16]. Mitotic figures are numerous [14]. Often, haloes surround tumor cells, and the neoplasm contains chicken-wire vasculature or even microcalcifications, features overlapping with anaplastic oligodendrogliomas [14], therefore 1p/19q studies are often necessary [14, 16, 17]. Absence of *IDH* mutations in small cell glioblastomas also helps elucidate the diagnosis [14, 16–18]. In some cases, vague perivascular pseudorosettes may be seen, mimicking ependymoma [1]. Unlike small cell GBM, ependymomas are discrete [1] and display little (if any) Olig-2 positivity [19–21]. The differential diagnosis also includes the primitive

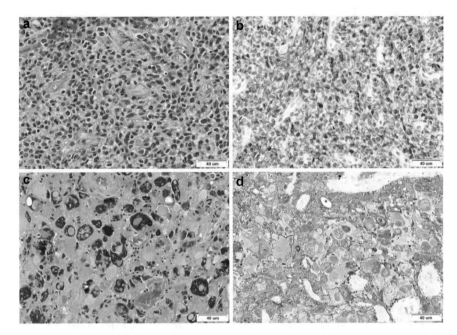

Fig. 5.2 Glioblastoma, small cell subtype. (**a**) Relative cellular uniformity is apparent, as well as frequent mitotic figures. Note how many cells display haloes (**b**) GFAP staining is strongly positive within tumor cells. Glioblastoma, giant cell subtype. (**c**) Bizarre extremes of cell size and shape, highlighted with (**d**) GFAP stain

neuroectodermal tumor (PNET) component of a glioma. Unlike PNET, small cell GBM retains fibrillary processes between cells, as well as staining for glial markers (Fig. 5.2b).

Giant Cell GBM

Giant cell GBM is an extremely rare variant of *IDH*-wildtype GBM [2], accounting for perhaps 1% of adult and 3% of childhood GBMs [22, 23]. Clinically, they can be confused with metastatic tumors, due to their superficial location and deceptive circumscription [2]. Histopathologically, the subtype is defined by tumor cells with gross extremes in size and shape, abundant, eosinophilic cytoplasm, and numerous nuclei [23–25] (Fig. 5.2c, d). Reticulin deposition may be abundant, a trait shared in common with gliosarcomas [26, 27]. Unlike most glioblastomas, prominent nucleoli are often seen, and microvascular proliferation is unusual [2]. Despite, the ugly, grotesque appearance of this neoplasm, the prognosis is believed to be somewhat better than other glioblastoma variants, with more patients surviving to 5-years post diagnosis [23, 26].

Gliosarcoma

Gliosarcomas (GSMs) are biphasic neoplasms, at one point thought to be a collision tumor between a glioblastoma and a sarcoma [28, 29]. Molecular studies have now demonstrated that both components are part of an *IDH*-wildtype glioblastoma, with metaplastic transformation of glial elements [2, 30–32]. Accounting for 2–8% of all glioblastomas, they are almost always seen in adults (40–60 years) and only rarely in children [32–35]. Clinically, they can be superficial and well-demarcated (especially with a dominance of the sarcomatous component) and can be confused for metastasis or even meningioma [2, 36]. Additionally, this variant has a propensity to invade the skull or even disseminate systemically [2, 32, 37]. Histopathologically, a marbling of the tumor is seen, with more typical glioblastoma elements intermingled with sarcomatoid elements [2] (Fig. 5.3a–c). The sarcoma component can appear fibrosarcomatous, or show specific mesenchymal differentiation, including osteosarcoma, chondrosarcoma, rhabdomyosarcoma, or angiosarcoma [1, 33] (Fig. 5.3d, e). Rarely, PNET elements are seen [38–40]. The two contrasting components can be distinguished with reticulin staining (for the sarcomatous component) and GFAP staining (for the gliomatous component) [1, 2] (Fig. 5.3b, c).

Epithelioid GBM

Epithelioid glioblastomas lack *IDH* mutations, and are diagnosed most frequently in children and young adults (<30 years of age) [2, 41, 42]. The tumor is particularly aggressive with a prognosis generally worse than other glioblastomas [41, 43, 44].

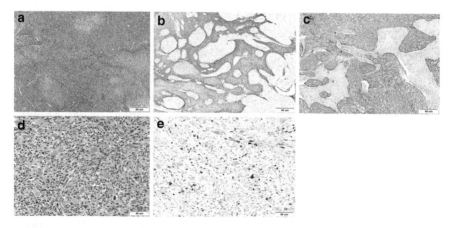

Fig. 5.3 Gliosarcoma. (**a**) interdigitating of the glial and collagen-rich sarcomatoid elements is seen. (**b**) GFAP highlights the GBM components, whereas the sarcomatoid elements (**c**) are reticulin rich. (**d**) Here, Eosinophilic cells with eccentric nuclei are highlighted with myogenin (**e**) a marker of rhabdomyosarcomatous differentiation

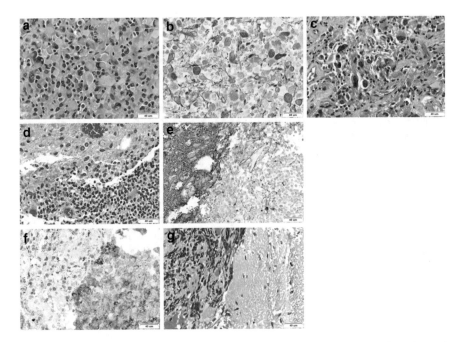

Fig. 5.4 Glioblastoma, epithelioid subtype. (**a**) The tumor cells have discrete cell borders and abundant, eosinophilic cytoplasm. Note the absence of fibrillary processes between cells. (**b**) The tumor cells stain strongly with GFAP stain (**c**) Pleomorphic xanthoastrocytoma, with scattered, large bizarre cells and frequent eosinophilic granular bodies (EGBs). Glioblastoma with PNET component (**d**) contrast the archetypical GBM component (top) with the PNET component (bottom). Mitotic activity and apoptotic bodies are numerous within the PNET component (**e**) GFAP stains the GBM component while synaptophysin (**f**) is strongly positive within the PNET component (**g**) The PNET component forms a sharp interface with adjacent, reactive brain parenchyma

Histopathology reveals a fairly uniform population of cells with discrete cell borders ("epithelioid"), prominent nucleoli, abundant, eosinophilic cytoplasm, discohesion, and a lack of fibrillar processes between cells [2, 17, 42, 45] (Fig. 5.4a, b). These features frequently enable to confuse this neoplasm with a metastasis of carcinoma or melanoma [1, 42]. Cytokeratin and EMA expression may also be present [41, 43, 46]. Often, at least some of the epithelioid cells display a "rhabdoid-like" morphology: eccentric nuclei, prominent nucleoli, and intracytoplasmic filamentous whorls [1, 41]. However, markers of myogenic differentiation are absent [43]. Focally, like in AT/RT, INI-1 staining can be lost [1]. Necrosis is invariably present, but usually not of the pseudo-palisading type [2]. Microvascular proliferation may be present [41, 47]. The tumor bears somewhat of a resemblance to pleomorphic xanthoastrocytoma (PXA); however, larger, bizarre cells are absent and the former also lacks eosinophilic granular bodies (EGBs) [2, 48] (Fig. 5.4c). In exceptional cases, the distinction is quite difficult [49].

GBM with Primitive Neuronal (PN) Component

Primitive neuronal component (PN) component can be seen in glioblastomas of any age, but are much more common in children [50–53]. It is an extremely rare pattern, seen in less than 1% of all GBMs [52]. Clinically, this applies only to supratentorial tumors, to distinguish from the molecularly (and prognostically distinct) infratentorial medulloblastomas [54]. Histopathologically, in addition to archetypal GBM features, this pattern consists of areas of primitive, densely cellular tumor with very high nuclear to cytoplasmic ratios, and speckled, ("salt and pepper") neuroendocrine-type chromatin. Mitotic activity is brisk, and apoptotic bodies are frequent [2, 55] (Fig. 5.4d–g). Occasionally, tumor cells form Homer-Wright rosettes, consisting of a circle of cells surrounding radially-oriented fibrillary processes [2, 50]. Often, these nodules of "small blue cells" appear well-circumscribed from adjacent, reactive, brain parenchyma [50], raising consideration of other entities, including metastatic neuroendocrine carcinoma [40] (Fig. 5.4g). Recognition of a PNET component is critical, as they carry a high risk of cerebrospinal fluid (CSF) spread [2, 52, 56]. This assessment may further be complicated, if by, whether sampling error or other reason, only the PNET component is present on the resection specimen [40]. Frustratingly, the PNET component, while positive for synaptophysin, is generally negative for glial markers (GFAP and Olig2) [2, 50] (Fig. 5.4e, f). In those cases, integration with molecular findings becomes essential, as the presence of glioblastoma molecular aberrations (including *TERT* promoter mutations) within the PNET component supports a glioblastoma origin [40, 57].

Glioblastoma with Gemistocytes

Gemistocytic differentiation can be seen frequently in infiltrating astrocytic neoplasms of different grades [2, 58]. In lower grade tumors, a diagnosis of gemistocytic astrocytoma requires at least 20% of all neoplastic cells to be gemistocytes [2] and is seen in around a tenth of diffuse astrocytomas and are *IDH*-mutant [59]. Patients tend to be diagnosed in their 40s [60, 61]. Histopathologically, gemistocytic tumor cells have abundant, rounded to somewhat angulated, finely granular eosinophilic cytoplasm, and eccentric nuclei with inconspicuous nucleoli [2, 1] (Fig. 5.5a, b). Like granular cell GBM, perivascular lymphocytes are common, and low proliferation indexes are seen [1, 2]. Unlike granular cell GBM, the cytoplasm is less coarse [1, 2] and fibrillary processes connect the tumor cells [17]. Previously, it was thought gemistocytic astrocytomas were more likely to progress to secondary GBMs than other diffuse astrocytoma subtypes [62]; more recent research suggests this may not be the case [58, 63, 64].

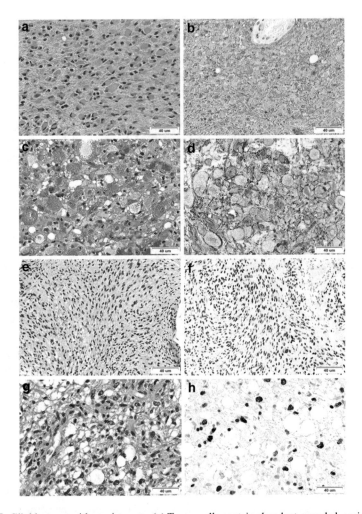

Fig. 5.5 Glioblastoma with gemistocytes (**a**) Tumor cells contain abundant, rounded, eosinophilic cytoplasm and eccentric nuclei. The presence of fibrillar processes between cells helps exclude other diagnostic possibilities, including granular cell glioblastoma and epithelioid glioblastoma. Nuclei are also inconspicuous (**b**) GFAP staining is strong and robust. Glioblastoma, granular cell subtype (**c**) Tumor cells are large, polygonal, with coarsely granular, eosinophilic cytoplasm in this case, GFAP (**d**) is diffusely positive. Glioblastoma, fascicular subtype: (**e**) Tumor cells are arranged in parallel bundles (**f**) Olig-2 is strongly positive, excluding a mesenchymal component. Glioblastoma, lipidized subtype (**g**) Tumor cells contain extensively vacuolated and clear cytoplasm, resembling adipose tissue (**h**) Staining with Olig-2 confirms their glial origin. Glioblastoma, with oligodendroglioma component (**i**) Within the oligodendroglioma areas, the tumor cells are round, rather uniformly-distributed, many with haloes (**j**) In other areas, oligo-like cells are intermixed with tumor cells of a more astrocytic phenotype. Glioblastoma, myxoid subtype (**k**) Malignant glial cells are embedded in a bluish-gray, amorphous matrix (**l**) Strong and robust GFAP staining excludes a mesenchymal component

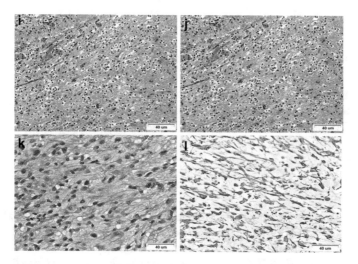

Fig. 5.5 (continued)

Granular Cell Glioblastoma

Granular cell astrocytoma/GBM is a rare, *IDH* wild-type tumor usually of middle to older adults [18, 65, 66]. Clinically, they present similarly to other GBMs, often with ring-enhancement on imaging [1, 65, 66]. Histopathologically, tumor cells obtain a large round to polygonal size, with abundant coarsely granular cytoplasm [2, 1, 18, 66] (Fig. 5.5c, d). Cells are often juxtaposed, with well-defined cell borders [1, 65]. Nuclei appear bland and small [1]. Perivascular lymphocytes are frequently prominent [65], a feature more commonly associated with low-grade glioma/glioneuronal tumors. Mitotic activity is restrained, with low Ki-67 proliferation indexes, similar to gemistocytic astrocytoma [1, 67]. Typically, microvascular proliferation and necrosis are absent [1]. The differential diagnosis includes macrophage-rich lesions, including demyelinating disease, or a cerebral infarction [2, 1]. With IHC, CD68 is often positive (due to rich lysosomal contents), but not CD163, a more specific marker of macrophage lineage [2, 1, 66]. At least partial GFAP and/or Olig-2 staining remains within granular cells [1, 18, 65]. The behavior of these tumors is distinct from other granular cell tumors of the CNS [68]: in spite of shared bland histopathology, these tumors behave malignantly, even in the absence of mitotic activity, necrosis, or microvascular proliferation [65, 66, 69]. Survival times mirror those of other GBM subtypes [2, 1, 65].

Other Patterns of GBM

Fascicular

In rare cases, GBMs can form compact, fascicular spindle cell arrangements, even mimicking a sarcoma [1, 70] (Fig. 5.5e, f). In contrast with gliosarcomas, these cells retain GFAP (and Olig-2) staining and lack reticulin.

Lipomatous

Lipidization of tumor cells in various tumors of the CNS is seen, but only rarely occurs in GBM [71–77]. The few cases described involved adults and the elderly [78]. The defining feature is cells with vacuolated, foamy or clear cytoplasm, resembling adipocytes [76, 78] (Fig. 5.5g, h). In cases where these lipidized cells are numerous or closely approximated, confusion with fat tissue is possible [2, 79], however, GFAP positivity reveals their true glial origin [1, 71, 79, 80].

Oligodendroglioma Component

Although rather uncommon, glioblastomas sometimes contain areas resembling classic oligodendroglioma [2, 81, 82] (Fig. 5.5i, j). These tumors may have a better prognosis than other glioblastoma subtypes [83–85], at least in part due to younger patient age at diagnosis [82–84, 86]. Some studies have also reported a higher frequency of *IDH* mutations [83, 86].

Myxoid

Myxoid change can be seen infrequently, in both GBMs and GSMs [2]. Grossly, if extensive, the tumor appears glistening and gelatinous. Histopathologically, the neoplastic spindle cells are embedded within a bluish-gray, amorphous, myxoid/mucoid matrix [1] (Fig. 5.5k, l). Unlike in gliosarcomas, the tumor cells retain GFAP positivity [2, 87–89].

Epithelial Differentiation

Epithelial metaplasia in GBMs is extremely rare, and may present as keratin pearls or glandular structures ("adenoid" glioblastomas) [1, 46]. The focal nature of these pockets of epithelial differentiation [2], in a sea of archetypal GBMs helps to avoid confusion with metastatic carcinomas. Expression of glial markers by immunohistochemistry is generally retained [46, 90, 91], though expression of cytokeratins is possible [92]. Epithelial differentiation can be seen in (and is more common in) gliosarcomas [1, 93].

Histopathology of GBM: Pediatric Versus Adult

As mentioned previously, GBMs can occur at any age, but are much more common in the adult population, particularly older adults [94, 95]. Often, these tumors at different ages are histopathologically indistinguishable [96]. However, differences do exist; some of these differences may be explained by the molecular drivers seen in these different cohorts. Mutations in chromatin and transcription regulation pathways occur commonly in children [2]. Pediatric tumors are more likely to be syndrome-associated (see below) [97]. Adolescent and young adults frequently have mutations in isocitrate dehydrogenase (*IDH1 or IDH2*) and the tumors typically begin as lower grade infiltrating astrocytomas and progress over time to GBM (i.e. secondary GBM). In middle aged and older adults, GBMs usually develop de novo (primary GBM), without an *IDH* mutation and frequently harbor a *TERT* promoter mutation [2].

Based on these molecular differences, the histopathology of GBMs can be categorized into three groups: pediatric GBMs, *IDH* mutant secondary GBMs of adolescents and younger adults, and *IDH* wild-type primary GBMs (the most common) of mostly elderly adults.

IDH Wild-Type GBMs in Children

From a histopathology perspective, pediatric GBMs mirror their adult counterparts [98]. The rarity of these tumors hitherto precludes an in-depth analysis. Nevertheless, according to one study, most tumors appeared to be of conventional subtypes [99]. Some variants more common in adults, are less frequently seen in children, including the small cell subtype [14, 15]. In contrast, the epithelioid subtype and PNET components are more common in the pediatric age group neoplasms [2, 41, 50–53]. Additionally, gliosarcomas, which are a relatively common unconventional variant in adults are distinctly uncommon in kids [32, 33]. In adults, the majority lower grade diffuse gliomas eventually progress to higher grade tumors; this is the exception in pediatric cases [43] (Fig. 5.6a, b).

IDH Wild-Type Primary GBMs (Mid-older Adults) Versus *IDH* Mutant Secondary GBMs (Adolescent-Younger Adults)

Over 90% of GBMs develop rapidly and *de novo* with no previous precursor lesion history and these are clinically referred to as 'primary GBMs'. These often occur in middle to elderly aged individuals with a median age of 62 years at diagnosis [100]. Among these, *IDH*-wildtype GBM accounts for about 90% with a mean age at diagnosis of 62 years. Conversely, *IDH1/2*-mutated tumors, commonly referred as secondary GBMs occur in younger individuals with median age of onset at ~45 years and typically have a previous history of a lower grade tumor, often present on the same side as the GBM (Fig. 5.6a, b). A multi-group collaborative effort in 2008, sequencing over 20,000 genes in 22 GBMs identified a common point mutation in 12% of the samples in the *IDH*1 gene [101]. Subsequently, further studies have found that ~80% of lower grade II-III gliomas and secondary GBMs harbor this mutation [101]. Mutations in *IDH*2 have also been identified and deemed to be much less common and being mutually exclusive to *IDH*1 mutations [102, 103]. The presence or absence of *IDH* mutations may help to explain some histopathological differences between primary and secondary GBMs. For example, some variants are described as being *IDH*-mutant subtypes (including gemistocytic) and would be expected to be seen in the younger adult patient population. Similarly, granular cell and gliosarcoma are *IDH* wild-type variants and tend to arise in older patients. The presence of a GBM with an oligodendroglial component is also more common in *IDH* mutant GBMs [104]. Despite these differences, they are largely indistinguishable histopathologically [96].

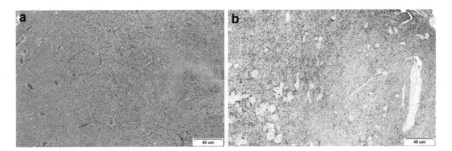

Fig. 5.6 Glioblastoma, secondary, with juxtaposed lower grade and higher-grade components. (**a**) The lower grade component (left) is noticeably less cellular and lacks high grade features of the high-grade component (right) (**b**) *IDH*-1 R132H is positive, supporting a progression of a lower-grade astrocytoma to higher grade

Genetic Susceptibility and Related Syndromes Associated with GBM

The etiology of most glioblastomas is largely unknown; however, several etiologic factors are discussed in further chapters. Only a very small proportion of GBM are seen in more than one family member or are inherited. Inherited tumor syndromes like Turcot syndrome (Type 1 or Brain tumor-polyposis syndrome 1 (BTP1) / Mismatch repair (MMR) cancer syndrome), Li-Fraumeni syndrome, Neurofibromatosis type I and rarer diseases like Ollier's disease / Mafucci syndrome [105] and L-2-hydroxyglutaric aciduria [106] are all associated with development of brain tumors, particularly gliomas. Moreover, there are five separate genome-wide association studies identifying eight specific heritable risk variants in seven genes (*TERT, CCDC26, EGFR, CDKN2B, TP53, PHLDB1*, and *RTEL1*) [107].

Neurofibromatosis Type I (NF1)

NF1 is an autosomal dominant disorder affecting 1 in 2500 to 3000 individuals [108]. Over half of the cases are familial and the remaining occur sporadically, de novo due to a mutation in the *NF1* tumor suppressor gene, located at chromosome 17q11.2 [109]. The mutation leads to loss or reduced production of the protein neurofibromin, which is involved in the RAS/MAPK pathway activity [110]. As a result, patients develop phenotypical features such as café-au-lait macules, neurofibromas, lisch nodules, iris hamartomas, freckling, optic glioma, and osseous lesions required for the diagnosis of NF1 as per the National Institutes of Health Consensus Development Conference Statement [111]. NF1 is associated with the risk of developing optic glioma is approximately 20% in children [112] and the risk for developing high grade glioma in adults is increased by 50–100 times [113]. In a large series of NF1-related tumors, a majority (49%) were pilocytic astrocytomas, 20% were WHO grade II and III gliomas and 7% were GBMs [114]. Specifically, there are several case reports and series illustrating occurrence of GBM in NF1 patients and it has been reported in all age groups from pediatric to older adults, and in both supra and infra-tentorial locations including brainstem and the cerebellum [115–119]. Histopathologically, various patterns have been described, including pleomorphic xanthoastrocytoma-like, epithelioid, adenoid, and giant cell [90, 117, 118, 120]. Almost all NF1 related GBMs were *IDH* wild type wherever data was available [117]. The overall survival associated with NF1 related GBMs were reported to be relatively longer compared to the non-NF1 GBMs [115, 117]. One report also suggested that NF1 GBMs in children might be less aggressive for reasons that are not well understood [115].

Turcot Syndrome

Turcot syndrome is an autosomal dominant disorder associated with two types of distinct cancer syndromes of brain tumors with gastrointestinal polyps. Brain tumor-polyposis syndrome 1 (BTP1)/Mismatch repair (MMR) cancer syndrome is associated with a bi-allelic mutation among one of the four mismatch repair genes (*MLH1, PMS2, MSH2* and *MSH6*) [121]. So far, more than 200 cases have been reported in the literature [122, 123]. Among brain tumors, malignant gliomas account for 25–40% of the cancers in this syndrome and appear within the first two decades of life [122, 123]. Histologically, most of these tumors are reminiscent of pleomorphic xanthoastrocytoma or giant cell glioblastoma with prominent nuclear pleomorphism and multinucleation [124]. Identification of these characteristic features may prompt immunohistochemical testing for MMR protein loss. Other gliomas like oligodendrogliomas, pleomorphic astrocytomas, other low-grade gliomas and medulloblastoma and primitive neuroectodermal tumors have also been described. Extraneural manifestations of this syndrome include, dermatological abnormalities (over 90%) including café-au-lait spots, hematological malignancies (30%) such as T-cell lymphoma and gastrointestinal polyps (almost all patients). Other cancers like sarcomas and urinary tract cancers have also been reported [122, 123]. Brain tumor-polyposis syndrome 2 (BTP2)/Familial adenomatous polyposis (FAP) is an autosomal dominant cancer syndrome due to heterozygous mutations in the *APC* tumor suppressor gene. Medulloblastomas are the main brain tumors reported in association with this cancer syndrome [125].

Li-Fraumeni Syndrome (LFS)

LFS is an autosomal dominant disorder associated with multiple primary cancers in children and young adults caused due to a germline mutation in the *TP53* tumor suppressor gene on chromosome 17p13 [126–128]. This gene encodes a protein that is a multifunctional transcription factor crucial in the control of cell cycle progression, DNA integrity and cell survival during exposures to DNA-damaging agents and non-genotoxic provocative factors like hypoxia. Activation of p53 protein during these situations causes transcriptional activation of genes responsible for the induction of cell cycle arrest or apoptosis [129, 130]. The predominant cancers encountered in LFS include soft tissue sarcomas, osteosarcoma, breast cancer, adreno-cortical carcinoma and brain tumors. The male to female ratio is 1.5:1 for brain tumors, occurring in 13% of the patients with LFS per the IARC TP53 Database (as of November 2013) [131]. The common brain tumors encountered in LFS are astrocytoma, GBM, medulloblastoma and choroid plexus papilloma. The incidence of these tumors shows a bimodal distribution with first peak in children, mostly with medulloblastomas and related primitive neuroectodermal tumors, choroid plexus tumors and ependymomas followed by a second peak in third and fourth decades, mainly with astrocytic gliomas, including diffuse astrocytomas, anaplastic astrocytomas and secondary GBMs [131, 132]. The tumor associated with *TP53* germline mutation tend to develop earlier than their sporadic counterparts with some marked organ-specific differences [132]. The *TP53* mutation in LFS substantially affects the acquisition of the subsequent *IDH1* mutation. The only *IDH1* mutation seen in the astrocytomas and secondary GBMs carrying a *TP53* germline mutation is the R132C (CGT->TGT) mutation that is uncommon in the sporadic cases [133]. This is an exception to the perception that *IDH* mutations are an early incident in gliomagenesis and the mutations persist even after progressing to a higher grade or *IDH*-mutant secondary GBM [134]. Thus, GBMs associated with LFS are always *IDH* mutant type.

L-2-Hydroxyglutaric Aciduria (L2-HGA)

L2-HGA is a rare neurometabolic, organic aciduria that is acquired in an autosomal recessive manner due to a mutation of the *L2HGDH* gene located at chromosome 14q22.1 [135]. The gene encodes for the enzyme L-2-HG dehydrogenase that catalyzes the conversion of L2-HG to alpha-ketoglutarate [136]. Accumulation of L2-HG, which is an oncometabolite may increase the risk of developing brain tumors in a mechanism similar to *IDH* mutant tumors, where there is accumulation of 2-HG (D-enantiomeric form). The exact mechanisms of the oncogenetic and myelinotoxic effects of the accumulated L2-HG and the potential carcinogenic level remains unclear [137]. Over 17 cases of different types of brain tumors have been reported in association with L2-HGA, with a typical age of onset of over 10 years. There were two case reports, where the age at presentation was under 10 years (a 3-year old child with medulloblastoma and a 9-year old child with a low-grade glioma) [138, 139]. The estimated prevalence of brain tumor in L2-HGA is <5%, taking into consideration the accrual bias due to the rarity of this condition [137], GBM has been reported in at least three cases. The location of GBM in these cases was in the left lateral ventricle (intraventricular location), temporal and temporoparietal lobes based on imaging [106, 138, 140]. Only one case had *IDH* mutation status assessment, reported as negative [140]. In one of the cases, the histopathological examination was consistent with GBM with regions morphologically resembling an oligodendroglioma [138].

Ollier's Disease (OD) / Maffucci Syndrome (MS)

These are rare non-inherited disorders characterized by development of enchrondromatosis due to post zygotic mutation in the *IDH* gene that results in mosaicism [141, 142]. In addition to enchondromatosis seen in OD, there is development of hemangiomata in MS. OD/MS are also associated with mutation in the type I receptor for parathyroid hormone and parathyroid hormone-related protein (*PTHR1*) on Chromosome 3p21.31 [143]. There is a higher risk of developing other malignancies like gliomas in OD. Most of the brain tumors reported in these disorders are gliomas, usually low grade and only few reports of GBM with histopathological evidence. Most of the OD/MS cases with gliomas were reported prior to the advent of the molecular characteristics [144, 145]. Almost all glioma cases reported recently harbored an *IDH* mutation, most commonly *IDH*R132H followed by *IDH*2R172S [146]. Not surprisingly, gliomas in OD/MS were frequently located in the frontal lobe similar to sporadic *IDH* mutated gliomas and mostly diffuse low-grade or anaplastic gliomas than GBMs [146]. These also presented at an earlier age (25.6 versus 44 years), were multicentric (32% versus 1%) and had a higher tendency to involve the brainstem (21% versus 1%) [146].

Conclusion

Glioblastomas are the most common and the deadliest infiltrating brain tumor. The diagnosis of GBM can pose a diagnostic challenge due to the veritable numerous histopathology patterns, even within the same tumor. Recognition of these inconsistencies, supplemented by ancillary testing can aid the practicing pathologist in correctly elucidating these neoplasms and providing crucial support to the rest of the patient care team in treatment decisions.

References

1. Burger PC, Scheithauer BW, editors. Neuropathology. Salt Lake City, UT: Amirsys; 2012. 800 p. (Diagnostic pathology).
2. Louis DN, Ohgaki H, Wiestler OD, Cavenee WK, editors. Weltgesundheitsorganisation. WHO classification of tumours of the central nervous system. Revised 4th ed. Lyon: International Agency for Research on Cancer; 2016. 408 p. (World Health Organization classification of tumours).
3. Louis DN, Wesseling P, Aldape K, Brat DJ, Capper D, Cree IA, et al. cIMPACT-NOW update 6: new entity and diagnostic principle recommendations of the cIMPACT-Utrecht meeting on future CNS tumor classification and grading. Brain Pathol. 2020;30(4):844–56.
4. Kaur B, Khwaja FW, Severson EA, Matheny SL, Brat DJ, Van Meir EG. Hypoxia and the hypoxia-inducible-factor pathway in glioma growth and angiogenesis. Neuro-Oncology. 2005;7(2):134–53.
5. Vallée A, Guillevin R, Vallée J-N. Vasculogenesis and angiogenesis initiation under normoxic conditions through Wnt/β-catenin pathway in gliomas. Rev Neurosci. 2018;29(1):71–91.
6. Shweiki D, Itin A, Soffer D, Keshet E. Vascular endothelial growth factor induced by hypoxia may mediate hypoxia-initiated angiogenesis. Nature. 1992;359(6398):843–5.
7. Haddad SF, Moore SA, Schelper RL, Goeken JA. Vascular smooth muscle hyperplasia underlies the formation of glomeruloid vascular structures of glioblastoma multiforme. J Neuropathol Exp Neurol. 1992;51(5):488–92.
8. Nagashima T, Hoshino T, Cho KG. Proliferative potential of vascular components in human glioblastoma multiforme. Acta Neuropathol. 1987;73(3):301–5.

9. Rodriguez FJ, Orr BA, Ligon KL, Eberhart CG. Neoplastic cells are a rare component in human glioblastoma microvasculature. Oncotarget. 2012;3(1):98–106.
10. Takeuchi H, Hashimoto N, Kitai R, Kubota T, Kikuta K. Proliferation of vascular smooth muscle cells in glioblastoma multiforme. J Neurosurg. 2010;113(2):218–24.
11. Burger PC, Heinz ER, Shibata T, Kleihues P. Topographic anatomy and CT correlations in the untreated glioblastoma multiforme. J Neurosurg. 1988;68(5):698–704.
12. Zagzag D, Esencay M, Mendez O, Yee H, Smirnova I, Huang Y, et al. Hypoxia- and vascular endothelial growth factor-induced stromal cell-derived factor-1alpha/CXCR4 expression in glioblastomas: one plausible explanation of Scherer's structures. Am J Pathol. 2008;173(2):545–60.
13. Alkhaibary A, Alassiri AH, AlSufiani F, Alharbi MA. Ki-67 labeling index in glioblastoma; does it really matter? Hematol Oncol Stem Cell Ther. 2019;12(2):82–8.
14. Perry A, Aldape KD, George DH, Burger PC. Small cell astrocytoma: an aggressive variant that is clinicopathologically and genetically distinct from anaplastic oligodendroglioma. Cancer. 2004;101(10):2318–26.
15. Kalogerak A, Tamiolakis D, Zoi I, Karvela-Kalogeraki I, Karvelas-Kalogerakis M, Segredakis J, et al. FNA Cytology in pediatric small cell glioblastoma. Acta Biomed. 2018;89(2):265–8.
16. Takeuchi H, Kitai R, Hosoda T, Yamada S, Hashimoto N, Kikuta K, et al. Clinicopathologic features of small cell glioblastomas. J Neuro-Oncol. 2016;127(2):337–44.
17. Gokden M. If it is not a glioblastoma, then what is it? A differential diagnostic review. Adv Anat Pathol. 2017;24(6):379–91.
18. Joseph NM, Phillips J, Dahiya S, Felicella MM, Tihan T, Brat DJ, et al. Diagnostic implications of IDH1-R132H and OLIG2 expression patterns in rare and challenging glioblastoma variants. Mod Pathol. 2013;26(3):315–26.
19. Ishizawa K, Komori T, Shimada S, Hirose T. Olig2 and CD99 are useful negative markers for the diagnosis of brain tumors. Clin Neuropathol. 2008;27(3):118–28.
20. Švajdler M, Rychlý B, Mezencev R, Fröhlichová L, Bednárová A, Pataky F, et al. SOX10 and Olig2 as negative markers for the diagnosis of ependymomas: an immunohistochemical study of 98 glial tumors. Histol Histopathol. 2016;31(1):95–102.
21. Otero JJ, Rowitch D, Vandenberg S. OLIG2 is differentially expressed in pediatric astrocytic and in ependymal neoplasms. J Neuro-Oncol. 2011;104(2):423–38.
22. Jin MC, Wu A, Xiang M, Azad TD, Soltys SG, Li G, et al. Prognostic factors and treatment patterns in the management of giant cell glioblastoma. World Neurosurg. 2019;128:e217–24.
23. Kozak KR, Moody JS. Giant cell glioblastoma: a glioblastoma subtype with distinct epidemiology and superior prognosis. Neuro-Oncology. 2009;11(6):833–41.
24. Borkar SA, Lakshmiprasad G, Subbarao KC, Sharma MC, Mahapatra AK. Giant cell glioblastoma in the pediatric age group: report of two cases. J Pediatr Neurosci. 2013;8(1):38–40.
25. Martinez-Diaz H, Kleinschmidt-DeMasters BK, Powell SZ, Yachnis AT. Giant cell glioblastoma and pleomorphic xanthoastrocytoma show different immunohistochemical profiles for neuronal antigens and p53 but share reactivity for class III beta-tubulin. Arch Pathol Lab Med. 2003;127(9):1187–91.
26. Figarella-Branger D, Bouvier C, Moroch J, Michalak S, Burel-Vandenbos F. Morphological classification of glioblastomas. Neurochirurgie. 2010;56(6):459–63.
27. Margetts JC, Kalyan-Raman UP. Giant-celled glioblastoma of brain. A clinico-pathological and radiological study of ten cases (including immunohistochemistry and ultrastructure). Cancer. 1989;63(3):524–31.
28. Feigin IH, Gross SW. Sarcoma arising in glioblastoma of the brain. Am J Pathol. 1955;31(4):633–53.
29. Feigin I, Allen LB, Lipkin L, Gross SW. The endothelial hyperplasia of the cerebral blood vessels with brain tumors, and its sarcomatous transformation. Cancer. 1958;11(2):264–77.
30. Boerman RH, Anderl K, Herath J, Borell T, Johnson N, Schaeffer-Klein J, et al. The glial and mesenchymal elements of gliosarcomas share similar genetic alterations. J Neuropathol Exp Neurol. 1996;55(9):973–81.

31. Reis RM, Könü-Leblebicioglu D, Lopes JM, Kleihues P, Ohgaki H. Genetic profile of glio-sarcomas. Am J Pathol. 2000;156(2):425–32.
32. Cachia D, Kamiya-Matsuoka C, Mandel JJ, Olar A, Cykowski MD, Armstrong TS, et al. Primary and secondary gliosarcomas: clinical, molecular and survival characteristics. J Neuro-Oncol. 2015;125(2):401–10.
33. Smith DR, Wu C-C, Saadatmand HJ, Isaacson SR, Cheng SK, Sisti MB, et al. Clinical and molecular characteristics of gliosarcoma and modern prognostic significance relative to conventional glioblastoma. J Neuro-Oncol. 2018;137(2):303–11.
34. Galanis E, Buckner JC, Dinapoli RP, Scheithauer BW, Jenkins RB, Wang CH, et al. Clinical outcome of gliosarcoma compared with glioblastoma multiforme: North Central Cancer Treatment Group results. J Neurosurg. 1998;89(3):425–30.
35. Karremann M, Rausche U, Fleischhack G, Nathrath M, Pietsch T, Kramm CM, et al. Clinical and epidemiological characteristics of pediatric gliosarcomas. J Neuro-Oncol. 2010;97(2):257–65.
36. Morantz RA, Feigin I, Ransohoff J. Clinical and pathological study of 24 cases of gliosarcoma. J Neurosurg. 1976;45(4):398–408.
37. Beaumont TL, Kupsky WJ, Barger GR, Sloan AE. Gliosarcoma with multiple extracranial metastases: case report and review of the literature. J Neuro-Oncol. 2007;83(1):39–46.
38. Shintaku M, Yoneda H, Hirato J, Nagaishi M, Okabe H. Gliosarcoma with ependymal and PNET-like differentiation. Clin Neuropathol. 2013;32(6):508–14.
39. Yao K, Qi X-L, Mei X, Jiang T. Gliosarcoma with primitive neuroectodermal, osseous, cartilage and adipocyte differentiation: a case report. Int J Clin Exp Pathol. 2015;8(2):2079–84.
40. McGahan BG, Toop N, Jones D, Kobalka PJ, Palmer J, Elder JB. Gliosarcoma with PNET component mimicking a neuroendocrine carcinoma with initially only PNET and sarcoma components: a case report. 2021 [In Press].
41. Sugimoto K, Ideguchi M, Kimura T, Kajiwara K, Imoto H, Sadahiro H, et al. Epithelioid/rhabdoid glioblastoma: a highly aggressive subtype of glioblastoma. Brain Tumor Pathol. 2016;33(2):137–46.
42. Kleinschmidt-DeMasters BK, Aisner DL, Birks DK, Foreman NK. Epithelioid GBMs show a high percentage of BRAF V600E mutation. Am J Surg Pathol. 2013;37(5):685–98.
43. Broniscer A, Tatevossian RG, Sabin ND, Klimo P, Dalton J, Lee R, et al. Clinical, radiological, histological and molecular characteristics of paediatric epithelioid glioblastoma. Neuropathol Appl Neurobiol. 2014;40(3):327–36.
44. Stupp R, Mason WP, van den Bent MJ, Weller M, Fisher B, Taphoorn MJB, et al. Radiotherapy plus concomitant and adjuvant temozolomide for glioblastoma. N Engl J Med. 2005;352(10):987–96.
45. Nitta N, Moritani S, Fukami T, Yoshimura Y, Hirai H, Nozaki K. Intraventricular epithelioid glioblastoma: a case report. World Neurosurg. 2018;112:257–63.
46. Rodriguez FJ, Scheithauer BW, Giannini C, Bryant SC, Jenkins RB. Epithelial and pseudo-epithelial differentiation in glioblastoma and gliosarcoma: a comparative morphologic and molecular genetic study. Cancer. 2008;113(10):2779–89.
47. Tanaka T, Kaijima M, Yonemasu Y, Cepeda C. Spontaneous secondarily generalized seizures induced by a single microinjection of kainic acid into unilateral amygdala in cats. Electroencephalogr Clin Neurophysiol. 1985;61(5):422–9.
48. Alexandrescu S, Korshunov A, Lai SH, Dabiri S, Patil S, Li R, et al. Epithelioid glioblastomas and anaplastic epithelioid pleomorphic xanthoastrocytomas--same entity or first cousins? Brain Pathol. 2016;26(2):215–23.
49. Furuta T, Miyoshi H, Komaki S, Arakawa F, Morioka M, Ohshima K, et al. Clinicopathological and genetic association between epithelioid glioblastoma and pleomorphic xanthoastrocytoma. Neuropathology. 2018;38(3):218–27.
50. Song X, Andrew Allen R, Terence Dunn S, Fung K-M, Farmer P, Gandhi S, et al. Glioblastoma with PNET-like components has a higher frequency of isocitrate dehydrogenase 1 (IDH1) mutation and likely a better prognosis than primary glioblastoma. Int J Clin Exp Pathol. 2011;4(7):651–60.

51. Kim DG, Lee DY, Paek SH, Chi JG, Choe G, Jung H-W. Supratentorial primitive neuroecto-dermal tumors in adults. J Neuro-Oncol. 2002;60(1):43–52.
52. Prelaj A, Rebuzzi SE, Caffarena G, Giròn Berrìos JR, Pecorari S, Fusto C, et al. Therapeutic approach in glioblastoma multiforme with primitive neuroectodermal tumor components: case report and review of the literature. Oncol Lett. 2018;15(5):6641–7.
53. Ohba S, Yoshida K, Hirose Y, Ikeda E, Kawase T. A supratentorial primitive neuro-ectodermal tumor in an adult: a case report and review of the literature. J Neuro-Oncol. 2008;86(2):217–24.
54. Kouyialis AT, Boviatsis EI, Karampelas IK, Korfias S, Korkolopoulou P, Sakas DE. Primitive supratentorial neuroectodermal tumor in an adult. J Clin Neurosci. 2005;12(4):492–5.
55. Xu G, Li JY. CDK4, CDK6, cyclin D1, p16(INK4a) and EGFR expression in glioblastoma with a primitive neuronal component. J Neuro-Oncol. 2018;136(3):445–52.
56. Vollmer K, Pantazis G, Añon J, Roelcke U, Schwyzer L. Spinal metastases of supratentorial glioblastoma with primitive neuronal component. World Neurosurg X. 2019;2:100019.
57. Yoshida Y, Ide M, Fujimaki H, Matsumura N, Nobusawa S, Ikota H, et al. Gliosarcoma with primitive neuronal, chondroid, osteoid and ependymal elements. Neuropathology. 2018;38(4):392–99.
58. Martins DC, Malheiros SM, Santiago LH, Stávale JN. Gemistocytes in astrocytomas: are they a significant prognostic factor? J Neuro-Oncol. 2006;80(1):49–55.
59. Heesters M, Molenaar W, Go GK. Radiotherapy in supratentorial gliomas. A study of 821 cases. Strahlenther Onkol. 2003;179(9):606–14.
60. Krouwer HG, Davis RL, Silver P, Prados M. Gemistocytic astrocytomas: a reappraisal. J Neurosurg. 1991;74(3):399–406.
61. Watanabe K, Peraud A, Gratas C, Wakai S, Kleihues P, Ohgaki H. p53 and PTEN gene muta-tions in gemistocytic astrocytomas. Acta Neuropathol. 1998;95(6):559–64.
62. Watanabe K, Tachibana O, Yonekawa Y, Kleihues P, Ohgaki H. Role of gemistocytes in astro-cytoma progression. Lab Investig. 1997;76(2):277–84.
63. Tihan T, Vohra P, Berger MS, Keles GE. Definition and diagnostic implications of gemisto-cytic astrocytomas: a pathological perspective. J Neuro-Oncol. 2006;76(2):175–83.
64. Yang HJ, Kim JE, Paek SH, Chi JG, Jung H-W, Kim DG. The significance of gemistocytes in astrocytoma. Acta Neurochir. 2003;145(12):1097–103; discussion 1103.
65. Brat DJ, Scheithauer BW, Medina-Flores R, Rosenblum MK, Burger PC. Infiltrative astro-cytomas with granular cell features (granular cell astrocytomas): a study of histopathologic features, grading, and outcome. Am J Surg Pathol. 2002;26(6):750–7.
66. Vizcaino MA, Palsgrove DN, Yuan M, Giannini C, Cabrera-Aldana EE, Pallavajjala A, et al. Granular cell astrocytoma: an aggressive IDH-wildtype diffuse glioma with molecular genetic features of primary glioblastoma. Brain Pathol. 2019;29(2):193–204.
67. Chorny JA, Evans LC, Kleinschmidt-DeMasters BK. Cerebral granular cell astrocytomas: a Mib-1, bcl-2, and telomerase study. Clin Neuropathol. 2000;19(4):170–9.
68. Caporalini C, Buccoliero AM, Scoccianti S, Moscardi S, Simoni A, Pansini L, et al. Granular cell astrocytoma: report of a case and review of the literature. Clin Neuropathol. 2016;35(4):186–93.
69. Schittenhelm J, Psaras T. Glioblastoma with granular cell astrocytoma features: a case report and literature review. Clin Neuropathol. 2010;29(5):323–9.
70. Porter BF, Summers BA, Leland MM, Hubbard GB. Glioblastoma multiforme in three baboons (Papio spp). Vet Pathol. 2004;41(4):424–8.
71. Roncaroli F, Scheithauer BW, Laeng RH, Cenacchi G, Abell-Aleff P, Moschopulos M. Lipomatous meningioma: a clinicopathologic study of 18 cases with special reference to the issue of metaplasia. Am J Surg Pathol. 2001;25(6):769–75.
72. Giangaspero F, Kaulich K, Cenacchi G, Cerasoli S, Lerch K-D, Breu H, et al. Lipoastrocytoma: a rare low-grade astrocytoma variant of pediatric age. Acta Neuropathol. 2002;103(2):152–6.
73. Garg N, Gaur K, Batra VV, Jagetia A. Pilocytic astrocytoma with adipocytic differentiation: a rare histological variation. J Pediatr Neurosci. 2018;13(2):260–3.

74. Aker FV, Ozkara S, Eren P, Peker O, Armağan S, Hakan T. Cerebellar liponeurocytoma/ lipidized medulloblastoma. J Neuro-Oncol. 2005;71(1):53–9.
75. Hamlat A, Le Strat A, Guegan Y, Ben-Hassel M, Saikali S. Cerebellar pleomorphic xanthoastrocytoma: case report and literature review. Surg Neurol. 2007;68(1):89–94; discussion 94–95.
76. Rickert CH, Riemenschneider MJ, Schachenmayr W, Richter H-P, Bockhorn J, Reifenberger G, et al. Glioblastoma with adipocyte-like tumor cell differentiation--histological and molecular features of a rare differentiation pattern. Brain Pathol. 2009;19(3):431–8.
77. Gupta K, Kalra I, Salunke P, Vasishta RK. Lipidized glioblastoma: a rare differentiation pattern. Neuropathology. 2011;31(1):93–7.
78. Gessi M, Gielen GH, Denkhaus D, Antonelli M, Giangaspero F, Zur Mühlen A, et al. Molecular heterogeneity characterizes glioblastoma with lipoblast/adipocyte-like cytology. Virchows Arch. 2015;467(1):105–9.
79. Johnson DR, Ma DJ, Buckner JC, Hammack JE. Conditional probability of long-term survival in glioblastoma: a population-based analysis. Cancer. 2012;118(22):5608–13.
80. Fukuda T, Yasumichi K, Suzuki T. Immunohistochemistry of gliosarcoma with liposarcomatous differentiation. Pathol Int. 2008;58(6):396–401.
81. Kelly MF, Parker PA, Scott RN. The application of neural networks to myoelectric signal analysis: a preliminary study. IEEE Trans Biomed Eng. 1990;37(3):221–30.
82. Laxton RC, Popov S, Doey L, Jury A, Bhangoo R, Gullan R, et al. Primary glioblastoma with oligodendroglial differentiation has better clinical outcome but no difference in common biological markers compared with other types of glioblastoma. Neuro-Oncology. 2013;15(12):1635–43.
83. Wang Y, Li S, Chen L, You G, Bao Z, Yan W, et al. Glioblastoma with an oligodendroglioma component: distinct clinical behavior, genetic alterations, and outcome. Neuro-Oncology. 2012;14(4):518–25.
84. Homma T, Fukushima T, Vaccarella S, Yonekawa Y, Di Patre PL, Franceschi S, et al. Correlation among pathology, genotype, and patient outcomes in glioblastoma. J Neuropathol Exp Neurol. 2006;65(9):846–54.
85. Kraus JA, Lamszus K, Glesmann N, Beck M, Wolter M, Sabel M, et al. Molecular genetic alterations in glioblastomas with oligodendroglial component. Acta Neuropathol. 2001;101(4):311–20.
86. Appin CL, Gao J, Chisolm C, Torian M, Alexis D, Vincentelli C, et al. Glioblastoma with oligodendroglioma component (GBM-O): molecular genetic and clinical characteristics. Brain Pathol. 2013;23(4):454–61.
87. Jie W, Bai J, Li B. An extracranial metastasis of glioblastoma mimicking mucoepidermoid carcinoma. World Neurosurg. 2018;116:352–6.
88. Kishikawa M, Tsuda N, Fujii H, Nishimori I, Yokoyama H, Kihara M. Glioblastoma with sarcomatous component associated with myxoid change. A histochemical, immunohistochemical and electron microscopic study. Acta Neuropathol. 1986;70(1):44–52.
89. Kepes JJ. Astrocytomas: old and newly recognized variants, their spectrum of morphology and antigen expression. Can J Neurol Sci. 1987;14(2):109–21.
90. Miyata S, Sugimoto T, Kodama T, Akiyama Y, Nakano S, Wakisaka S, et al. Adenoid glioblastoma arising in a patient with neurofibromatosis type-1. Pathol Int. 2005;55(6):348–52.
91. Kepes JJ, Fulling KH, Garcia JH. The clinical significance of "adenoid" formations of neoplastic astrocytes, imitating metastatic carcinoma, in gliosarcomas. A review of five cases. Clin Neuropathol. 1982;1(4):139–50.
92. Mørk SJ, Rubinstein LJ, Kepes JJ, Perentes E, Uphoff DF. Patterns of epithelial metaplasia in malignant gliomas. II. Squamous differentiation of epithelial-like formations in gliosarcomas and glioblastomas. J Neuropathol Exp Neurol. 1988;47(2):101–18.
93. Lopez Fernandez A. Osteoarticular tuberculosis in the child. Acta Pediatr Esp. 1956;14(162):486–7.
94. Tamimi AF, Juweid M. Epidemiology and outcome of glioblastoma. In: De Vleeschouwer S, editor. Glioblastoma [Internet]. Brisbane (AU): Codon Publications; 2017 [cited 2020 Aug 16]. Available from: http://www.ncbi.nlm.nih.gov/books/NBK470003/.

95. Arora RS, Alston RD, Eden TOB, Estlin EJ, Moran A, Birch JM. Age-incidence patterns of primary CNS tumors in children, adolescents, and adults in England. Neuro-Oncology. 2009;11(4):403–13.
96. Ohgaki H, Dessen P, Jourde B, Horstmann S, Nishikawa T, Di Patre P-L, et al. Genetic pathways to glioblastoma: a population-based study. Cancer Res. 2004;64(19):6892–9.
97. Liu M, Thakkar JP, Garcia CR, Dolecek TA, Wagner LM, Dressler EVM, et al. National cancer database analysis of outcomes in pediatric glioblastoma. Cancer Med. 2018;7(4):1151–9.
98. Suri V, Das P, Pathak P, Jain A, Sharma MC, Borkar SA, et al. Pediatric glioblastomas: a histopathological and molecular genetic study. Neuro-Oncology. 2009;11(3):274–80.
99. Das KK, Mehrotra A, Nair AP, Kumar S, Srivastava AK, Sahu RN, et al. Pediatric glioblastoma: clinico-radiological profile and factors affecting the outcome. Childs Nerv Syst. 2012;28(12):2055–62.
100. Ostrom QT, Patil N, Cioffi G, Waite K, Kruchko C, Barnholtz-Sloan JS. CBTRUS Statistical report: primary brain and other central nervous system tumors diagnosed in the United States in 2013–2017. Neuro Oncol. 2020;22(Suppl_1):iv1–96.
101. Parsons DW, Jones S, Zhang X, Lin JC-H, Leary RJ, Angenendt P, et al. An integrated genomic analysis of human glioblastoma multiforme. Science. 2008;321(5897):1807–12.
102. Yan H, Parsons DW, Jin G, McLendon R, Rasheed BA, Yuan W, et al. IDH1 and IDH2 mutations in gliomas. N Engl J Med. 2009;360(8):765–73.
103. Hartmann C, Meyer J, Balss J, Capper D, Mueller W, Christians A, et al. Type and frequency of IDH1 and IDH2 mutations are related to astrocytic and oligodendroglial differentiation and age: a study of 1,010 diffuse gliomas. Acta Neuropathol. 2009;118(4):469–74.
104. Nobusawa S, Watanabe T, Kleihues P, Ohgaki H. IDH1 mutations as molecular signature and predictive factor of secondary glioblastomas. Clin Cancer Res. 2009;15(19):6002–7.
105. Frappaz D, Ricci AC, Kohler R, Bret P, Mottolese C. Diffuse brain stem tumor in an adolescent with multiple enchondromatosis (Ollier's disease). Childs Nerv Syst. 1999;15(5):222–5.
106. Haliloglu G, Jobard F, Oguz KK, Anlar B, Akalan N, Coskun T, et al. L-2-hydroxyglutaric aciduria and brain tumors in children with mutations in the L2HGDH gene: neuroimaging findings. Neuropediatrics. 2008;39(2):119–22.
107. Ostrom QT, Bauchet L, Davis FG, Deltour I, Fisher JL, Langer CE, et al. The epidemiology of glioma in adults: a "state of the science" review. Neuro-Oncology. 2014;16(7):896–913.
108. Evans DG, Howard E, Giblin C, Clancy T, Spencer H, Huson SM, et al. Birth incidence and prevalence of tumor-prone syndromes: estimates from a UK family genetic register service. Am J Med Genet A. 2010;152A(2):327–32.
109. Gutmann DH, Ferner RE, Listernick RH, Korf BR, Wolters PL, Johnson KJ. Neurofibromatosis type 1. Nat Rev Dis Primers. 2017;3:17004.
110. Gutmann DH, Parada LF, Silva AJ, Ratner N. Neurofibromatosis type 1: modeling CNS dysfunction. J Neurosci. 2012;32(41):14087–93.
111. National Institutes of Health Consensus Development Conference Statement: neurofibromatosis. Bethesda, MD, USA, July 13–15, 1987. Neurofibromatosis. 1988;1(3):172–8.
112. Rasmussen SA, Friedman JM. NF1 gene and neurofibromatosis 1. Am J Epidemiol. 2000;151(1):33–40.
113. Gutmann DH, Rasmussen SA, Wolkenstein P, MacCollin MM, Guha A, Inskip PD, et al. Gliomas presenting after age 10 in individuals with neurofibromatosis type 1 (NF1). Neurology. 2002;59(5):759–61.
114. Rodriguez FJ, Perry A, Gutmann DH, O'Neill BP, Leonard J, Bryant S, et al. Gliomas in neurofibromatosis type 1: a clinicopathologic study of 100 patients. J Neuropathol Exp Neurol. 2008;67(3):240–9.
115. Huttner AJ, Kieran MW, Yao X, Cruz L, Ladner J, Quayle K, et al. Clinicopathologic study of glioblastoma in children with neurofibromatosis type 1. Pediatr Blood Cancer. 2010;54(7):890–6.
116. Fortunato JT, Reys B, Singh P, Pan E. Brainstem glioblastoma multiforme in a patient with NF1. Anticancer Res. 2018;38(8):4897–900.

117. Shibahara I, Sonoda Y, Suzuki H, Mayama A, Kanamori M, Saito R, et al. Glioblastoma in neurofibromatosis 1 patients without IDH1, BRAF V600E, and TERT promoter mutations. Brain Tumor Pathol. 2018;35(1):10–8.

118. Taraszewska A, Bogucki J, Powała A, Matyja E. Giant cell glioblastoma with unique bilateral cerebellopontine angle localization considered as extraaxial tumor growth in a patient with neurofibromatosis type 1. Clin Neuropathol. 2013;32(1):58–65.

119. Takahashi Y, Makino K, Nakamura H, Hide T, Yano S, Kamada H, et al. Clinical characteristics and pathogenesis of cerebellar glioblastoma. Mol Med Rep. 2014;10(5):2383–8.

120. Kroh H, Matyja E, Marchel A, Bojarski P. Heavily lipidized, calcified giant cell glioblastoma in an 8-year-old patient, associated with neurofibromatosis type 1 (NF1): report of a case with long-term survival. Clin Neuropathol. 2004;23(6):286–91.

121. Durno CA, Sherman PM, Aronson M, Malkin D, Hawkins C, Bakry D, et al. Phenotypic and genotypic characterisation of biallelic mismatch repair deficiency (BMMR-D) syndrome. Eur J Cancer. 2015;51(8):977–83.

122. Bakry D, Aronson M, Durno C, Rimawi H, Farah R, Alharbi QK, et al. Genetic and clinical determinants of constitutional mismatch repair deficiency syndrome: report from the constitutional mismatch repair deficiency consortium. Eur J Cancer. 2014;50(5):987–96.

123. Wimmer K, Kratz CP, Vasen HFA, Caron O, Colas C, Entz-Werle N, et al. Diagnostic criteria for constitutional mismatch repair deficiency syndrome: suggestions of the European consortium "care for CMMRD" (C4CMMRD). J Med Genet. 2014;51(6):355–65.

124. Erson-Omay EZ, Çağlayan AO, Schultz N, Weinhold N, Omay SB, Özduman K, et al. Somatic POLE mutations cause an ultramutated giant cell high-grade glioma subtype with better prognosis. Neuro-Oncology. 2015;17(10):1356–64.

125. Leoz ML, Carballal S, Moreira L, Ocaña T, Balaguer F. The genetic basis of familial adenomatous polyposis and its implications for clinical practice and risk management. Appl Clin Genet. 2015;8:95–107.

126. Malkin D, Li FP, Strong LC, Fraumeni JF, Nelson CE, Kim DH, et al. Germ line p53 mutations in a familial syndrome of breast cancer, sarcomas, and other neoplasms. Science. 1990;250(4985):1233–8.

127. Frebourg T, Barbier N, Yan YX, Garber JE, Dreyfus M, Fraumeni J, et al. Germ-line p53 mutations in 15 families with Li-Fraumeni syndrome. Am J Hum Genet. 1995;56(3):608–15.

128. Varley JM, McGown G, Thorncroft M, Santibanez-Koref MF, Kelsey AM, Tricker KJ, et al. Germ-line mutations of TP53 in Li-Fraumeni families: an extended study of 39 families. Cancer Res. 1997;57(15):3245–52.

129. Levine AJ. p53, the cellular gatekeeper for growth and division. Cell. 1997;88(3):323–31.

130. Ko LJ, Prives C. p53: puzzle and paradigm. Genes Dev. 1996;10(9):1054–72.

131. Olivier M, Goldgar DE, Sodha N, Ohgaki H, Kleihues P, Hainaut P, et al. Li-Fraumeni and related syndromes: correlation between tumor type, family structure, and TP53 genotype. Cancer Res. 2003;63(20):6643–50.

132. Kleihues P, Schäuble B, zur Hausen A, Estève J, Ohgaki H. Tumors associated with p53 germline mutations: a synopsis of 91 families. Am J Pathol. 1997;150(1):1–13.

133. Watanabe T, Vital A, Nobusawa S, Kleihues P, Ohgaki H. Selective acquisition of IDH1 R132C mutations in astrocytomas associated with Li-Fraumeni syndrome. Acta Neuropathol. 2009;117(6):653–6.

134. Watanabe T, Nobusawa S, Kleihues P, Ohgaki H. IDH1 mutations are early events in the development of astrocytomas and oligodendrogliomas. Am J Pathol. 2009;174(4):1149–53.

135. Topçu M, Jobard F, Halliez S, Coskun T, Yalçinkayal C, Gerceker FO, et al. L-2-Hydroxyglutaric aciduria: identification of a mutant gene C14orf160, localized on chromosome 14q22.1. Hum Mol Genet. 2004;13(22):2803–11.

136. Rzem R, Van Schaftingen E, Veiga-da-Cunha M. The gene mutated in l-2-hydroxyglutaric aciduria encodes l-2-hydroxyglutarate dehydrogenase. Biochimie. 2006;88(1):113–6.

137. Patay Z, Mills JC, Löbel U, Lambert A, Sablauer A, Ellison DW. Cerebral neoplasms in L-2 hydroxyglutaric aciduria: 3 new cases and meta-analysis of literature data. AJNR Am J Neuroradiol. 2012;33(5):940–3.

138. Moroni I, Bugiani M, D'Incerti L, Maccagnano C, Rimoldi M, Bissola L, et al. L-2-hydroxyglutaric aciduria and brain malignant tumors: a predisposing condition? Neurology. 2004;62(10):1882–4.
139. Wanders RJ, Vilarinho L, Hartung HP, Hoffmann GF, Mooijer PA, Jansen GA, et al. L-2-Hydroxyglutaric aciduria: normal L-2-hydroxyglutarate dehydrogenase activity in liver from two new patients. J Inherit Metab Dis. 1997;20(5):725–6.
140. Tan AP, Mankad K. Intraventricular glioblastoma multiforme in a child with L2-hydroxyglutaric aciduria. World Neurosurg. 2018;110:288–90.
141. Pansuriya TC, van Eijk R, d'Adamo P, van Ruler MAJH, Kuijjer ML, Oosting J, et al. Somatic mosaic IDH1 and IDH2 mutations are associated with enchondroma and spindle cell hemangioma in Ollier disease and Maffucci syndrome. Nat Genet. 2011;43(12):1256–61.
142. Amary MF, Bacsi K, Maggiani F, Damato S, Halai D, Berisha F, et al. IDH1 and IDH2 mutations are frequent events in central chondrosarcoma and central and periosteal chondromas but not in other mesenchymal tumours. J Pathol. 2011;224(3):334–43.
143. Hopyan S, Gokgoz N, Poon R, Gensure RC, Yu C, Cole WG, et al. A mutant PTH/PTHrP type I receptor in enchondromatosis. Nat Genet. 2002;30(3):306–10.
144. Chang S, Prados MD. Identical twins with Ollier's disease and intracranial gliomas: case report. Neurosurgery. 1994;34(5):903–6; discussion 906.
145. Ranger A, Szymczak A, Hammond RR, Zelcer S. Pediatric thalamic glioblastoma associated with Ollier disease (multiple enchondromatosis): a rare case of concurrence. J Neurosurg Pediatr. 2009;4(4):363–7.
146. Bonnet C, Thomas L, Psimaras D, Bielle F, Vauléon E, Loiseau H, et al. Characteristics of gliomas in patients with somatic IDH mosaicism. Acta Neuropathol Commun. 2016;4:31.

Chapter 6
Principles of Radiation Therapy for Glioblastoma Patients

Sasha Beyer and Arnab Chakravarti

Introduction

Glioblastoma (GBM) is the most common malignant primary brain tumor in adults. GBMs are aggressive tumors with diffusely infiltrating microscopic disease that extends into the brain parenchyma and, despite years of ongoing research, the prognosis remains poor. With both diagnostic and therapeutic implications, surgical resection is the primary treatment modality for GBM and the extent of resection has been shown to be related to patient prognosis [1]. However, complete surgical resection of GBM is uncommon due to the diffuse, infiltrative nature of the disease and maximal safe resection alone results in high rates of local recurrence [2]. Post-operative radiation therapy (60 Gy in 30 daily fractions) is essential in controlling this unresectable microscopic disease and has been shown to significantly increase median survival compared to surgery alone [2–5].

In 2004, a randomized phase III trial by the European Organization for Research and Treatment of Cancer (EORTC) 26981-22981/National Cancer Institute of Canada Clinical Trials Group (NCIC CTG) established the widely adopted current standard of care for GBM. This landmark study showed a survival benefit with the addition of concurrent and adjuvant temozolomide (TMZ), an oral alkylating chemotherapy, to maximal safe resection and post-operative radiation therapy. Indeed, overall survival increased to 9.8% at 5 years with the addition of TMZ to radiation therapy compared to 1.9% OS at 5 years with radiotherapy alone [6, 7]. Moreover, patients in the chemotherapy arm had an increased median survival of 14.6 months compared to 12.1 months for the radiation alone arm [7]. Since this landmark study

S. Beyer · A. Chakravarti (✉)
Department of Radiation Oncology, Arthur G. James Hospital/The Ohio State University Comprehensive Cancer Center, Columbus, OH, USA
e-mail: Arnab.Chakravarti@osumc.edu

J. J. Otero, A. P. Becker (eds.), *Precision Molecular Pathology of Glioblastoma*, Molecular Pathology Library, https://doi.org/10.1007/978-3-030-69170-7_6

in 2004, the standard of care for the management of GBM remains maximal safe resection followed by concurrent chemoradiation and adjuvant chemotherapy.

In contrast to other malignancies, GBM tend to recur locally rather than at distant areas of the central nervous system (CNS) [2]. Indeed, the majority of recurrences occur within the previous high dose radiation field, further emphasizing the need for improving the efficacy of radiation therapy. While the standard of care for treatment of GBM has not significantly changed since the landmark EORTC/NCIC CTG study [7], radiation therapy techniques have evolved over the past 15 years with the hopes of increasing local control and survival in these patients. In this chapter, we will explore the principles of radiation therapy, radiation techniques that have been studied as potential approaches for increasing the efficacy of radiation as well as a more recent focus toward identifying molecular biomarkers that may help radiosensitize glioblastoma cells and predict response to radiation.

Basics of Radiation Therapy

External beam radiation therapy has long been an essential part of treatment for GBM patients. Therapeutic X-rays (photons) are produced by linear accelerators and form the basis of external beam radiation therapy. The biologic effects of X-rays may be caused by direct action (by directly ionizing the target molecule) or by indirect action (by interacting with water to produce free radicals that in turn interact with the target molecule). In most cases, X-rays are indirectly ionizing by transferring their energy to free radicals that in turn damage DNA. When the DNA damage is unrepairable, radiation leads to death of the cancer cell [8]. TMZ chemotherapy is believed to facilitate this process by producing cytotoxic lesions, such as methylation of O^6-methylguanine, that stabilize and further delay repair of RT-induced double strand breaks [9–11].

Radiation Planning Techniques

Involved field radiation therapy is the current standard approach for adjuvant RT in patients with GBMs and the involved area is defined by radiographic MRI abnormalities. In order to precisely locate the area of interest to be covered and minimize errors in daily setup, computed tomography (CT) simulation for radiation planning is necessary. The patient is immobilized in supine treatment position with a custom-fitted thermoplastic mask (Fig. 6.1a). A CT scan of the head is done once the patient is immobilized in treatment position. This planning CT scan is used for radiation planning and registered with the post-operative MRI brain (both T1 contrast enhancing and T2-weighted MRI on a fluid-attenuated inversion recover (FLAIR) series are helpful for defining targets). As shown in Fig. 6.1b, c, the radiation oncologist will use both the CT and MRI to define and delineate volumes for tumor targets and

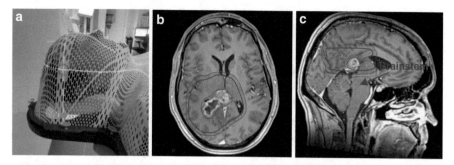

Fig. 6.1 (**a**) A thermoplastic mask conforms to the patient's head for immobilization during the CT simulation for radiation planning. (**b**) Axial T1-enhancing MRI is fused to the planning CT scan in order to delineate tumor volumes and critical surrounding structures. (**c**) Brainstem, in close proximity to tumor volumes, is shown on the sagittal view

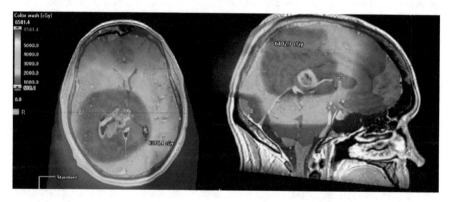

Fig. 6.2 A 3-arc VMAT radiation plan for glioblastoma. The 60 Gy treatment volume shown in red includes the glioblastoma resection cavity with a margin on both axial and sagittal views

surrounding normal structures (such as the optic chiasm, optic nerves, retina, lens and brainstem).

Intensity-modulated radiation therapy (IMRT) and Volumetric modulation arc therapy (VMAT) are commonly used in the treatment of GBM. IMRT is an advanced technology that allows several photon radiation beams from different angles to be manipulated in order to conform to the shape of the GBM target. The shape and dose intensity of the beams can be varied across the treatment field in order to better target the tumor and at the same time avoid critical structures. This is especially important in radiation planning for patients in which tumors are in close proximity to critical structures. Typically IMRT utilizes five, seven or nine stationary radiation beams, each from different angles. VMAT is a type of IMRT in which the head of the linear accelerator continues to move in an arc around the patient while delivering the radiation treatment (Fig. 6.2).

Radiation Toxicity

The toxicity of radiation depends on multiple factors, including the volume of brain treated, radiation dose, fractionation schedule, as well as any chemotherapies or targeted agents being delivered concurrently with radiation. Toxicity following radiation can be grouped into three phases, including early toxicity (days to weeks), early delayed toxicity (1–6 months) and late toxicity (>6 months to years).

Acute toxicities of intracranial radiation may occur days to weeks after radiation and are often managed with supportive care. General symptoms include fatigue, headache, nausea, vomiting, dermatitis and alopecia. Transient worsening of pre-treatment neurologic symptoms and seizures may also occur due to radiation-related edema, which often responds to dexamethasone steroids [12]. In contrast, late toxicities can develop months to years after radiation and are often progressive and irreversible. There can be a risk of cognitive decline and memory impairment depending on the location and size of the radiation field. Treatment of lesions near the optic pathways, cochlea, sensory or motor cortex may cause focal neurologic deficits if radiation dose constraints are not respected. Radiation necrosis is a complication of radiation that may cause mass effect and/or neurologic symptoms. Radiation necrosis is a complex process that may be related to vascular endothelial cell injury, white matter damage and immune mechanisms [13]. Differentiating progressive or recurrent tumor from radiation necrosis by imaging is often challenging.

The Evolution of Radiation Therapy for GBMs

As we previously discussed, GBM recur locally rather than at distant CNS sites, therefore emphasizing the importance of increasing local control by optimizing radiation therapy [2]. Since the landmark EORTC/NCIC CTG study in 2004 [6, 7], extensive research has explored different approaches for increasing radiation dose and efficacy against the tumor as well as minimizing radiation toxicity.

Dose Escalation Studies

In a disease where distant spread is uncommon and most recurrences occur within the previous radiation field, dose intensification clinical studies were conducted to better understand the radiation dose that provides the best local control with minimal toxicity [14]. The Brain Tumor Study group examined adjuvant radiation doses among 621 patients with malignant gliomas after surgery and found that patients with 50 Gy adjuvant radiation had a median survival of 36 weeks compared to the median survival of 42 weeks of those patients with 60 Gy of adjuvant radiation [15]. Therefore, the median survival significantly improved by approximately 1.3 times when increasing the dose from 50 to 60 Gy [15]. Another randomized trial by the Medical Research Council also concluded that increasing the radiation dose to 60 Gy improved survival outcomes when two common GBM radiation dose regimens of 45 Gy in 20 fractions and 60 Gy in 30 fractions were compared [16]. While these initial dose-escalation studies showed promise for improving outcomes in GBM patients, a subsequent study showed that further dose escalation from 70 to 90 Gy increased toxicity with no survival benefit [17]. Together, these studies confirmed 60 Gy in 30 daily fractions to be the standard radiation dosing for GBM.

Multiple studies have also examined dose escalation with a stereotactic boost as another approach for increasing radiation dose and local control with minimal toxicity. Stereotactic radiosurgery is a highly precise technique in which ablative doses of radiation are delivered focally within a single fraction with a very sharp dose fall off such that critical structures are avoided at the same time. Initially, Loeffler et al. (1992) reported benefit to stereotactic radiosurgery (SRS) as part of the initial treatment of malignant gliomas [18]. Moreover, Sarkaria et al. (1995) found a median survival benefit and an increase in 2-year overall survival with stereotactic treatment of newly diagnosed GBMs in addition to conventional radiation and surgery [19]. However, the Phase III randomized Radiation Oncology Therapy Group (RTOG) 9305 later evaluated dose escalation with an upfront SRS boost in addition to conventional radiation therapy and BCNU in newly diagnosed GBMs. Unfortunately, there was no survival benefit (median survival of 13.5 months in the SRS arm versus 13.6 months in the standard arm), no changes in local failure and no changes in quality of life with the addition of an SRS boost compared to conventional radiation and BCNU alone [20]. Currently, there is no strong evidence for using SRS in the management of newly diagnosed GBMs, although it is often used in the recurrent glioblastoma setting.

Hyperfractionation, also studied as a method for increasing radiation dose, refers to the more frequent administration of smaller than standard radiation therapy doses. This often involves two doses of radiation daily, each dose occurring at least 6 hours apart. Hyperfractionation was believed to offer increased local control by preventing tumor cells from repopulating between radiation treatments and at the same time reducing late radiation injury. RTOG 8302 initially evaluated 64.8 Gy vs. 72 Gy hyperfractionated twice per day radiation in the presence of BCNU and found no significant difference in survival or toxicity with conventional radiation [21]. RTOG 9006 was a Phase III randomized study comparing a hyperfractionated radiation regimen of 72 Gy in 60 fractions given twice per day with the standard regimen of 60 Gy in 30 daily fractions (both arms receiving concurrent BCNU) and found no benefit to survival or toxicity outcomes with hyperfractionation [22].

Protons have also been studied as a way to get more dose to the tumor tissue but at the same time spare surrounding normal structures. Protons are charged particles that have the ability to concentrate the majority of their dose at the end of their finite path length (Bragg peak), thus resulting in a sharper dose fall off and better ability to avoid surrounding normal tissue [8]. Fitzek conducted a Phase II trial treating GBM with a photon-proton mixture to a 90 gray cobalt equivalent (CBE) in order to minimize toxicity with escalated dosing and found that survival was increased to

20 months [23]. Mizomuto et al. conducted a Phase II trial in which patients with GBM were treated with conventional photon radiation followed by an evening (>6 hours later) proton boost to a prescribed dose of 96.6 Gy in 56 twice daily fractions with concurrent nimustine chemotherapy [24]. Median survival was 22 months and 2-year survival was 45% [24], suggesting that more clinical trials with proton treatment of GBM are warranted due to these promising results. There is an ongoing Phase II clinical trial, NRG BN001, comparing dose-escalated protons and IMRT photons to conventional photon radiation (NCT02179086), which is estimated to be completed by 2026.

Decreasing Radiation Volumes to Minimize Toxicity

Before CT and MRI imaging, radiation therapy for GBMs was delivered as whole brain radiation therapy [25], in which large, opposed lateral fields were utilized to cover the entire brain volume. However, now involved-field partial brain radiation is the standard of care as studies have demonstrated that radiation field volumes can be decreased from whole brain radiation and still provide disease control with less toxicity. In fact, Ramsey and Brand (1973) found that GBM patients treated with limited field radiation therapy compared to whole brain radiation therapy had significantly increased overall survival, which was believed to be due to reduced toxicity of sensitive areas of the brain [26]. Moreover, in the Brain Tumor Cooperative Group Trial (BTCG) 80-01, patients receiving whole brain radiation to 60.2 Gy had no significant survival advantage compared to patients receiving 43 Gy to the whole brain plus an additional 17.2 Gy radiation to the tumor volume [27].

Since these studies, involved field conformal brain radiation has become the standard adjuvant treatment for GBM. Historically, many have delineated the target as gross tumor volume and resection cavity along with a 2 cm margin in the radiation field, which has been influenced by multiple studies. Indeed, after the advent of CT imaging, Hochberg and Pruitt (1980) used CT scans to show that more than 90% of GBM cases recurred within 2 cm of the primary tumor [28]. Wallner et al. reported that 78% of 32 GBMs recurred within 2.0 cm of the initial tumor margin [25]. Kelly et al. (1987) evaluated 40 untreated GBMs by CT and MRI-guided stereotactic biopsies and found that T1 contrast enhancement corresponded to gross GBM tissue and that isolated GBM cells extended at least as far as the edema or T2 FLAIR signal [29]. As a result of these studies, the inclusion of all radiographic MRI evidence of GBM and associated edema with large 2 cm margins became widely adopted.

However, even today there is no consensus regarding optimal radiation volumes for maintaining local control in GBMs yet at the same time avoiding treatment-associated toxicity. In Radiation Oncology, recommended radiation treatment volumes and margins depend on the specific pathology of tumor. For GBM, the gross tumor volume, referred to as GTV, corresponds to any residual gross tumor after surgery and the resection cavity. The clinical target volume (CTV) is a margin on the GTV that accounts for the estimated extent of microscopic or subclinical disease. The planning treatment volume (PTV) is an additional margin on the CTV that accounts for uncertainties in set up and radiation delivery (Fig. 6.1). While the GTV is more straightforward, there continues to be wide variation in radiation volumes, especially CTV and the inclusion of peri-tumoral edema, included in the radiation field [30–40].

While further investigation is warranted for identifying the best margin for radiation volumes, studies provide evidence that decreased margins may improve survival by minimizing toxicity without compromising recurrence patterns [31]. Kumar et al. (2019) recently reported that while two common contouring consensus guidelines resulted in similar recurrence rates, there was significantly improved survival and quality of life in patients treated with smaller radiation volumes [41]. One hypothesis is that reduced radiation volumes may decrease the incidence of severe lymphopenia in GBM patients, possibly by reducing the irradiated circulating blood volume (reviewed in [31, 42]). Huang et al. showed that increased brain volumes receiving 25 Gy was an independent predictor of severe lymphopenia and those patients developing severe lymphopenia had significantly worse median survival of 12.5 months compared to 20.2 months in those without lymphopenia [43]. While the exact mechanism of lymphopenia-related decreases in overall survival is uncertain, many hypothesize that reduced lymphocyte counts cause the immune system to be less effective at removing malignant GBM cells from the body.

Molecular Biomarkers and Radiation Therapy in GBM

Along with the World Health Organization's (WHO) update on the classification of gliomas to incorporate molecular markers [44], researchers have also evaluated the ability of molecular markers to predict patient response to treatments in order to facilitate clinical decision making. While GBM is associated with poor prognoses, a small subset of patients have been shown to experience longer survival, suggesting some heterogeneity among GBMs. As a tool for predicting prognosis of GBM patients, initial recursive partitioning analyses (RPA) identified clinical non-molecular based prognostic factors, such as age, histology, performance status, mental status, extent of surgery, and radiation dose [45–47]. However, with our improved understanding of molecular pathways involved in GBM pathogenesis, a revised RTOG GBM RPA included both clinical and molecular biomarkers to better stratify GBM patient outcomes. Indeed, Bell et al. [48] evaluated expression of more than 12 proteins by immunohistochemical staining of tissue microarrays from patients enrolled on the RTOG 0525 clinical trial, a phase III randomized trial comparing conventional adjuvant TMZ to dose-dense TMZ [49]. This revised RPA model, including c-MET and MGMT protein levels, resulted in improved outcome stratification in GBM patients treated with radiation and TMZ compared with earlier RPA models [48]. Importantly, their results also reported MGMT protein expression to have better prognostic significance than the more commonly reported

MGMT promoter methylation. As previously mentioned, MGMT protein expression has also been shown to be related to increased radiation response in pre-clinical studies [10]. Future studies on identifying additional molecular biomarkers to predict response to radiation and increase sensitivity to radiation are ongoing.

Hypofractionated Radiation Therapy in Elderly Patients

Almost half of all GBMs occur in patients greater than 65 years old and these patients often have worse outcomes than the younger cohorts [50]. Moreover, patients older than 70 years old were excluded from the EORTC/NCIC CTG study that developed the current standard of care for treatment of patients with GBM [6, 7]. Considering the poor prognosis associated with newly diagnosed GBM in elderly and frail patients, multiple studies have investigated the role for more tolerable treatment regimens in this patient population. Keime-Guibert et al. (2007) reported patients >70 years old and Karnofsky performance status (KPS) >70 with anaplastic astrocytoma/GBM had improved median survival when receiving 50.4 Gy of conventional radiation in 28 fractions compared to supportive care alone (29.1 weeks vs. 16.9 weeks) without a decline in quality of life or cognition [51], providing support for the benefit of radiation therapy in the elderly GBM population. Multiple trials have shown that hypofractionated (shortened) radiation schedules yield the same survival outcomes as conventional radiation, yet also reduce morbidity with shorter treatment times for patients enduring a terminal illness. Hypofractionation of radiation treatments refers to the use of a fewer number of higher dose radiation treatments in order to reduce the overall treatment time. Roa et al. (2004) compared GBM patients >60 years old receiving hypofractionated radiation schedule (40 Gy in 15 fractions) to the conventional fractionation schedule (60 Gy in 30 fractions) without concurrent chemotherapy and found no difference in survival (5.6 months vs. 5.1 months) between the two radiation schedules [52]. Moreover, Roa et al. (2015) reported that a hypofractionated radiation regimen of 25 Gy in 5 fractions had non-inferior overall survival compared to 40 Gy in 15 fractions in elderly and frail patients with newly diagnosed GBM not receiving chemotherapy [53].

The Phase III randomized EORTC 26062 trial later evaluated whether there was benefit to adding TMZ chemotherapy to 40 Gy in 15 fraction hypofractionated radiation in patients >60 years old with newly diagnosed GBM. They reported an overall survival benefit with the addition of TMZ to hypofractionated radiation compared to radiation alone (9.3 vs. 7.6 months) [54]. Moreover, Ammirati et al. (2015) demonstrated that GBM patients receiving hypofractionated radiation (52.5 Gy in 15 fractions) with concurrent TMZ tolerated the treatment well [55]. In summary, these studies generated support for combined modality therapy in older patients, especially those with *MGMT* hypermethylation. However, hypofractionated radiation alone can be an effective treatment in elderly patients with GBM who are not candidates for TMZ due to poor functional status or medical co-morbidities, especially those patients with GBM that are not *MGMT* hypermethylated [56].

Re-irradiation of GBM

Despite standard aggressive therapies, nearly all GBM recur within months to years following initial therapy. Most recurrences are located within or adjacent to the high dose radiation field. Since radiation necrosis and recurrent GBM have similar appearances on MRI imaging, determining the diagnosis of recurrent GBM can be challenging. While there is no standard of care treatment for recurrent GBMs in the United States, potential treatment options include re-resection, re-irradiation, systemic therapy, best supportive care or a combination of these palliative treatment modalities. The treatment plan for each patient should be individualized with close consideration of age, performance status, time since initial treatment, extent of recurrence and tumor location (any involvement of eloquent areas of the brain).

Re-irradiation is increasingly being used in the treatment of recurrent GBMs and is often recommended for patients, especially those who are not candidates for re-resection and have minimal systemic options available to them. The patient's performance status and how the potential toxicities of re-irradiation may impact the patient's quality of life should be heavily weighed before proceeding with re-irradiation. Moreover, radiation dose, fractionation and treatment volume should be carefully planned in order to minimize radiation necrosis and other serious toxicities. Stereotactic radiation has been used for focal recurrent GBMs in order to avoid wide margins that may increase the risk of toxicity [57–60]. However, in cases of multifocal or large recurrent tumors, conventional external beam radiation with smaller dose per fraction may offer local control of larger treatment volumes with less toxicity. Various radiation dose and fractionation regimens for external beam radiation therapy have been reported, however, at this time, there is not enough data to recommend a standard regimen [30]. TMZ, bevacizumab and immune modulators are systemic therapies that have been the most commonly studied in the re-irradiation setting [61–65]. While many retrospective studies have shown encouraging survival outcomes, these studies are difficult to interpret and compare due to inconsistencies in treatment technique, dose, and volumes treated (reviewed in [30, 66, 67]). More prospective clinical trials are warranted for direct comparisons of radiation regimens.

Summary and Conclusions

In summary, GBM is an aggressive tumor that most commonly recurs within or adjacent to the previous high dose radiation field, further emphasizing the need for improving the efficacy of radiation therapy. Radiation therapy techniques have been studied over time in order to increase local control but minimize radiation toxicity with some success. Further pre-clinical and clinical studies are needed to not only improve the efficacy of radiation therapy, but also identify molecular biomarkers that may help predict response to radiation and prognosis in GBM patients.

References

1. Lacroix M, Abi-Said D, Fourney DR, Gokaslan ZL, Shi W, DeMonte F, et al. A multivariate analysis of 416 patients with glioblastoma multiforme: prognosis, extent of resection, and survival. J Neurosurg. 2001;95(2):190–8.
2. Laperriere N, Zuraw L, Cairncross G, Cancer Care Ontario Practice Guidelines Initiative Neuro-Oncology Disease Site G. Radiotherapy for newly diagnosed malignant glioma in adults: a systematic review. Radiother Oncol. 2002;64(3):259–73.
3. Walker MD, Green SB, Byar DP, Alexander E Jr, Batzdorf U, Brooks WH, et al. Randomized comparisons of radiotherapy and nitrosoureas for the treatment of malignant glioma after surgery. N Engl J Med. 1980;303(23):1323–9.
4. Walker MD, Alexander E Jr, Hunt WE, MacCarty CS, Mahaley MS Jr, Mealey J Jr, et al. Evaluation of BCNU and/or radiotherapy in the treatment of anaplastic gliomas. A cooperative clinical trial. J Neurosurg. 1978;49(3):333–43.
5. Kristiansen K, Hagen S, Kollevold T, Torvik A, Holme I, Nesbakken R, et al. Combined modality therapy of operated astrocytomas grade III and IV. Confirmation of the value of postoperative irradiation and lack of potentiation of bleomycin on survival time: a prospective multicenter trial of the Scandinavian Glioblastoma Study Group. Cancer. 1981;47(4):649–52.
6. Stupp R, Hegi ME, Mason WP, van den Bent MJ, Taphoorn MJ, Janzer RC, et al. Effects of radiotherapy with concomitant and adjuvant temozolomide versus radiotherapy alone on survival in glioblastoma in a randomised phase III study: 5-year analysis of the EORTC-NCIC trial. Lancet Oncol. 2009;10(5):459–66.
7. Stupp R, Mason WP, van den Bent MJ, Weller M, Fisher B, Taphoorn MJ, et al. Radiotherapy plus concomitant and adjuvant temozolomide for glioblastoma. N Engl J Med. 2005;352(10):987–96.
8. Hall EJ, Giaccia AJ. Radiobiology for the radiologist. 8th ed. Philadelphia: Wolters Kluwer; 2019. vii, 597 p.
9. Tentori L, Graziani G. Pharmacological strategies to increase the antitumor activity of methylating agents. Curr Med Chem. 2002;9(13):1285–301.
10. Chakravarti A, Erkkinen MG, Nestler U, Stupp R, Mehta M, Aldape K, et al. Temozolomide-mediated radiation enhancement in glioblastoma: a report on underlying mechanisms. Clin Cancer Res. 2006;12(15):4738–46.
11. van Rijn J, Heimans JJ, van den Berg J, van der Valk P, Slotman BJ. Survival of human glioma cells treated with various combination of temozolomide and X-rays. Int J Radiat Oncol Biol Phys. 2000;47(3):779–84.
12. Halperin EC, Perez CA, Brady LW. Perez and Brady's principles and practice of radiation oncology. 5th ed. Philadelphia: Wolters Kluwer Health/Lippincott Williams & Wilkins; 2008. xxxii, 2106 p.
13. Rahmathulla G, Marko NF, Weil RJ. Cerebral radiation necrosis: a review of the pathobiology, diagnosis and management considerations. J Clin Neurosci. 2013;20(4):485–502.
14. Parsa A, Raizer J; Ohio Library and Information Network. Current understanding and treatment of gliomas [text]. Cham: Springer; 2015. Available from: OhioLINK http://rave.ohiolink.edu/ebooks/ebc/9783319120485 Connect to resource SpringerLink http://link.springer.com/10.1007/978-3-319-12048-5 Connect to resource SpringerLink http://proxy.ohiolink.edu:9099/login?url=http://link.springer.com/10.1007/978-3-319-12048-5 Connect to resource (off-campus).
15. Walker MD, Strike TA, Sheline GE. An analysis of dose-effect relationship in the radiotherapy of malignant gliomas. Int J Radiat Oncol Biol Phys. 1979;5(10):1725–31.
16. Bleehen NM, Stenning SP. A Medical Research Council trial of two radiotherapy doses in the treatment of grades 3 and 4 astrocytoma. The Medical Research Council Brain Tumour Working Party. Br J Cancer. 1991;64(4):769–74.
17. Nelson DF, Diener-West M, Horton J, Chang CH, Schoenfeld D, Nelson JS. Combined modality approach to treatment of malignant gliomas--re-evaluation of RTOG 7401/ECOG 1374

with long-term follow-up: a joint study of the Radiation Therapy Oncology Group and the Eastern Cooperative Oncology Group. NCI Monogr. 1988;6:279–84.

18. Loeffler JS, Alexander E 3rd, Shea WM, Wen PY, Fine HA, Kooy HM, et al. Radiosurgery as part of the initial management of patients with malignant gliomas. J Clin Oncol. 1992;10(9):1379–85.

19. Sarkaria JN, Mehta MP, Loeffler JS, Buatti JM, Chappell RJ, Levin AB, et al. Radiosurgery in the initial management of malignant gliomas: survival comparison with the RTOG recursive partitioning analysis. Radiation Therapy Oncology Group. Int J Radiat Oncol Biol Phys. 1995;32(4):931–41.

20. Souhami L, Seiferheld W, Brachman D, Podgorsak EB, Werner-Wasik M, Lustig R, et al. Randomized comparison of stereotactic radiosurgery followed by conventional radiotherapy with carmustine to conventional radiotherapy with carmustine for patients with glioblastoma multiforme: report of Radiation Therapy Oncology Group 93-05 protocol. Int J Radiat Oncol Biol Phys. 2004;60(3):853–60.

21. Nelson DF, Curran WJ Jr, Scott C, Nelson JS, Weinstein AS, Ahmad K, et al. Hyperfractionated radiation therapy and bis-chlorethyl nitrosourea in the treatment of malignant glioma--possible advantage observed at 72.0 Gy in 1.2 Gy B.I.D. fractions: report of the Radiation Therapy Oncology Group Protocol 8302. Int J Radiat Oncol Biol Phys. 1993;25(2):193–207.

22. Ali AN, Zhang P, Yung WKA, Chen Y, Movsas B, Urtasun RC, et al. NRG oncology RTOG 9006: a phase III randomized trial of hyperfractionated radiotherapy (RT) and BCNU versus standard RT and BCNU for malignant glioma patients. J Neuro-Oncol. 2018;137(1):39–47.

23. Fitzek MM, Thornton AF, Rabinov JD, Lev MH, Pardo FS, Munzenrider JE, et al. Accelerated fractionated proton/photon irradiation to 90 cobalt gray equivalent for glioblastoma multiforme: results of a phase II prospective trial. J Neurosurg. 1999;91(2):251–60.

24. Mizumoto M, Yamamoto T, Takano S, Ishikawa E, Matsumura A, Ishikawa H, et al. Long-term survival after treatment of glioblastoma multiforme with hyperfractionated concomitant boost proton beam therapy. Pract Radiat Oncol. 2015;5(1):e9–16.

25. Wallner KE, Galicich JH, Krol G, Arbit E, Malkin MG. Patterns of failure following treatment for glioblastoma multiforme and anaplastic astrocytoma. Int J Radiat Oncol Biol Phys. 1989;16(6):1405–9.

26. Ramsey RG, Brand WN. Radiotherapy of glioblastoma multiforme. J Neurosurg. 1973;39(2):197–202.

27. Shapiro WR, Green SB, Burger PC, Mahaley MS Jr, Selker RG, VanGilder JC, et al. Randomized trial of three chemotherapy regimens and two radiotherapy regimens and two radiotherapy regimens in postoperative treatment of malignant glioma. Brain Tumor Cooperative Group Trial 8001. J Neurosurg. 1989;71(1):1–9.

28. Hochberg FH, Pruitt A. Assumptions in the radiotherapy of glioblastoma. Neurology. 1980;30(9):907–11.

29. Kelly PJ, Daumas-Duport C, Kispert DB, Kall BA, Scheithauer BW, Illig JJ. Imaging-based stereotaxic serial biopsies in untreated intracranial glial neoplasms. J Neurosurg. 1987;66(6):865–74.

30. Cabrera AR, Kirkpatrick JP, Fiveash JB, Shih HA, Koay EJ, Lutz S, et al. Radiation therapy for glioblastoma: executive summary of an American Society for Radiation Oncology evidence-based clinical practice guideline. Pract Radiat Oncol. 2016;6(4):217–25.

31. Wernicke AG, Smith AW, Taube S, Mehta MP. Glioblastoma: radiation treatment margins, how small is large enough? Pract Radiat Oncol. 2016;6(5):298–305.

32. Niyazi M, Brada M, Chalmers AJ, Combs SE, Erridge SC, Fiorentino A, et al. ESTRO-ACROP guideline "target delineation of glioblastomas". Radiother Oncol. 2016;118(1):35–42.

33. Wee CW, Sung W, Kang HC, Cho KH, Han TJ, Jeong BK, et al. Evaluation of variability in target volume delineation for newly diagnosed glioblastoma: a multi-institutional study from the Korean Radiation Oncology Group. Radiat Oncol. 2015;10:137.

34. Farace P, Giri MG, Meliado G, Amelio D, Widesott L, Ricciardi GK, et al. Clinical target volume delineation in glioblastomas: pre-operative versus post-operative/pre-radiotherapy MRI. Br J Radiol. 2011;84(999):271–8.
35. Chang EL, Akyurek S, Avalos T, Rebueno N, Spicer C, Garcia J, et al. Evaluation of peritumoral edema in the delineation of radiotherapy clinical target volumes for glioblastoma. Int J Radiat Oncol Biol Phys. 2007;68(1):144–50.
36. Gebhardt BJ, Dobelbower MC, Ennis WH, Bag AK, Markert JM, Fiveash JB. Patterns of failure for glioblastoma multiforme following limited-margin radiation and concurrent temozolomide. Radiat Oncol. 2014;9:130.
37. Dobelbower MC, Burnett Iii OL, Nordal RA, Nabors LB, Markert JM, Hyatt MD, et al. Patterns of failure for glioblastoma multiforme following concurrent radiation and temozolomide. J Med Imaging Radiat Oncol. 2011;55(1):77–81.
38. Mason WP, Maestro RD, Eisenstat D, Forsyth P, Fulton D, Laperriere N, et al. Canadian recommendations for the treatment of glioblastoma multiforme. Curr Oncol. 2007;14(3):110–7.
39. Easaw JC, Mason WP, Perry J, Laperriere N, Eisenstat DD, Del Maestro R, et al. Canadian recommendations for the treatment of recurrent or progressive glioblastoma multiforme. Curr Oncol. 2011;18(3):e126–36.
40. McDonald MW, Shu HK, Curran WJ Jr, Crocker IR. Pattern of failure after limited margin radiotherapy and temozolomide for glioblastoma. Int J Radiat Oncol Biol Phys. 2011;79(1):130–6.
41. Kumar N, Kumar R, Sharma SC, Mukherjee A, Khandelwal N, Tripathi M, et al. Impact of volume of irradiation on survival and quality of life in glioblastoma: a prospective, phase 2, randomized comparison of RTOG and MDACC protocols. Neurooncol Pract. 2020;7(1):86–93.
42. Yovino S, Grossman SA. Severity, etiology and possible consequences of treatment-related lymphopenia in patients with newly diagnosed high-grade gliomas. CNS Oncol. 2012;1(2):149–54.
43. Huang J, DeWees TA, Badiyan SN, Speirs CK, Mullen DF, Fergus S, et al. Clinical and dosimetric predictors of acute severe lymphopenia during radiation therapy and concurrent temozolomide for high-grade glioma. Int J Radiat Oncol Biol Phys. 2015;92(5):1000–7.
44. Louis DN, Perry A, Reifenberger G, von Deimling A, Figarella-Branger D, Cavenee WK, et al. The 2016 World Health Organization classification of tumors of the central nervous system: a summary. Acta Neuropathol. 2016;131(6):803–20.
45. Curran WJ Jr, Scott CB, Horton J, Nelson JS, Weinstein AS, Fischbach AJ, et al. Recursive partitioning analysis of prognostic factors in three Radiation Therapy Oncology Group malignant glioma trials. J Natl Cancer Inst. 1993;85(9):704–10.
46. Li J, Wang M, Won M, Shaw EG, Coughlin C, Curran WJ Jr, et al. Validation and simplification of the Radiation Therapy Oncology Group recursive partitioning analysis classification for glioblastoma. Int J Radiat Oncol Biol Phys. 2011;81(3):623–30.
47. Gorlia T, van den Bent MJ, Hegi ME, Mirimanoff RO, Weller M, Cairncross JG, et al. Nomograms for predicting survival of patients with newly diagnosed glioblastoma: prognostic factor analysis of EORTC and NCIC trial 26981-22981/CE.3. Lancet Oncol. 2008;9(1):29–38.
48. Bell EH, Pugh SL, McElroy JP, Gilbert MR, Mehta M, Klimowicz AC, et al. Molecular-based recursive partitioning analysis model for glioblastoma in the temozolomide era: a correlative analysis based on NRG Oncology RTOG 0525. JAMA Oncol. 2017;3(6):784–92.
49. Gilbert MR, Wang M, Aldape KD, Stupp R, Hegi ME, Jaeckle KA, et al. Dose-dense temozolomide for newly diagnosed glioblastoma: a randomized phase III clinical trial. J Clin Oncol. 2013;31(32):4085–91.
50. Buckner JC. Factors influencing survival in high-grade gliomas. Semin Oncol. 2003;30(6 Suppl 19):10–4.
51. Keime-Guibert F, Chinot O, Taillandier L, Cartalat-Carel S, Frenay M, Kantor G, et al. Radiotherapy for glioblastoma in the elderly. N Engl J Med. 2007;356(15):1527–35.
52. Roa W, Brasher PM, Bauman G, Anthes M, Bruera E, Chan A, et al. Abbreviated course of radiation therapy in older patients with glioblastoma multiforme: a prospective randomized clinical trial. J Clin Oncol. 2004;22(9):1583–8.

53. Roa W, Kepka L, Kumar N, Sinaika V, Matiello J, Lomidze D, et al. International Atomic Energy Agency randomized phase III study of radiation therapy in elderly and/or frail patients with newly diagnosed glioblastoma multiforme. J Clin Oncol. 2015;33(35):4145–50.
54. Perry JR, Laperriere N, O'Callaghan CJ, Brandes AA, Menten J, Phillips C, et al. Short-course radiation plus temozolomide in elderly patients with glioblastoma. N Engl J Med. 2017;376(11):1027–37.
55. Ammirati M, Chotai S, Newton H, Lamki T, Wei L, Grecula J. Hypofractionated intensity modulated radiotherapy with temozolomide in newly diagnosed glioblastoma multiforme. J Clin Neurosci. 2014;21(4):633–7.
56. Wick W, Platten M, Meisner C, Felsberg J, Tabatabai G, Simon M, et al. Temozolomide chemotherapy alone versus radiotherapy alone for malignant astrocytoma in the elderly: the NOA-08 randomised, phase 3 trial. Lancet Oncol. 2012;13(7):707–15.
57. Koga T, Maruyama K, Tanaka M, Ino Y, Saito N, Nakagawa K, et al. Extended field stereotactic radiosurgery for recurrent glioblastoma. Cancer. 2012;118(17):4193–200.
58. Sharma M, Schroeder JL, Elson P, Meola A, Barnett GH, Vogelbaum MA, et al. Outcomes and prognostic stratification of patients with recurrent glioblastoma treated with salvage stereotactic radiosurgery. J Neurosurg. 2018;131(2):489–99.
59. Combs SE, Widmer V, Thilmann C, Hof H, Debus J, Schulz-Ertner D. Stereotactic radiosurgery (SRS): treatment option for recurrent glioblastoma multiforme (GBM). Cancer. 2005;104(10):2168–73.
60. Holt DE, Bernard ME, Quan K, Clump DA, Engh JA, Burton SA, et al. Salvage stereotactic radiosurgery for recurrent glioblastoma multiforme with prior radiation therapy. J Cancer Res Ther. 2016;12(4):1243–8.
61. Combs SE, Bischof M, Welzel T, Hof H, Oertel S, Debus J, et al. Radiochemotherapy with temozolomide as re-irradiation using high precision fractionated stereotactic radiotherapy (FSRT) in patients with recurrent gliomas. J Neuro-Oncol. 2008;89(2):205–10.
62. Osman MA. Phase II trial of temozolomide and reirradiation using conformal 3D-radiotherapy in recurrent brain gliomas. Ann Transl Med. 2014;2(5):44.
63. Greenspoon JN, Sharieff W, Hirte H, Overholt A, Devillers R, Gunnarsson T, et al. Fractionated stereotactic radiosurgery with concurrent temozolomide chemotherapy for locally recurrent glioblastoma multiforme: a prospective cohort study. Onco Targets Ther. 2014;7:485–90.
64. Gutin PH, Iwamoto FM, Beal K, Mohile NA, Karimi S, Hou BL, et al. Safety and efficacy of bevacizumab with hypofractionated stereotactic irradiation for recurrent malignant gliomas. Int J Radiat Oncol Biol Phys. 2009;75(1):156–63.
65. Cabrera AR, Cuneo KC, Desjardins A, Sampson JH, McSherry F, Herndon JE 2nd, et al. Concurrent stereotactic radiosurgery and bevacizumab in recurrent malignant gliomas: a prospective trial. Int J Radiat Oncol Biol Phys. 2013;86(5):873–9.
66. Barney C, Shukla G, Bhamidipati D, Palmer JD. Re-irradiation for recurrent glioblastoma multiforme. Chin Clin Oncol. 2017;6(4):36.
67. Kim MS, Lim J, Shin HS, Cho KG. Re-irradiation and its contribution to good prognosis in recurrent glioblastoma patients. Brain Tumor Res Treat. 2020;8(1):29–35.

Chapter 7
Implementing Molecular Pathology in a Developing Country

Marcus M. Matsushita

Developed Countries and Developing Countries

The main criterion used to distinguish developed and developing countries is related to their gross domestic product (GDP) per capita. GDP summarizes in US dollars the sum of all goods and services produced in a country over the course of a year. The quotient of a country's GDP by its population results in GDP per capita (GDP,PPP) (Fig. 7.1). Although there is no official figure, a country with a GDPPP greater than US$12,000–25,000 is considered a developed country [1]. However, this isolated criterion may not be sufficient to classify a country as developed and causes distortions. Another frequently used index is the Human Development Index (HDI), which was developed by the United Nations and uses criteria such as life expectancy, education and income (Fig. 7.2). Again, there is no defined criterion for considering a country as developed. In general, nations with an HDI greater than 0.8 are considered developed [2]. Thus, developed countries have high level of industrialization, stable rates of births and deaths, low rates of infant mortality, life expectancy over 70–80 years, more women working in high executive positions, high consumption of gas, electricity and oil, and high financing and debt [3]. In turn, developing nations share low real per capita income, high rates of population growth, high unemployment rates, high dependence on the primary sectors of production and export of commodities [4]. Another crucial aspect common to many developing nations is its poor quality of teaching and education. Although in some of these countries there is a growing awareness of the need for quality education for

M. M. Matsushita (✉)
Department of Pathology, Barretos Cancer Hospital, São Paulo, Brazil

© The Author(s), under exclusive license to Springer Nature
Switzerland AG 2021
J. J. Otero, A. P. Becker (eds.), *Precision Molecular Pathology of Glioblastoma*,
Molecular Pathology Library, https://doi.org/10.1007/978-3-030-69170-7_7

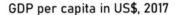

GDP per capita in US$, 2017

Gross domestic product per capita adjusted for price changes over time (inflation) and expressed in US-Dollars.

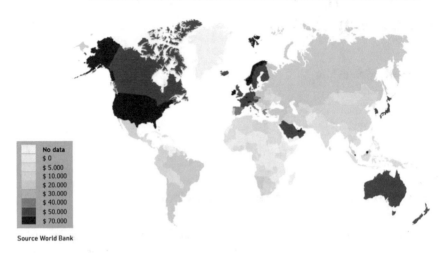

No data
$ 0
$ 5.000
$ 10.000
$ 20.000
$ 30.000
$ 40.000
$ 50.000
$ 70.000

Source World Bank

Fig. 7.1 Gross domestic product per capita in US dollars – 2017. (Source: World Bank)

Human Development Index, 2017

The Human Development Index (HDI) is a summary measure of key dimensions of human development; a long
and healthy life, a good education, and having a decent standard of living.

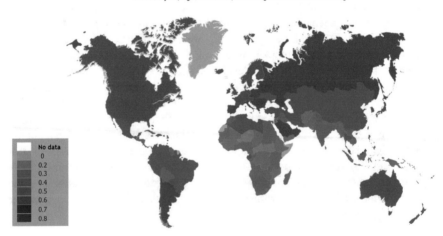

No data
0
0.2
0.3
0.4
0.5
0.6
0.7
0.8

Fig. 7.2 Human Development Index around the world – 2017. (UNDP (2018))

economic development, general public education is precarious. For most of the
population, going to college means working all day to be able to afford an evening
course. Still, expectations of income improvement through higher education are not
very encouraging. Full-time courses such as medicine are difficult to access for

students coming from public schools, who are highly dependent on the family's ability to support the student throughout the course and still often pay the high fees and tuitions of a college of this type [5–8].

South America and Brazil

The South American subcontinent is a vast piece of land with an incredible geographical, political, economic and cultural variety. The entire territory of South America has an area of more than 6.8 million square miles (+17.8 million square kilometers) irregularly distributed in 12 countries, most of them with Spanish as an official language, but also Portuguese (the most spoken language on the continent), English, French, Dutch, and many indigenous languages (Quechua and Guarani) that are still spoken in several countries [9, 10]. In Economics, South America presents enormous contrasts. Chile, for example, has a GDP-PPP of US$22,337.00, HDI 0.82, life expectancy of 75 years, infant mortality rate of 7/1000 live births and, since 2010 has been part of the Organization for Economic Co-operation and Development (OECD). Based on these data, Chile is the only developed country in South America. At the other extreme, Venezuela and Bolivia dispute the unhonorable position of poorer countries, with GDP-PPP of US$3,374.00 and US$3,683.00 respectively [11].

Many discouraging characteristics afflict most South American countries such as political instability, fragile institutions, corruption and large income inequality [12]. At the turn of the millennium, a growing trend towards improvement in different socioeconomic indices was reversed in many countries. Populist governments and serious economic crises have affected to a greater or lesser extent almost all countries, with a major impact on health. Venezuela, for instance, was one of the South American countries that showed the most substantial improvements in infant mortality rates between the years 1950 and 2000. Since then there has been a great deterioration in this indicator and the infant mortality rate in this country is currently estimated to be of 21 deaths per 1000 live births [13]. Similarly, at the beginning of the last century Argentina had better economic conditions than several European countries. It was one of the most important world exporters of grains and meat. Its GDP represented 50% of all Hispanic America, occupying the 10th place in the world economy and its trade totaled 7% of the world total. Currently, Argentina has high inflation rates, above 50%, and has enormous financial volatility with rapid depreciation of its currency, peso, against the US dollar [14–17]. The infant mortality rate in the country is 9.9 per 1000 live births, almost double that of most developed nations. There are large areas in Argentina where residents do not have access to clean drinking water, healthy food or adequate medical assistance [18]. Thus, Argentina, despite having better rates than several developing countries (HDI 0.83, GDP-PPP US $12,500), is still not considered a developed country [3].

Brazil is the largest country and the largest economy in South America. Its territorial extension has more than 3.2 million square miles (8.5 million km^2), which represents almost half of all South American territory and about 20% of the territory of the Americas [19]. The current population of Brazil is 212 million people, 87% of whom live in an urban environment, with an average age of 33.5 years, life expectancy of 76.57 years and an infant mortality rate of 11 deaths per 1000 live births [20]. With an HDI of 0.75 and a GDP-PPP of US$8,727.00, Brazil is still a developing country [3]. However, the overall analysis of the entire nation hides very large intrinsic disparities. The state of São Paulo, for example, the richest state in the country, has an HDI of 0.805, a population of 11 million people, 99% of the urban population, with more than 99% of households with electricity, treated water, sewage and garbage collection. At the other extreme, the state of Maranhão is the poorest in the federation, with an HDI of 0.639, and a population of 6.5 million people, almost 37% of whom live in rural areas. About 30% of homes in that state do not have running water, 15% do not have garbage collection and 2.7% do not have electricity [21]. Despite these contrasts, the country as a whole suffers from huge bureaucratic obstacles, serious infrastructure problems and legislative instability. There have been major projects and investments in recent decades in Brazil with the aim of modernizing the country. However, the objectives initially proposed were not achieved, largely due to the lack of institutional leadership, low technical capacity and low efficiency of regulatory bodies. In addition, populist governments have been involved in huge corruption scandals involving the the country's largest infrastructure companies [22].

The Revolutions of Pathology

Two silent revolutions from the beginning of this century are underway in pathology and will forever change the pathologist's way of working: digital pathology and molecular pathology [23, 24]. Since Virchow described in 1858 that most diseases had a morphological substrate in his work *Die Cellularpathologie in Ihrer Begründung Auf Physiologische Und Pathologische Gewebelehere* thus founding histopathology, pathologists continued to work in a way with little alterations until the late 1980s. In fact, techniques of tissue fixation, sampling, processing, paraffin embedding, sectioning and staining are basically the same since the beginning, in an incredibly handcrafted process by the current standards of other medical areas. Histochemical stains still in use in all pathology laboratories around the world use the same stains used for more than a century and a half [25]. Likewise, the traditional anatomopathological diagnostic method has remained the same since Virchow, basically identifying cellular and architectural morphological changes and trying, by similarity, to approximate a certain morphological pattern to other previously described. Most of the equipment used until the end of the last century was mechanical or electromechanical with little added technology. In addition, in some countries many pathologists often work in isolation, outside the hospital environment, with little information about the material sent to them for analysis, without much contact with other medical specialties [26].

In general, the examination of anatomic pathology is a low-cost procedure, despite the enormous impact that this examination has on the patients' lives and treatment choices [27]. Waiting for the result of a pathological diagnosis often causes great anxiety and expectation to the patient, greater than most other tests, and even than the treatment itself [28]. The diagnosis determines whether a patient will have a mutilating surgical procedure, expensive chemo and/or radiotherapy treatments and what is the prognostic expectation of a certain condition. The pathology report is often seen from a dualistic and fatalistic perspective by the patient: death sentence or salvation, yet costs with anatomic pathology represent, on average, only 3–4% of the total health expenditure, even in developed nations [27].

Despite the determinant nature of histopathology, most people would be surprised with the subjectiveness of this analysis. Many characteristics observed in different diseases are overlapping, making the correct diagnosis extremely difficult in various situations, requiring patience, common sense and many years of pathologist practice. Even so, several studies show that there is great inter-observer and even intra-observer diagnostic variability within pathology [29–31]. In addition to the traditional stain with hematoxylin and eosin (H&E), immunohistochemistry (IHC) started to be used routinely in the 90s and, although it advanced the identification of biological markers, it did not represent a significant change in how a pathologist works. Immunohistochemistry is a form of staining that uses antibodies targeting certain antigens that are desired to be investigated in a tissue sample. In fact, although the antibodies used are far from representing an insignificant expense, the basic structure of a laboratory does not necessarily need major investments in structure or equipment to accommodate immunohistochemistry, immunohistochemistry can be performed manually [32], and, similar to histology, analyzed using a conventional optical microscope. Thus, even the interpretation of an immunohistochemical examination can also be subject to considerable variation, both inter- and intra-observer [33–36].

On the other hand, medical sciences continued to evolve and required increasingly less subjective assessments and specific diagnoses. In particular, cancer treatments have introduced a new generation of target therapies in clinical practice, combined with the assessment of cellular and tissue biomarkers of specific molecular pathways, permiting the oncologist to predict the response to expensive drugs [37, 38]. In response to this, from the beginnig of 2000s, the WHO began to gradually and progressively associate molecular aspects with anatomopathological diagnoses in its classification of tumors, especially of hematological and central nervous system (CNS) neoplasms, for example, which is certainly a path of no return [39, 40]. Currently, several CNS neoplasms require molecular evaluation for their final diagnosis. For example, *IDH* mutations are the main splitting factor for infiltrative gliomas classification; the diagnosis of oligodendrogliomas demands evaluation of chromosomal 1p and 19q co-deletions screening; C19MC-altered and H3F3A mutation are essential for the diagnosis of Embryonal Tumor with Multilayered Rosettes (ETMR) and Diffuse Midline Glioma, respectively; *BRAF* V600E mutation observed in Gangliogliomas and Pleomorphic Xanthoastrocytomas [40, 41] may expand the treatment options for these tumors.

Importantly, neoplasms grouped presenting similar morphological aspects can be subclassified from their molecular profile, as is the case of Glioblastomas, Ependymomas and Medulloblastomas, with important impacts on their treatments and prognosis. In fact, the consortium C-IMPACT-NOW has increased the importance of molecular changes for pediatric and adult glioma, making the final diagnosis of these tumors extremely limited without the use of molecular diagnostic tools [42].

All molecular tests require a completely new structure, with expensive equipment, which also uses costly inputs, in addition to specialized labor. The pathologist now needs to maintain more intimate contact with surgeons and oncologists and to better understand clinical and radiological aspects to indicate the most appropriate molecular tests in each case. In parallel, morphometric analyzes more precise than the mere estimatives with which pathologists have become accustomed to work begin to have increasingly significant impacts on diagnoses and therapeutic approaches, such as evaluation of cell proliferation by Ki-67 to classify neuroendocrine tumors or Combined Positive Score (CPS) score in PDL1 [36, 43–46]. A new horizon is opening up to supply these demands with digital pathology and new possibilities that are even more refined using metric tools and, furthermore, artificial intelligence algorithms will complement the next generation of pathologists [47, 48]. The digitalization of pathology also requires a new and costly technology park in pathology laboratories. As an inevitable consequence, pathology is becoming a more expensive procedure.

The Dilemmas of Pathology in Brazil, as an Example of Developing Country

Considering the South American countries, different countries represent very different realities as already explained above. The only country considered developed in the region is Chile, all the others are considered to be in development, including Argentina, whose characterization is so complex that the Nobel Laureat in Economics Simon Kuznets famously stated that there were four economies: developed, undeveloped, Argentina, and Japan. Within South America, if there is a country that portrays this huge contrast, that country is Brazil, with cities like São Caetano do Sul presenting an HDI of 0.862, almost as high as European countries, in contrast to 0.418 in the municipality of Melgaço, comparable to the least developed countries in Asia and Africa [21].

Heterogeneous Distribution of Health Care Professionals and Structure

Specifically in Brazil, the distribution of doctors across the country follows these contrasts. The country as a whole has 2.11 doctors / 1000 inhabitants, a number not far from countries like the United States (2.61) for example [49, 50] This distribution, however, is extremely irregular. The Southeastern region, the richest in the country and where the states of São Paulo and Rio de Janeiro are located, have a ratio of 2.81 doctors / 1000 inhabitants. In the North of the country, the poorest region where the states of Amazonia and Pará are located, has only 1.16 doctors per 1000 inhabitants. The consequences of these disparities are observed in the long waiting times in public health systems for simple medical consultation, state bureaucracy and administrative inefficiency [51]. In a survey by the Brazilian federal board regulator of Medicine (*Conselho Federal de Medicina* - CFM), 746 patients were waiting more than 10 years for an elective surgery in the public health system in 2017 [52].

The small number of pathologists is a phenomenon that occurs worldwide, including the most developed countries, and the potential problems resulting from it are an open topic for debate [53, 54]. The distribution of pathologists in Brazil is as irregular as that observed for doctors in general (Fig. 7.3). According to a 2018 census, approximately 60% of Brazilian doctors have specialty registrations, with only 0.8% registered as pathologists. Out of the 3,210 Brazilian pathologists, 54% are located in the Southeastern region, mainly in the states capital cities (Fig. 7.4).

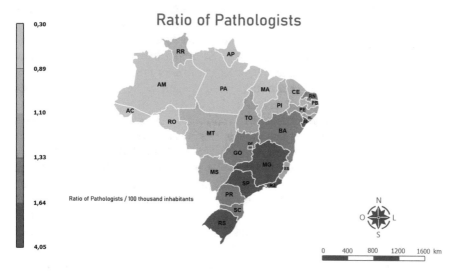

Fig. 7.3 Brazilian ratio of pathologists/100 thousand inhabitants – 2018. (Modified from Scheffer et al. [50])

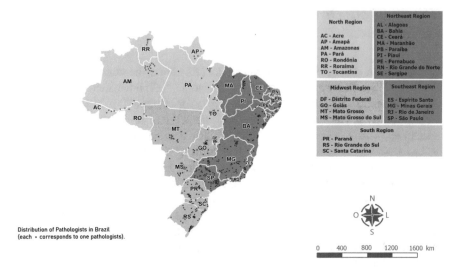

Distribution of Pathologists in Brazil
(each • corresponds to one pathologists).

Fig. 7.4 Distribution of Pathologists in Brazil – 2018. (Modified from Scheffer et al. [50])

The average age of a Brazilian pathologist is 50 years, and the age curves show that they are mostly over the age of 60 and under the age of 40 [50]. Although there are no official figures, the vast majority of pathologists are generalists, with few cases in which some pathologists focus on two or three subspecialties.

Distant from large urban centers and capital cities, most pathology laboratories in Brazil are medium and small. There are no accurate records, but it can be said that the vast majority of these laboratories do not even have their own IHC service, nor any molecular test available. Generally these services are outsourced to a few other larger laboratories or to public educational institutions that end up performing those services. In fact, many Brazilian pathology laboratories rely only on routine (H&E) and specific stains, as well as material processing and staining methods performed manually, with few equipment and old technology.

It cannot be said, however, that Brazil still suffers from a large number of cases of contagious infectious diseases, or that it does not have centers of excellence in the treatment of complex oncological diseases. The number of hospital admissions due to lack of sanitation fell from 184.7 people per 100,000 inhabitants in 2009 to 65.6 in 2018 [55]. On the other hand, according to the National Cancer Institute (INCA), it is estimated that in 2020 Brazil will have 626,000 new cases of cancer, including about 10,000 new cases of tumors of the CNS [56]. To this end, the country also has large cancer treatment centers, both for care in the public health system and in the private sector [57, 58]. In this scenario, it is quite evident that there is a demand for the detection of molecular markers in tumors diagnosed in the country.

About 80% of the Brazilian population depends exclusively on a public health plan (Sistema Único de Saúde - SUS) for all medical care. According to the Brazilian constitution itself, the state is responsible for health care. This involves everything from basic health care, such as disease prevention, to complex treatments for chronic and oncological diseases. In some cases, SUS maintains free distribution of any necessary medication, including high-cost medications for chronic diseases and emerging immunotherapy [59]. Of course, for a country like Brazil, the costs involved can quickly become expensive and choices need to be made. What is the best way to use finite resources for health? Serve a larger population with more basic health programs or a smaller percentage with expensive procedures? There is still no answer to that. Until the answer arrives, apparently the solution found was to develop complex and time-consuming bureaucratic mechanisms to better select who will receive a certain treatment [51, 52]. The result of this is that SUS is a long way from achieving the proposed objectives, both in quantitative and qualitative terms, although some outsourced institutions act as a notable exception. Therefore, those who can end up paying for private health care system.

In Brazil, there are two forms of private health plans. Those for individuals and those for legal entities. Currently, most plans aimed at individuals operate as medical cooperatives. Once their prices are controlled by the Brazilian national supplemental health care agency (Agência Nacional de Saúde Suplementar - ANS), they are a cheaper option [60]. However, many healthcare operators end their activities in this field over time due to financial infeasibility since they could not adjust their values according to the needs of the market [61–63]. Others end up creating their own bureaucratic mechanisms to delay or prevent the performance or remuneration of more expensive procedures. Even so, they are a better option than SUS and about 17% of the Brazilian population opt for them [60]. Finally, a third option is to pay a health plan through a legal entity. This modality does not have its adjustments controlled by ANS and therefore has better conditions to meet the modern demands of medicine, obviously at a higher cost for its users.

Pathology laboratories are part of this system. Governments maintain some public laboratories in some public hospitals and colleges. In others, the service is outsourced to private laboratories. These in turn can simultaneously attend private health plans and a few private cases in which the patient pays directly for the anatomopathological examination. In general, examinations are poorly remunareted except perhaps in cases where the patient pays for his own examination. In some cases, such as a pap smear, for example, the SUS tables (currently priced at around US$1.5) barely cover the costs of the exam supplies [64], let alone medical fees. Still, some private laboratories carry out these exams because they are part of a package that includes more profitable ones. However, this results in a great workload for the pathologist, much greater than that observed in his colleagues from more developed nations.

The Need of Different Techniques and Assays for the Integrated Diagnosis of CNS Tumors

Implementing a costly routine, which requires expensive equipment and consumables, operated by highly qualified labor, comes up against several barriers. The first and most important is the amount of investment required. Some molecular markers,

Table 7.1 Comparison between performance and cost benefit of manual and automated immunohistochemistry (IHC)

Parameter	Manual IHC	Automated IHC
Cost per reaction	Lower	Higher
Investment in equipment	Lower	Higher
Fixed assets on antibodies	Higher	Lower
Risk of loss due to expiration date	Higher	Lower
Need for skilled labor	Higher	Lower
Specialized maintenance dependency	Lower	Higher
Standardization	More difficult	Easier

such as IDH1 R132H, BRAF V600E can be initially evaluated by IHC. But even IHC, as already mentioned, is not part of the routine of many pathology laboratories in Brazil. Furthermore, IHC was not even part of the training of older pathologists (>60 years old) during their medical residency. Of the laboratories that have IHC, most of it is still performed using manual, rather than automatized methods, which cost almost twice as much as the manual procedure in the country. This is if there is no loss of unused antibodies by the expiration date, because the volume of antibodies purchased for manual reactions is greater and less diluted than those used in automated processes. If there is not enough volume to use a certain antibody before its expiration, the laboratory will be forced to discard material, which represents a lost investment (Table 7.1).

Another aspect of this form of work is the impact caused by a large sum of money immobilized in the form of antibodies for a long period of time until it is gradually converted into income as the stock is slowly being used. But IHC is just the beginning of a molecular investigation. The complete evaluation of *IDH* and *BRAF* mutations may require further evaluation with polymerase chain reaction (PCR) or DNA sequencing in certain cases [65–67]. Likewise, the molecular classification of medulloblastomas may require RNA evaluation; the diagnosis of oligodendrogliomas require 1p19q co-deletion evaluation by Fluorescence in Situ Hybridization (FISH) or single-nucleotide polymorphism (SNP) array, just to name a few situations in which the thorough analysis of a neoplasm of the CNS goes beyond histochemical and immunohistochemical stains [68–70]. All these up-to-date procedures require a completely new technology park, very different from the one that pathological anatomy laboratories are used to working with.

Cost of Equipment and Reagents

We must also consider that all reagents and antibodies used for IHC and molecular assays are quoted in US dollars, but the exams themselves are charged in local currency. Only exchange rate fluctuation, therefore, can represent a substantial and abrupt increase in the costs involved in such procedures, without this having an impact on the amount charged for the examination. At the beginning of the year 2020, a dollar cost about R$4.00 (Brazilian currency, Real), but in mid-May this value was already close to R$6.00, accumulating an increase of almost 50% in less than 5 months [71]. This increase was driven mainly by the pandemic COVID19, but it represents neither an isolated factor nor the biggest increase in the American currency in the country. In 2002, for electoral reasons, there was an increase of almost 70% in a similar period of time. Exchange rate fluctuation is a constant in the country's economy and several factors, both in the always turbulent domestic environment, and as a result of global factors, affect the daily exchange rate of the American currency [72].

Health insurance companies in Brazil have repeatedly treated pathology as a low-cost specialty and are reluctant to pay for molecular tests. Most of the molecular tests necessary for the integrated diagnosis in neuropathology are included in the Brazilian Hierarchical Classification of Medical Procedures (CBHPM), which is used by the supplementary health system (insurance/health plan operators) and was designed by the main national medical entities such as Associação Médica Brasileira (AMB), CFM and Federação Nacional dos Médicos (FENAM), beside state entities and Societies of Specialties [73]. Despite that, many operators are reluctant to authorize such tests for a crescent number of patients. Some of those operators even centralize exams in their own or third-party laboratories in an attempt to avoid popularization. Medium and smaller laboratories are, therefore, reluctant to perform the molecular tests for fear of not being reimbursed and not having a return on investment.

Specialized Work Force Needed for Molecular Pathology

Finding skilled labor force is another obstacle to overcome in developing countries. This difficulty is greater in locations more distant from large urban centers and capital cities. In recent years, there has been a huge increase in the number of students receiving higher education courses in Brazil. Even so, the percentage of people attending college is much lower than that seen in developed countries [74]. In addition to these courses being more concentrated in large cities, job opportunities are also greater in large urban centers. Smaller cities are less attractive, both professionally and culturally, and these are major factors that limit the emigration of more qualified people to the interior of the country, exactly where the most deprived areas of specialized professionals are located. In addition to the superior education being quantitatively inferior, elementary and middle level education is also largely inferior in quality, especially in public schools. This is a fact that is common to South American countries (Chile is one of the South American countries that does best) and in developing contries in general [75]. This means that students from the failed school systems have great difficulty in understanding what they read and are fairly motivated to follow apparently meaningless protocols, which are usually written in English. This is also true for technicians in equipment maintenance, which usually generates a large number of visits until the solution of a defect is solved in a satisfactory way.

Experience from a Large Cancer Center in Brazil

Therefore, the available solution (though not the best) is to concentrate more complex exams in few and larger laboratories, thus outsourcing molecular exams, which is the current reality. However, this ends up further limiting the access of molecular tests to a large number of the public. In addition, smaller laboratories do not always use good quality reagents or process their tests in the best way. In our institution [57], the molecular laboratory performs exams both internal and from other services. In our experience, there is a much higher proportion of inconclusive tests in external cases. Electrocautery artifacts, material processed at an inadequate temperature, poor quality reagents and dyes are frequent. Samples that require DNA extraction show lower yield. The reality is that many laboratories are forced to reduce costs due to the low remuneration of health plans and end up sacrificing the quality of their processes. For routine diagnostic evaluation of most cases, this may not represent a major problem, but in cases where more sensitive tests are needed, this practice may render a molecular test and a sample unfeasible.

A developing country's own poor infrastructure is a complicating factor. The long distances between laboratories make it difficult transfer materials. Although some Brazilian states have decent highways and infra-structure, for most of the territory the reality is quite different. The country does not have a well-distributed railway structure, and the airport system has a network concentrated in large cities and capital cities. Equipment maintenance itself ends up being hampered by the difficulty to access certain regions of the country and equipment remains inoperative for weeks, if not months, waiting for technical support. Finally, the import of reagents needed to carry out the tests are still held in the government's bureaucratic mechanisms waiting for release. Reagents take several weeks to reach their destination, which implies an important reduction in the time of their use.

In an attempt to keep the country updated in molecular exams Brazilian major educational institutions and philanthropic institutions have made a great effort [57, 58]. Specifically our institution (Barretos Cancer Hospital) has raised funds earmarked for this purpose coming largely from research projects financed by funding agencies (Fundacao da Amparo à Pesquisa do Estado de São Paulo – FAPESP) or even through individual and corporate donations. Thus, the more expensive exams can be extended to at least a part of the needy population, which, however, does not guarantee the sustainability of the process in more troubled times and for a long period of time. Neither the model of private funding is a constant in the country for the vast majority of cancer centers.

In short, developing countries are able to implement the molecular diagnosis necessary to apply integrated diagnostics as recommended by WHO. However, this implementation may be slightly slower and less available to low-income populations than in developed countries. The challenges are many, but ensuring that the entire population has access to advances in molecular biology is the main barrier to be overcome.

References

1. Chappelow J. Gross domestic product—GDP 2020. 2020 June 1 [cited 2020 April 6]. Available from: www.investopedia.com/terms/g/gdp.asp.
2. United Nations Development Programme. Human development data (1990–2017). [cited 2020 July 20]. Available from: http://hdr.undp.org/en/data.
3. Top 25 developed and developing countries. 2019 [cited 2020 July 20]. Available from: https://www.investopedia.com/updates/top-developing-countries/#citation-20.
4. Agarwal P. Characteristics of developing economies. 2017 [cited 2020 July 21]. Available from: https://www.intelligenteconomist.com/characteristics-of-developing-economies/.
5. Epstein MJ, Yuthas K. Redefining education in the developing world. 2012 [cited 2020 July 20]. Available from: https://ssir.org/articles/entry/redefining_education_in_the_developing_world.
6. King EMH, Anne M. Women's education in developing countries.
7. 15 Facts on education in developing countries. 2014 [cited 2020 July 20]. Available from: https://acei-global.blog/2014/03/06/15-facts-on-education-in-developing-countries/.
8. Guardia ER, et al. Aspectos Fiscais da Educação no Brasil. In: S.d.T. Nacional, editor. Tesouro Nacional; 2018.
9. Avila HF. South Ameria. 2020 [cited 2020 July 21]. Available from: https://www.britannica.com/place/South-America.
10. Official and spoken languages of the countries of the Americas and the Caribbean. Available from: https://www.nationsonline.org/oneworld/american_languages.htm.
11. Nag OS. The poorest countries in South America. 2019 [cited 2020 July 21]. Available from: https://www.worldatlas.com/articles/the-poorest-countries-in-south-america.html.
12. Zovatto D. The rapidly deteriorating quality of democracy in Latin America. 2020 [cited 2020 July 21]. Available from: https://www.brookings.edu/blog/order-from-chaos/2020/02/28/the-rapidly-deteriorating-quality-of-democracy-in-latin-america/.
13. Garcia J, Correa G, Rousset B. Trends in infant mortality in Venezuela between 1985 and 2016: a systematic analysis of demographic data. Lancet Glob Health. 2019;7(3):e331–6.
14. Cohen L. Argentina's economic crisis explained in five charts. 2018 [cited 2020 July 22]. Available from: https://www.reuters.com/article/us-argentina-economy/argentinas-economic-crisis-explained-in-five-charts-idUSKCN1LD1S7.
15. Gillespie P. Why Argentina keeps finding itself in a debt crisis. Bloomberg Businessweek. 2019.
16. How Argentina and Japan continued to confound macroeconomists. The Economist. 2019.
17. Hamilton JIG. Historical Reflections On The Splendor And Decline Of Argentina. Cato Journal. 2005;25(3):521–40.
18. UNICEF. Argentina: key demographics indicators. 2020 [cited 2020 July 21]. Available from: https://data.unicef.org/country/arg/#.
19. The World Bank. 2020 [cited 2020 July 21]. Available from: https://data.worldbank.org/indicator/AG.LND.TOTL.K2?locations=BR.
20. Worldometer. 2020 [cited 2020 July 22]. Available from: https://www.worldometers.info/world-population/brazil-population.

21. Atlas do desenvolvimento humano no Brasil. 2020 [cited 2020 July 22]. Available from: http://www.atlasbrasil.org.br/2013/pt/.
22. Amann E, et al. Infrastructure and its role in Brazil's development process. Q Rev Econ Finance. 2016;62:66–73.
23. Salto-Tellez M, Maxwell P, Hamilton P. Artificial intelligence-the third revolution in pathology. Histopathology. 2019;74(3):372–6.
24. Fassan M. Molecular diagnostics in pathology: time for a next-generation pathologist? Arch Pathol Lab Med. 2018;142(3):313–20.
25. Titford M. The long history of hematoxylin. Biotech Histochem. 2005;80(2):73–8.
26. Nakhleh RE, Gephardt G, Zarbo RJ. Necessity of clinical information in surgical pathology. Arch Pathol Lab Med. 1999;123(7):615–9.
27. Fleming KA, et al. An essential pathology package for low- and middle-income countries. Am J Clin Pathol. 2017;147(1):15–32.
28. Pope TP. The anxiety of the biopsy. 2009 [cited 2020 July 20]. Available from: https://well.blogs.nytimes.com/2009/02/24/the-anxiety-of-the-biopsy/.
29. Gomes DS, et al. Inter-observer variability between general pathologists and a specialist in breast pathology in the diagnosis of lobular neoplasia, columnar cell lesions, atypical ductal hyperplasia and ductal carcinoma in situ of the breast. Diagn Pathol. 2014;9:121.
30. Montgomery E. Is there a way for pathologists to decrease interobserver variability in the diagnosis of dysplasia? Arch Pathol Lab Med. 2005;129(2):174–6.
31. Fukunaga M, et al. Interobserver and intraobserver variability in the diagnosis of hydatidiform mole. Am J Surg Pathol. 2005;29(7):942–7.
32. Prichard JW. Overview of automated immunohistochemistry. Arch Pathol Lab Med. 2014;138(12):1578–82.
33. Gavrielides MA, et al. Observer variability in the interpretation of HER2/neu immunohistochemical expression with unaided and computer-aided digital microscopy. Arch Pathol Lab Med. 2011;135(2):233–42.
34. Thomson TA, et al. HER-2/neu in breast cancer: interobserver variability and performance of immunohistochemistry with 4 antibodies compared with fluorescent in situ hybridization. Mod Pathol. 2001;14(11):1079–86.
35. Nielsen LAG, et al. Evaluation of the proliferation marker Ki-67 in gliomas: interobserver variability and digital quantification. Diagn Pathol. 2018;13(1):38.
36. Varga Z, et al. How reliable is Ki-67 immunohistochemistry in grade 2 breast carcinomas? A QA study of the Swiss Working Group of Breast- and Gynecopathologists. PLoS One. 2012;7(5):e37379.
37. Dietel M, et al. Predictive molecular pathology and its role in targeted cancer therapy: a review focussing on clinical relevance. Cancer Gene Ther. 2013;20(4):211–21.
38. Harris TJ, McCormick F. The molecular pathology of cancer. Nat Rev Clin Oncol. 2010;7(5):251–65.
39. Swerdlow SH, et al. The 2016 revision of the World Health Organization classification of lymphoid neoplasms. Blood. 2016;127(20):2375–90.
40. Wen PY, Huse JT. 2016 World Health Organization classification of central nervous system tumors. Continuum (Minneap Minn). 2017;23(6, Neuro-oncology):1531–47.
41. Behling F, Schittenhelm J. Oncogenic BRAF alterations and their role in brain tumors. Cancers (Basel). 2019;11(6):794.
42. Louis DN, et al. cIMPACT-NOW: a practical summary of diagnostic points from Round 1 updates. Brain Pathol. 2019;29(4):469–72.
43. Bera K, et al. Artificial intelligence in digital pathology – new tools for diagnosis and precision oncology. Nat Rev Clin Oncol. 2019;16(11):703–15.
44. El Hallani S, et al. Evaluation of quantitative digital pathology in the assessment of Barrett esophagus-associated dysplasia. Am J Clin Pathol. 2015;144(1):151–64.

45. Humphries MP, et al. Automated tumour recognition and digital pathology scoring unravels new role for PD-L1 in predicting good outcome in ER-/HER2+ breast cancer. J Oncol. 2018;2018:2937012.
46. Volynskaya Z, et al. Ki67 quantitative interpretation: insights using image analysis. J Pathol Inform. 2019;10:8.
47. Acs B, Hartman J. Next generation pathology: artificial intelligence enhances histopathology practice. J Pathol. 2020;250(1):7–8.
48. Niazi MKK, Parwani AV, Gurcan MN. Digital pathology and artificial intelligence. Lancet Oncol. 2019;20(5):e253–61.
49. The World Bank. [cited 2020 July]. Available from: https://data.worldbank.org/indicator/.
50. Scheffer M, et al. Demografia médica no Brasil 2018. FMUSP; 2018.
51. CFM entrega dados sobre filas de cirurgia. 2018 [cited 2020 July 28]. Available from: https://portal.cfm.org.br/index.php?option=com_content&view=article&id=27414: cfm-entrega-dados-sobre-filas-de-cirurgia&catid=3.
52. Crise no SUS: pacientes aguardam mais de 10 anos na fila de espera. 2017 [cited 2020 July 28]. Available from: https://portal.cfm.org.br/index.php?option=com_content&view=article& id=27317:crise-no-sus-pacientes-aguardam-mais-de-10-anos-na-fila-de-espera&catid=3.
53. Metter DM, et al. Trends in the US and Canadian pathologist workforces from 2007 to 2017. JAMA Netw Open. 2019;2(5):e194337.
54. Pathologists, R.C.o. Meeting pathology demand: histopathology workforce census. London: Royal College of Pathologists; 2018.
55. Lopes A, Pachedo E. O saneamento básico no Brasil em 6 gráficos. 2019. Available from: https://www.saneamentobasico.com.br/saneamento-basico-brasil-graficos/.
56. INCA – Instituto Nacional do Câncer. 08/05/2020 [cited 2020 July 27]. Available from: https://www.inca.gov.br/numeros-de-cancer.
57. Barretos Cancer Hospital (Hospital de Amor). [cited 2020 July 27]. Available from: http://www.hcancerbarretos.com.br/en/.
58. A. C. Camargo Center. [cited 2020 July 27]. Available from: https://www.accamargo.org.br/.
59. Mais Saúde Direito de Todos. In: S.E. Ministério da Saúde, editor. Ministério da Saúde; 2010.
60. Agência Nacional de Saúde Suplementar. 2020 [cited 2020 Sept 2]. Available from: http://www.ans.gov.br/.
61. Gavras D, Brandão R. Após perda de 3 milhões de clientes, cem planos de saúde fecham as portas. In: Estadão. Economia & Negócios; 2018.
62. Castro M. Planos de saúde acabam sem aviso aos usuários. In: Estado de Minas. Economia; 2018.
63. Vieira E. Controle de preços inviabilizou planos de saúde individuais, diz presidente da FenaSaúde. In: JC. Universo Online: Consumidor; 2015.
64. Ministério da Saúde, G.d.M. Portaria n° 3.388, de 30 de dezembro de 2013. 2015 [cited 2020 Sept 2]. Available from: http://bvsms.saude.gov.br/bvs/saudelegis/gm/2013/ prt3388_30_12_2013.html.
65. Catteau A, et al. A new sensitive PCR assay for one-step detection of 12 IDH1/2 mutations in glioma. Acta Neuropathol Commun. 2014;2:58.
66. Colomba E, et al. Detection of BRAF p.V600E mutations in melanomas: comparison of four methods argues for sequential use of immunohistochemistry and pyrosequencing. J Mol Diagn. 2013;15(1):94–100.
67. Felsberg J, et al. Rapid and sensitive assessment of the IDH1 and IDH2 mutation status in cerebral gliomas based on DNA pyrosequencing. Acta Neuropathol. 2010;119(4):501–7.
68. Woehrer A, et al. FISH-based detection of 1p 19q codeletion in oligodendroglial tumors: procedures and protocols for neuropathological practice – a publication under the auspices of the Research Committee of the European Confederation of Neuropathological Societies (Euro-CNS). Clin Neuropathol. 2011;30(2):47–55.

69. Northcott PA, et al. Rapid, reliable, and reproducible molecular sub-grouping of clinical medulloblastoma samples. Acta Neuropathol. 2012;123(4):615–26.
70. Dubbink HJ, et al. Diagnostic detection of allelic losses and imbalances by next-generation sequencing: 1p/19q co-deletion analysis of gliomas. J Mol Diagn. 2016;18(5):775–86.
71. Dolar Comercial. Uol economia 2020 [cited 2020 July 29]. Available from: https://economia. uol.com.br/cotacoes/cambio/dolar-comercial-estados-unidos/.
72. Dolar Comercial Oficial. 2002 [cited 2020 July 30]. Available from: http://www.yahii.com.br/ dolardiario02.html.
73. Filho, FdAC, Zilli EC. Classificação brasileira hierarquizada de procedimentos médicos. Associação Médica Brasileira; 2012.
74. INEP. Censo da educação superior 2017. In: M.d.E.e.C. (MEC), editor. Diretoria de Estatísticas Educacionais – Deed. Brasília, DF; 2017.
75. Programme for international student assessment. 2018 [cited 2020 July 30]. Available from: http://www.oecd.org/pisa/.

Part II
Molecular Pathology of Glioblastoma

Chapter 8
Molecular Stratification of Adult and Pediatric High Grade Gliomas

Yuanfan Yang, Huifang Dai, and Giselle Y. López

Introduction

Glioblastoma is the most common primary malignant brain tumor in adults, with an incidence of over 10,000 cases per year in the United States [1]. They most commonly occur in adults, in the cerebral hemispheres [1]. While less common in children, high grade glial and glioneuronal tumors are diagnosed in over 1000 pediatric patients per year in the United States [1]. Given the marked advances in massively parallel sequencing over the last two decades, combined with advances in epigenetic studies such as methylation profiling, we now have a better understanding of the molecular features underlying and driving these tumors. Herein, we describe the genetic characteristics of the most common high grade glial and glioneuronal tumors in adults and children.

Y. Yang
Department of Pathology, Duke University School of Medicine, Durham, NC, USA

The Preston Robert Tisch Brain Tumor Center, Duke University School of Medicine, Durham, NC, USA
e-mail: yuanfan.yang@duke.edu

H. Dai
Department of Pathology, Duke University School of Medicine, Durham, NC, USA
e-mail: huifang.dai@duke.edu

G. Y. López (✉)
Department of Pathology, Duke University School of Medicine, Durham, NC, USA

The Preston Robert Tisch Brain Tumor Center, Duke University School of Medicine, Durham, NC, USA

Duke Cancer Institute, Duke University School of Medicine, Durham, NC, USA
e-mail: giselle.lopez@duke.edu

© The Author(s), under exclusive license to Springer Nature Switzerland AG 2021
J. J. Otero, A. P. Becker (eds.), *Precision Molecular Pathology of Glioblastoma*, Molecular Pathology Library, https://doi.org/10.1007/978-3-030-69170-7_8

Glioblastoma, *IDH* Wildtype, WHO Grade 4

Background

Diffuse gliomas are primary brain tumors which, in adults, are most commonly found in the cerebral hemispheres [1]. These tumors were traditionally graded based on histologic features, from grade 1 to grade 4. Glioblastomas are among the most aggressive gliomas and are considered grade 4 tumors [2]. Glioblastomas are classified as astrocytomas, or brain tumors with cells resembling astrocytes. Prior to the use of molecular characteristics, glioblastomas were defined as infiltrative gliomas with atypical nuclei and the presence of either microvascular proliferation or necrosis [2] (Fig. 8.1). While histologic features can be used to stratify infiltrative glial tumors, there is interobserver variability [3], and the histology does not always align with behavior, limiting its usefulness for risk stratification. Our understanding of the molecular features of glioblastomas has expanded significantly since the turn of the century. It is now known that glioblastomas largely arise from two distinct molecular pathways, which can be broadly divided into (1) those without *IDH* mutations and which most often arise *de novo*, and (2) those with *IDH* mutations and which most often arise from a prior lower grade astrocytoma (i.e. progressive or secondary gliomas) (Fig. 8.2) [2, 4]. Distinguishing these two groups proved to be so important, that within a decade after the identification of *IDH* mutation as a key driver in

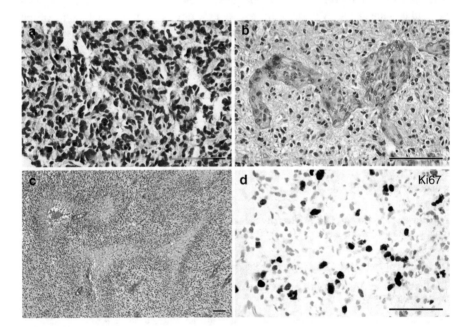

Fig. 8.1 Histologic features of glioblastoma. Glioblastomas are characterized by (**a**) hypercellularity and hyperchromatic, atypical nuclei, (**b**) microvascular proliferation, (**c**) palisading necrosis, and (**d**) elevated proliferation index, as highlighted on this Ki-67 immunohistochemical stain. Scale bars = 100 microns

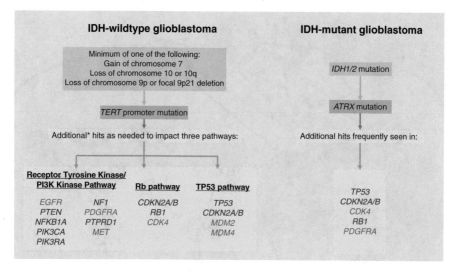

Fig. 8.2 Adult glioblastoma and *IDH*-mutant astrocytoma genetic characteristics. Genes shown represent common genetic alterations, but the lists are not exhaustive. Green box = common driver alterations. Blue box = telomere-maintaining alteration. Yellow box = additional genetic alterations commonly observed. Genes in red are activated, either through mutation, fusion, or amplification. Genes in blue are suppressed, either through mutation or deletion. *TERT* promoter mutation leads to increased *TERT* expression, while *ATRX* mutation leads to inactivation of *ATRX*. *In most cases one or more of the three pathways has already been impacted by earlier genetic alterations. For example, Chromosome 10 loss (a common early event) leads to loss of one copy of *PTEN*, and focal 9p21 deep deletion leads to loss of *CDKN2A*

progressive gliomas, the mutational status of this gene was integrated into the 2016 World Health Organization (WHO) classification of gliomas [2]. The molecular integrated diagnosis is supported by clinical evidence suggesting they are distinct clinical entities: *IDH*-mutant glioblastomas occur in younger patients (often 30s to 50s) with an average survival of 2–3 years, while *IDH*-wildtype glioblastomas tend to occur in older patients (often over age 50, with a median of 65 years of age in the United States [1]) with an average survival of only 1–1.5 years [4, 5]. Histologic features cannot safely distinguish between the two entities. This molecular integrated classification has been shown to have a profound impact on the understanding of the pathogenesis of glioblastoma, on the prognosis and management of glioblastoma in patients, and has provided the opportunity to gain further insights into their genomic subtypes, and the histologic correlates.

Defining Mutations

Glioblastomas that are primary or "de novo" usually arise in older patients without a history of prior lower-grade glioma, whereas secondary or "progressive" glioblastomas arise from a previously diagnosed lower grade glioma. The majority of

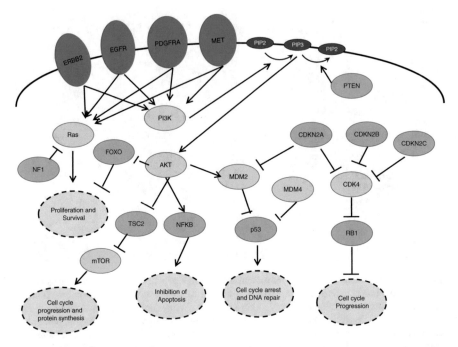

Fig. 8.3 Signaling pathways frequently altered in adult high grade gliomas. Red = receptor tyrosine kinases. Yellow = oncogenes. Blue = tumor suppressors. Dashed lines with gray = downstream pathways impacted. Purple = membrane phospholipids phosphatidylinositol (4,5)-bisphosphate (PIP2), and phosphatidylinositol (3,4,5)-triphosphate (PIP3)

glioblastomas are primary (>90%), and most of those (>90%) are *IDH*-wild type [4, 5]. *IDH*-wildtype glioblastomas lack a single defining mutation like the *IDH*-mutant glioblastomas. However, studies based on mutation analysis, mRNA expression, and DNA copy number alterations have revealed three key genetic pathways almost always altered in *IDH*-wildtype glioblastomas: mutations in 1) the p53 pathway, 2) the RB pathway, and 3) activation of the receptor tyrosine kinase (RTK)/Ras/PI3K pathway [5, 6]. These pathways have some degree of overlap (Fig. 8.3), and some genes which are discussed in detail under one pathway also play roles in other pathways.

RTK/PI3K/AKT *Pathway*

Among the three main molecular pathways, the RTK/PI3K/AKT pathway is most commonly altered in *IDH*-wildtype glioblastoma (altered in 88%), and the most common targets are Epidermal Growth Factor Receptor (*EGFR*) and *PTEN* [5–7]. *EGFR* is a key driver oncogene behind the development of adult *IDH*-wildtype glioblastoma [8]. Its amplification or overexpression occurs in greater than 40% of *IDH*-wildtype glioblastomas [9]. *EGFR*vIII is a constitutively activated mutant variant of this receptor that, when present, is often found together with *EGFR* amplification in glioblastoma [6, 10, 11]. *EGFR*vIII serves as a ligand-independent mechanism to activate the downstream PI3K/AKT pathway and cell proliferation [12]. *EGFR* amplification and mutation are characteristic of adult *IDH*-wildtype glioblastoma, but are very rare in pediatric high grade gliomas. Amplification or overexpression of another receptor tyrosine kinase, *PDGFRA*, has also been described [5, 6, 13]. A negative regulator of the pathway, *PTEN* (phosphatase and tensin homology) encodes a phosphatase that inactivates phosphatidylinositol (3,4,5)-triphosphate (PIP_3) through conversion to phosphatidylinositol (4,5)-bisphosphate (PIP2) (Fig. 8.3). *PTEN* mutation/alteration thus facilitates pathway activation and also regulates cell migration and invasion [14]. *PTEN* mutation or deletion is found in over 25% of *IDH*-wildtype glioblastomas [5–7, 15]. Other genes in the RTK pathway have also been found to be altered in glioblastomas at varying frequencies, including but not limited to *PIK3CA*, *PIK3R1*, and *NF1* [5, 6]. Mutations in this pathway appear to converge on pathways leading to increased proliferation and survival.

TP53/ MDM2/MDM4/CDKN2A *Pathway*

TP53 is a well-known tumor suppressor gene involved in cell cycle arrest and apoptosis in response to DNA damage and stress. When activated under these conditions, it works as a transcription factor to stop uncontrolled proliferation. Inactivating mutations of *TP53* are found in approximately one third of *IDH*-wildtype glioblastomas [5, 6], compared to about two-thirds of *IDH*-mutant astrocytomas [7]. While *IDH*-mutant astrocytomas typically have hotspot *TP53* mutations, *TP53* mutations in *IDH*-wildtype glioblastomas occur at more widespread loci, possibly due to increased genomic instability in *IDH*-wildtype glioblastomas [7]. *MDM2* amplification is found in 10–14% of glioblastomas [16], and likely serves as another regulator of this pathway. MDM2 is an inhibitor of p53 [17], mediating p53 degradation and thereby promoting tumorgenesis [18]. *MDM2* amplification is mutually exclusive with *TP53* mutation [19]. *MDM4* amplification has a similar role in this pathway, and is present in 4% of glioblastomas [20].

RB/CDK4/CDKN2A-p16^{INK4a} *Pathway*

In quiescent cells, Rb protein acts as a cell cycle checkpoint for entry into S-phase when phosphorylated by CDK4/cyclin D1. This growth inhibition mechanism is often found defective in glioblastoma, most commonly through alterations in *RB1*, *CDK4* and *CDKN2A*, with *CDKN2A* homozygous deletion being most common (present in over half of cases) [5, 6, 21, 22]. These alterations lead to dysregulated cell cycle and uncontrolled proliferation [6]. Genetic alterations impacting *RB1*, *p16^{INK4a}* and *CDK4* seems to affect both *IDH*-wildtype glioblastomas and grade 4 *IDH*-mutant astrocytomas [23].

Telomere Maintenance

In addition to recurrent alterations in the above three pathways, alterations have also been identified which aid in maintaining telomere length. Telomeres are DNA repeats that sit at the ends of chromosomes [24]. As cells divide, these repeats gradually shorten, and upon reaching a certain length, the cells cease dividing and undergo replicative senescence [25, 26]. Therefore, tumors often find a mechanism to avoid this shortening of the telomeres. In *IDH*-wildtype glioblastomas, the most common mechanism for achieving this goal is *TERT* promoter mutation [27]. *TERT* encodes the catalytic subunit of telomerase, a protein that maintains telomeres [28–30]. The most common oncogenic mutations in *TERT* occur in the promoter at C228 and C250, or less commonly C229 [27]. The mutations lead to a novel binding site for the transcription factor GA-binding protein (GABP), leading to increased transcription, and avoidance of replicative senescence [31]. In glioblastomas lacking *TERT* promoter mutations, a subset instead display complex chromosomal rearrangements involving regions upstream of *TERT*, leading to telomere activation [32].

However, there remained a subset of glioblastomas (less than 20%) [32] demonstrating no identifiable *TERT* alterations. This cohort was found to have abnormally long telomeres [32], a phenomenon referred to as the alternative lengthening of telomeres (ALT) phenotype [33, 34]. Of these IDH-wildtype glioblastomas demonstrating alternative lengthening of telomeres, a subset demonstrated loss-of-function *SMARCAL1* mutations [32], while another subset demonstrated mutations in α-thalassemia/mental retardation syndrome X-linked (*ATRX*) [32], which will be discussed in more detail in the section on IDH-mutant astrocytomas. Between all of the genetic alterations, the vast majority of glioblastomas have an identified genetic alteration leading to maintenance of telomeres, stressing the importance of this process to the growth of glioblastomas.

Other Genetic and Epigenetic Alterations

Additional chromosomal changes accumulate during glioblastoma pathogenesis. The clinical and pathological relevance are being studied. Loss of chromosome 10 and gain of chromosome 7 have been identified as early initiating events in a common evolutionary trajectory of *IDH*-wildtype glioblastomas, while *TERT* promoter mutations occur later (Fig. 8.2) [8]. Molecular profiling has identified chromosome

19/20 co-gain to be significantly associated with improved long term survival in patients with *IDH*-wildtype glioblastoma [35].

Promoter methylation serves as another mechanism to regulate genes expression in glioma. O^6-methylguanine-DNA methyltransferase (*MGMT*) encodes an enzyme to repair DNA from damage induced by alkylating agents. Promoter methylation and downregulation of *MGMT* thus predicts better therapy response to temozolomide chemotherapy, and it is more commonly observed in *IDH*-mutant high grade astrocytomas than in *IDH*-wildtype glioblastomas [36]. It has become the next step in the standard workup of glioblastoma after learning *IDH* mutational status, and lack of both *IDH* mutation and *MGMT* methylation has been associated with particularly poor outcome in *IDH*-wildtype glioblastoma [37].

Glioblastoma Variants

With the ability to explore the molecular features of glioblastoma, we are now in a better position to characterize some rare glioblastoma variants. Gliosarcoma, giant cell glioblastoma, and epithelioid glioblastoma, are placed under *IDH*-wildtype glioblastoma umbrella in the 2016 WHO classification.

Epithelioid glioblastoma is characterized by its histological features of epithelioid cells, but the genetic features are variable [38–41]. Combined epigenetic and cytogenetic clustering suggests that, instead of being a distinct entity, the majority of histologically-defined epithelioid glioblastomas fall into three previously defined entities: anaplastic pleomorphic xanthoastrocytomas, *IDH*-wildtype glioblastoma, and pediatric-type glioblastoma of RTK1 type [40]. Those which fall into the anaplastic pleomorphic xanthoastrocytomas subtype tended to occur in children or young adults, and were more likely to have *BRAF* V600E mutations and *CDKN2A* homozygous deleton [40]. Those that clustered with adult *IDH*-wildtype glioblastoma were more likely to be adults (median age of 50 years at diagnosis), and to have the genetic profile described above for *IDH*-wildtype glioblastoma [40]. The last cohort were more likely to occur in children or young adults, and were more likely to have *PDGFRA* amplification, sometimes with *MYCN* amplification [40]; this cohort of pediatric high-grade gliomas will be described in more detail in a later section. As additional studies are performed, this classification may undergo further refinement.

Gliosarcoma is a variant of glioblastoma in which a portion of the tumor has histologic features of sarcoma, often characterized by spindled cells and increased collagen. A key distinction from sarcoma is the biphasic appearance- while portions of the tumor appear sarcomatous, these regions are interwoven with regions demonstrating both histologic and immunohistochemical features of classic *IDH*-wildtype glioblastoma [2]. Some genetic features frequently seen in *IDH*-wildtype glioblastomas are enriched in this particular variant, including *TERT* promoter mutations, *PTEN* mutation or deletion, and *CDKN2A* homozygous deletion [42]. On the other hand, *EGFR* amplification is rare [42].

Giant cell glioblastoma is a variant of glioblastoma demonstrating frequent cells with large, bizarre-appearing nuclei. Compared to *IDH*-wildtype glioblastomas as a whole, giant cell glioblastomas appear to have a somewhat better prognosis, with patients surviving a few months longer than *IDH*-wildtype glioblastomas patients as a whole [43], although they are still very aggressive tumors. While *IDH* mutations are rare in this cohort, the spectrum of genetic alterations differs somewhat from those seen in *IDH*-wildtype glioblastomas [2]. While *TERT* promoter mutations are common in *IDH*-wildtype glioblastomas, they are present in less than one-quarter of giant cell glioblastomas [42, 44, 45]. Additionally, a subset of giant cell glioblastomas without *TERT* promoter mutations demonstrate loss of expression of *ATRX* [42, 44]. On the other hand, *TP53* mutations are common, present in 40–84% of giant cell glioblastomas [42, 45]. However, while *ATRX* and *TP53* mutations are common in giant cell glioblastomas, *IDH* mutations are rare [42]. Additionally, *EGFR* amplification [42, 45] and *CDKN2A* homozygous deletion are uncommon [42]. Copy number alterations frequently seen in giant cell glioblastoma include the commonly identified chromosome 7 gain and chromosome 10 loss [45]. Additional copy number changes seen in giant cell glioblastoma include chromosome 20 gain and loss of chromosome arm 22q [45].

Gene Expression Profiling and Genomic Subtypes

The emergence of gene microarray has allowed for high-throughput gene expression profiling of glioblastomas. This system-based analysis of gene expression pattern has revealed several distinct molecular subgroups of glioblastoma with prognostic and therapeutic significance [46–49]. When combining gene expression profiles with patterns of known gene mutations, an integrated molecular classification consisting of classic, mesenchymal, and proneural subtypes are proposed [13]. The classic subtype displays a profile supporting high proliferation, and it is most commonly associated with *EGFR* amplification, loss chromosome 10 (with *PTEN* mutation/alteration), and homozygous deletion of *CDKN2A* [13]. On the other hand, the proneural subtype is associated with *IDH*-mutant glioblastoma and a better outcome [13]. Interestingly, single cell data has revealed that most tumors contain cells which individually would be classified under the different subtypes, even in tumors for which the bulk data clearly places the overall tumor into one subtype [50]. This finding supports the presence of intratumoral heterogeneity with regards to gene expression patterns and cell types. Likewise, glioblastomas can be categorized based on the methylation profiles [51]. These methylation profiles are generated by looking at the epigenetic changes, namely modifications to DNA that are used to regulate gene expression patterns. As with gene expression patterns, studies looking at different regions of the tumor with methylation profiling demonstrate intratumoral heterogeneity [52], confirming that while tumors may have overarching patterns, there is a great deal of intratumoral heterogenetiy with regards to methylation and expression patterns [50, 52].

Astrocytoma, IDH-Mutant, WHO Grade 4

Background

The histological classification of glioma is increasingly refined by advances in genetics. The identification of *Isocitrate Dehydrogenase* (*IDH*) mutations in a subset of what we had considered glioblastomas has drastically changed our understanding of this tumor [4]. *IDH1* mutations, or less commonly, *IDH2* mutations, were identified in a subset of glioblastoma, predominantly those which arose from lower grade astrocytomas [4]. Because these glioblastomas appear to arise from a distinct pathway compared to their *IDH*-wildtype counterparts and represent a distinct tumor type, they are now referred to as "Astrocytoma, IDH-mutant, grade 4," rather than glioblastoma [53, 54]. This integrated diagnosis, incorporating the *IDH* status, is now used to categorize and define all diffuse astrocytomas across WHO grades 2–4 [2, 54]. *IDH*-mutant grade 4 astrocytomas are associated with younger age of onset and better survival than *IDH*-wildtype glioblastoma [4, 55, 56]. Whereas *IDH*-wildtype glioblastomas appear to occur throughout all lobes of the brain, *IDH*-mutant astrocytomas seem to occur a higher frequency in the frontal and temporal lobes [57]. Here, we focus on the grade 4 *IDH*-mutant astrocytomas (as opposed to the grade 2–3); these tumors are defined by presence of microvascular proliferation, necrosis, or homozygous deletion of *CDKN2A* [54].

IDH1/2 Mutation

Genomic studies initially identified recurrent heterozygous mutations in *IDH1* (or rarely *IDH2*) in 3–10% of glioblastomas [4, 5]. The most common mutation in *IDH1* results in the specific amino acid substitution R132H (arginine to histidine), but numerous other mutations have been identified at this codon, or in the analogous codon in *IDH2* [4, 58]. *IDH1/2* mutation is considered an early event in gliomagenesis, as it is always among the earliest genetic alterations identified in diffuse astrocytomas of all grades [57, 59]. As a class, isocitrate dehydrogenases are enzymes involved in glucose metabolism, where dysregulation can result in widespread impacts. Whereas wildtype IDH1/2 function to convert isocitrate to α-ketoglutarate, mutant IDH1/2 instead converts α-ketoglutarate to an oncogenic metabolite, (*R*)-2-hydroxyglutarate (2-HG) [60, 61]. This oncometabolite induces a characteristic epigenetic pattern called the glioma CpG island methylator phenotype (G-CIMP) [60, 62], via inhibition TET family of hydroxylase and histone lysine demethylase involved in DNA demethylation [63]. By changing the way in which DNA and histones are methylated (i.e. epigenetic changes), *IDH* mutations are able to lead to changes in gene expression patterns that are pro-tumorigenic [63–65]. Some of the changes appear to lead to a more stem-like state for the tumor cells [65]. The epigenetic pattern leads to a distinct gene expression pattern including *platelet-derived growth factor receptor alpha (PDGFRA)* oncogene activation [64]. 2-HG also creates a tumorigenic microenvironment by inhibiting T cell-mediated immune surveillance in *IDH* mutant tumors [66].

Genetic Landscape of IDH-Mutant Astrocytomas, WHO Grade 4

Concurrent *TP53* and *ATRX* mutations are often found together with *IDH* mutations in diffuse astrocytomas of all grades (Fig. 8.4). While *ATRX* mutation is present in the majority of *IDH*-mutant astrocytomas, it is rare in *IDH*-wildtype glioblastomas [67, 68]. The presence of *ATRX* mutation is highly associated with the alternative lengthening of telomeres (ALT) phenotype [67, 69, 70]. Studies appear to show that *ATRX* does not accomplish this ALT phenotype independently [71], but rather works in concert with mutant *IDH*, leading to ALT [72]. *TP53* mutation is present in 83% of *IDH*-mutant astrocytomas, compared to 23–27% of *IDH*-wild-type glioblastomas [4, 5].

Genetic alterations impacting genes in the *RB* pathway are frequently observed in *IDH*-mutant grade 4 astrocytomas, with the most common alterations being *CDKN2A/B* homozygous deletion, *CDK4* amplification and *RB1* mutation [70, 73]. In

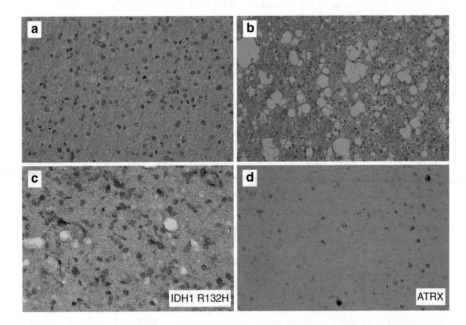

Fig. 8.4 Astrocytoma, *IDH*-mutant. (**a**) H&E-stained section in a region of lower cellularity, containing mitoses and moderate atypia. (**b**) Different region containing frequent microcysts, a common features in *IDH*-mutant gliomas. (**c**) Immunohistochemical staining against IDH1 R132H mutant protein. (**d**) Immunohistochemical stain against ATRX, demonstrating loss of nuclear expression in tumor cells

particular, *CDKN2A/B* deletion is common among *IDH* mutant grade 4 astrocytomas (43% in one study [73]) and are associated with aggressive behavior [73–76]. The other two mutations are potential factors for risk stratification [75], although research is ongoing to determine the clinical significance of the presence of these mutations.

Gene Expression Profiling

Gene expression profiling studies suggest that glioblastomas and *IDH*-mutant astrocytomas have distinct molecular subclasses [70, 77]. Most *IDH*-mutant glioblastomas fall into the category of proneural subtype, characterized by *IDH/TP53* mutations, *PDGFRA* gain, and a lack of *EGFR* mutation [57, 77]. The G-CIMP epigenetic phenotype induced by *IDH* mutation is likewise associated with proneural subtype [57]. Loss of the G-CIMP phenotype can occur in *IDH*-mutant astrocytomas; this tends to happen more in grade 3 and grade 4 tumors, and is associated with a worse survival compared to those with retained G-CIMP phenotype [70].

Diffuse Midline Glioma, H3 K27M-Mutant, WHO Grade 4

Background

Clinicians have long noted the presence of a diffuse high-grade glioma which occurs at higher frequencies in children and most commonly involves the pons. Sampling of these "diffuse intrinsic pontine gliomas" was discouraged due to the location and unresectability [78]. With the onset of stereotactic biopsies and improved techniques, sampling became available [79]. It was quickly realized that these tumors were characterized by recurrent mutations in one of the Histone 3 variant genes: *H3F3A, H3F3B, HIST1H3B,* or *HIST1H3C* [80–85].

Further studies revealed that, in addition to pontine tumors (where H3 K27M mutation is present in 80% of pediatric pontine gliomas) [82], H3 K27M mutations were also identified at a high frequency in other pediatric midline high grade gliomas, including those involving the thalamus, midbrain, medulla, cerebellum, and spinal cord locations [80, 83, 85–91]. While they usually arise in children and young adults, they can also be found in adults of all ages [92, 93]. This unique tumor group was formally recognized by the WHO 2016 classification, as "diffuse midline gliomas, H3 K27M-mutant, WHO grade 4" [2, 94]. This entity includes most of the brain stem high grade astrocytomas previously called diffuse intrinsic pontine glioma, and additionally incorporates other diffuse midline gliomas bearing this mutation [2, 94]. Classifying H3 M27M-mutant diffuse midline gliomas as their own tumor type serves an important prognostic value: H3 K27M mutation defines a clinically distinct subgroup of diffuse midline glioma with more aggressive biological behaviors [80], compared to pediatric midline gliomas with wild-type H3 [89].

The H3 K27M-mutant diffuse midline gliomas are considered high-grade gliomas (WHO grade 4) regardless of their histological appearance [2, 94]. They generally have a poor prognosis, with a lower overall survival for pediatric high grade gliomas with the H3 K27M mutation compared to tumors in similar locations without such mutations [80, 89, 95, 96], and a 2-year survival rate of less than 10% under current therapy [87, 89].

H3 K27M Mutation

Histone H3 is the major histone variant to be loaded on chromatin scaffolding. Histone H3 K27 trimethylation is normally established by recruitment of Polycomb Repressive Complex 2 (PRC2), which contains an H3 K27-specific histone methyltransferase subunit EZH2 [97]. H3 K27M missense mutation causes a methionine substitution at a key site, binding to the active site of the SET domain of the PRC2 complex and thereby stalling it [98], blocking the ability of PRC to put inhibitory trimethylation on histone H3 [98, 99]. In high grade gliomas bearing a heterozygous H3 K27M mutation, this leads to a specific loss of tri-methylated lysine in H3 (H3K27me3) [100, 101], (Fig. 8.5) a repressive histone epigenetic modification

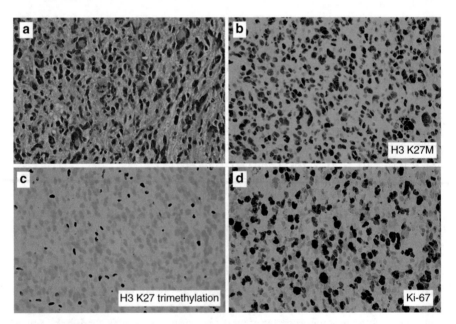

Fig. 8.5 Diffuse midline glioma, H3 K27M-mutant. (**a**) H&E-stained section demonstrating hypercellularity, marked nuclear atypia, and atypical mitoses. (**b**) Immunohistochemical stain against H3 K27M is positive in the tumor nuclei. (**c**) Immunohistochemical stain against trimethylation of H3 K27 shows loss of nuclear staining in tumor cells. (**d**) Ki-67 immunohistochemical stain highlights the brisk mitotic activity of the tumor

[99], while other key histone marks are spared [100]. Mechanistically, in vitro studies have shown a dominant negative effect of heterozygous H3 K27M mutation on global ablation of H3 K27me3 across the genome, regardless of the mutant histone H3 variant [101]. This aberrant binding leads to global DNA demethylation [102] and focal gain of H3K27me3 at certain loci (e.g. *CDK6*), exemplifying epigenetic regulation of gene expression involved in development and tumorigenesis [81, 103].

Mutations of *ATRX* are also present in approximately one third of H3 K27M mutant pediatric diffuse gliomas [81]. *ATRX* mutations are mutually exclusive with *TOP3A* alterations [104], suggesting increased *TOP3A* expression may serve as an alternate mechanism of telomere maintenance in H3 K27M-mutant diffuse midline gliomas without *ATRX* mutations.

Genetic Landscape of Diffuse Midline Gliomas

A few co-existing mutations have been identified by whole-genome or whole-exome sequencing, including *Activin Receptor Type 1* (*ACVR1*), and *Fibroblast Growth Factor Receptor 1* (*FGFR1*) [104, 105]. Concurrent *ACVR1* mutation primarily occurs in pontine tumors with H3.1 mutation, while *FGFR1* mutations or fusions occur predominantly in thalamic tumors in conjunction with H3.3 mutation [104, 105]. *ACVR1* mutation, present in up to 30% of pediatric diffuse midline glioma, is associated with younger patient age and longer overall survival [84]. *ACVR1* encodes a bone morphogenetic protein (BMP) type 1 receptor *ALK2*, and its mutation results in constitutive activation of BMP-TGFβ signaling pathway, with phosphorylation of downstream effectors like SMAD and ID proteins [83, 106]. *ACVR1* mutation has been found to drive tumorigenesis in one mouse model [107], and inhibitors of ACVR1 and antagonists of BMP signaling [108] are being tested as targeted therapy in preclinical models. *TP53* and *PPM1D* mutation also occur frequently in diffuse midline gliomas, often in combination with H3.3 K27M variant [85, 109], and both are proteins involved in DNA damage response [109]. *MYCN* or *MYC* amplifications are also observed in some diffuse midline gliomas with H3 K27M mutations [110].

Mutations in the receptor tyrosine kinase/PI3K signaling pathway are common in diffuse midline glioma, although the specific alterations appear to differ between diffuse midline gliomas with H3.3-mutant and H3.1-mutant [104]. *PDGFRA* is involved upstream in the receptor tyrosine kinase-PI3K signaling pathway, and is more common in diffuse midline gliomas with H3.3 mutations [85, 104]. Downstream in the PI3K pathway, mutation in *PIK3CA* [95, 111] and deletion of *PTEN* [112] also occur, and are often associated with concurrent *ACVR1* mutation and a malignant phenotype [105]. Intragenic copy number breakpoints are also more commonly identified in H3 K27M mutant pediatric gliomas compared to wild-type gliomas or H3 G34R/V tumors [113].

H3 K27M Mutations in Other Tumor Types

H3 K27M mutation is also present, albeit rarely, in other types of gliomas, including ependymomas [114–116], pilocytic astrocytomas [117–120], and gangliogliomas [121, 122], but the prognostic value of this mutation in these tumors types is not as clear, and studies suggest that at least some of these may have a better prognosis than infiltrative midline gliomas with H3 K27M [123]. In pediatric supratentorial non-midline diffuse high grade gliomas, the most common *H3F3A* mutation is G34V/R [124], while H3 K27M mutation is exceptionally rare [125]. Because of the uncertainty regarding the implications of H3 K27M mutations in unusual locations (non-midline) or non-infiltrative tumor types, the diagnosis of "diffuse midline glioma, H3 K27M-mutant" is restricted to tumors which are (1) diffuse, (2) involve midline structures, and (3) have an H3 K27M mutation [94].

High Grade Gliomas with H3 G34R/V Mutation, WHO Grade 4

Background

Gliomas are the most common central nervous system tumor in children [126] and nearly half of them are high grade gliomas [1]. Epigenetic modifications of histone play an important role in the pathogenesis and classification of pediatric high grade gliomas. In 2012, two groups independently reported the first highly recurrent mutation in the genes encoding histone 3 variant H3.3 (*H3F3A*) and H3.1 (*HIST1H3B*) in association with pediatric high grade gliomas [81, 82]. H3 is one of four core histones highly conserved in evolution and is critical for maintaining chromatin structure. These mutations occur specifically at two hotspots resulting in amino acid substitution K27M or G34R/V [81, 82]. These two missense mutations have a unique spatial distribution; as previously mentioned, K27M is found in diffuse gliomas involving the midline (i.e., thalamus, brainstem, spinal cord), while G34R/V-driven tumors more often reside in the cerebral hemispheres [81, 82] (Fig. 8.6). Here, we focus on the H3 G34R/V high grade gliomas. They have a better prognosis (2 year survival of 10–30%) than H3 K27M-mutant diffuse midline gliomas, but worse prognosis than IDH-mutant astrocytomas [110, 127].

H3 G34R/V Mutation

The landmark genomic study identified 15 of 48 pediatric high grade gliomas harbor heterozygous H3.3 mutation, with 40% being H3 G34R/V mutation and the rest of them being H3 K27M mutation [81]. H3 G34R/V mutation is found almost

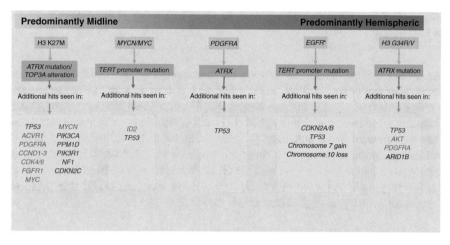

Fig. 8.6 Pediatric high grade glioma genetic characteristics. Genes shown represent common genetic alterations, but the lists are not exhaustive. Green box = common driver alterations. Blue box = most common telomere-maintaining alteration identified to date. Yellow box = additional genetic alterations seen. *EGFR* dinucleotide alterations appear to be limited to bithalamic gliomas and represent a distinct subtype from hemispheric tumors with *EGFR* amplification

exclusively in supratentorial glioblastomas [82, 128], with only rare cases with a non-canonical H3 G34W identified in the spinal cord [85]. The fact that H3 G34R/V-associated high grade gliomas arise in the cerebral hemispheres and mostly in adolescents (median age 18), whereas H3 K27M-associated high grade gliomas arise in midline structures and predominantly in children, suggests a distinct oncogenic mechanism and glioma niche compared to H3 K27M-mutant diffuse midline gliomas [124].

Compared to the H3 K27M mutation, the role of H3 G34R/V is less defined, but its close interaction with lysine 36 (H3K36) has shed light on the pathogenesis. Some studies have suggested that H3 G34R/V mutation leads to decreased tri-methylation of H3K36 (H3K36me3) by inhibiting its specific methyltransferase SETD2 [99, 101], although other studies have had conflicting results [81]. This epigenetic change resulted in a distinct gene expression pattern from that of H3 K27M-mutant gliomas and normal brain [81]. In particular, H3 G34R/V-mutant gliomas demonstrate upregulation of oncogene *MYCN* [129] and a few genes involved in brain development [81]. Loss of *SETD2*, as an alternative mechanism leading to H3K36 hypo-methylation, is also found in pediatric hemispheric high grade gliomas, but not in midline gliomas [128]. Whole-exome sequencing of 35 pediatric hemispheric high grade gliomas revealed 17% harbor G34R/V mutation, and 26% with *SETD2* mutation, with the two genetic alterations being mutually exclusive, raising the possibility that they may play similar roles in the development of these tumors [128].

Genetic Landscape of High Grade Gliomas with H3 G34R/V Mutations

ATRX inactivating mutations are present in the majority of H3 G34R/V-mutant hemispheric gliomas [81, 104], and this finding is correlated with alternative lengthening of telomeres (ALT) in these tumors [80, 81], consistent with the role of ATRX in maintaining telomere stability [130, 131]. H3 G34R/V-mutant gliomas also demonstrate frequent *TP53* mutations [81, 104]. Similar to H3 K27M mutant diffuse midline gliomas, copy number variation involving *PDGFR* amplification is also frequently observed in gliomas with H3 G34R/V mutation [81]. High expression of epidermal growth factor receptor (*EGFR*) is also common, but *EGFR* amplification (typical of primary adult glioblastoma) is rare [132].

Pediatric High Grade Gliomas, Other

Background

Approximately half of pediatric high grade gliomas can be characterized by mutations in H3 [104]. However, the remaining H3-wildtype tumors are highly heterogeneous and harbor genetic alterations that show some overlap with each other. Recent studies based on genome-wide molecular profiling have identified three main molecular subtypes among H3-wildtype and IDH-wildtype pediatric high grade gliomas [133], which can be broadly characterized by the distinct patterns of copy number alterations that are enriched for in each group: *MYCN/MYC* amplification, *PDGFRA* amplification, and *EGFR* amplification [104, 134].

PDGFRA-*Driven*

Platelet-Derived Growth Factor Alpha (PDGFRA) is a receptor upstream of the PI3K signaling pathway, and alterations in *PDGFRA* are seen in approximately 9% of pediatric high grade gliomas [104]. In the absence of H3 mutations, this results in activation of the PI3K and MAPK signaling pathways [111]. *PDGFRA* amplification is somewhat more common in pediatric high grade gliomas from the midline [135, 136], especially in the pons [104], whereas *PDGFRA* mutations are more common in the hemispheres [136]. *PDGFRA* mutations (as opposed to amplification) are more common in older pediatric patients, and patients with *PDGFRA* mutations have a poor prognosis, with an average of less than 2 year-survival [136].

MYCN/MYC-*Driven*

MYCN and *MYC* have been recognized as driver mutations in a large subset of pediatric gliomas lacking H3 mutations [133]. While these tumors are predominantly hemispheric, they can occur in the midline [137, 138]. Histologically and radiologically, these tumors appear largely solid, with only minimal infiltration at the periphery [137, 138]. *MYCN*-amplified tumors shows worse outcomes compared to diffuse midline glioma, H3 K27M-mutant [138]. Among the H3-wildtype pediatric high grade gliomas, *MYCN*-amplified tumors also carry a worse prognosis [133]. Co-amplification of the nearby *ID2* is seen in over half of these tumors [137, 138]. Additional genetic alterations seen in pediatric high grade gliomas with *MYCN* or *MYC* amplification include *TP53* mutations [138]. Interestingly, when pediatric high grade gliomas are divided by methylation profiling patterns, only about half of the tumors in its cluster demonstrate *MYCN* amplification [133], suggesting other genetic or epigenetic alterations may lead to similar methylation profiles and clinical behavior.

EGFR-*Driven*

Whereas *EGFR* amplification is a characteristic copy number alteration of adult glioblastoma, it is rare in pediatric high grade glioma (0–5% *vs* 36–40%) [132, 139]. *EGFR* amplification is found in less than 10% of pediatric high grade gliomas [132, 140], and in a large multi-institutional cohort of pediatric high grade gliomas, only 3% of tumors harbor *EGFR* amplification [141]. However *EGFR* overexpression is present in 80% of these tumors through other mechanisms [140, 142]. It is worth noting that although *EGFR* amplification and mutation are risk factors for poor outcome in adult glioblastoma, its amplification is associated with a longer survival in pediatric high grade gliomas compared to tumors without *EGFR* amplification [133].

Infantile High Grade Gliomas

Rarely, high grade gliomas (as defined by histologic features) occur in infants under 1 year of age. These tumors often demonstrate genetic alterations in the receptor tyrosine kinase/PI3K signaling pathways as driver events. *NTRK* fusions are rare genetic alterations in high grade gliomas, and occur most commonly in infants [104]. Additional alterations that appear to occur more frequently in infants with high grade gliomas include other genes in the receptor tyrosine kinase signaling pathway, including *ALK*, *ROS1*, and *MET* [143]. These tumors are almost always hemispheric, typically occur in children under 1 year of age, and are driven by fusion/amplification, rather than point mutations [143]. Within this group, *ROS1* alterations carry the worst prognosis, with a 5-year survival of 25%, compared to over 40% for patients with *ALK* or *NTRK*-driven tumors [143].

Germline-Mutations Associated with High Grade Glioma Susceptibility

There are several germline mutations that are associated with increased risk of high grade gliomas, predominantly in children and young adults. Below, we describe some of the genetic features of glioblastomas in the better-characterized tumor syndromes, including neurofibromatosis type 1, constitutional mismatch repair deficiency, and Li-Fraumeni syndrome. Additional tumor syndromes associated with high grade gliomas (among other tumors) include tuberous sclerosis (*TSC1* or *TSC2*) [144–146], Ollier disease/Maffucci syndrome (*IDH1* or *IDH2*) [147, 148], and L-2-hydroxyglutaric aciduria (*L2HGDH*) [149, 150].

Neurofibromatosis Type 1

Neurofibromatosis type 1 is driven by mutations in *NF1*. Approximately half of the mutations are germline, and half appear de novo [151]. Inactivation of *NF1* leads to activation of signaling through Ras (Fig. 8.3). While low grade gliomas are more common in this cohort and tend to occur in children, high grade gliomas can occur [152], with a median age of 39 years [153]. When patients with neurofibromatosis type 1 develop high grade gliomas, these tumors demonstrate (in addition to *NF1* mutation) frequent homozygous deletion of *CDKN2A*, seen in over half of these tumors [153]. Additional findings include mutations in T*P53*, as well as mutations in *ATRX*, or less commonly, *TERT* promoter mutations [153].

Li-Fraumeni Syndrome

Li-Fraumeni syndrome was initially identified as a familial syndrome with increased sarcomas, leukemia, and multiple kinds of carcinomas [154]. The syndrome is defined by the presence of germline mutations in *TP53* [155]. Subsequent studies found increased rates of bone and soft tissue neoplasms, breast cancers, brain tumors, leukemias, and adrenocortical tumors [155], although numerous other tumor types have also been described in these families [156]. With regards to the brain tumors, patient with Li-Fraumeni syndrome are at increased risk of diffuse gliomas, choroid plexus carcinomas, medulloblastomas, ependymomas, and other high grade neuroepithelial tumors [157]. When gliomas develop in these patients, they can develop with or without *IDH1/2* mutations [157–159]. When these tumors have *IDH* mutations, the tumors are often lower grade, and demonstrate less common *IDH1/2* mutations, such as R132C or R132G [157, 158]. Glioblastomas were more often *IDH*-wildtype, and demonstrated a larger spectrum of genetic alterations, with frequent *NF1* biallelic inactivation, and some tumors demonstrating alterations in cell cycle and proliferation genes, including *CDKN2A* homozygous deletion, *MYCN* amplification, or *CDK6* amplification [159].

Constitutional Mismatch Repair Deficiency/Turcot Syndrome Type 1

Constitutional mismatch repair deficiency was initially described as a familial tumors syndrome with high rates of familial polyposis and tumors of the central nervous system [160]. This tumor syndrome is also referred to Turcot syndrome type 1, and it is characterized by biallelic germline mutations in one of the mismatch repair genes, *MLH1, PMS2, MSH2,* or *MSH6* [2]. For patients with biallelic germline mutations in one of the mismatch repair genes, the rarity of these tumors means limited samples for genetic studies. In small cohorts, glioblastomas in patients with constitutional mismatch repair deficiency demonstrate frequent *TP53* mutation and homozygous deletion of *CDKN2A* [161]. One case reported concurrent *IDH*-wildtype and *IDH*-mutant tumors within the same pediatric patient [162]. These tumors also create a large number of mutations, and subsequently neo-epitopes, which may make them more responsive to immune checkpoint inhibitors [163–166].

References

1. Ostrom QT, Cioffi G, Gittleman H, et al. CBTRUS statistical report: primary brain and other central nervous system tumors diagnosed in the United States in 2012–2016. Neuro-Oncology. 2019;21(Suppl 5):V1–V100. https://doi.org/10.1093/neuonc/noz150.
2. Louis DN, Ohgaki H, Wiestler OD, et al., editors. WHO classification of tumours of the central nervous system. 4th ed. Lyon: International Agency for Research on Cancer; 2016.
3. Van Den Bent MJ. Interobserver variation of the histopathological diagnosis in clinical trials on glioma: a clinician's perspective. Acta Neuropathol. 2010;120(3):297–304. https://doi.org/10.1007/s00401-010-0725-7.
4. Yan H, Parsons DW, Jin G, et al. IDH1 and IDH2 mutations in gliomas. N Engl J Med. 2009;360(8):765–73. https://doi.org/10.1056/NEJMoa0808710.
5. Parsons DW, Jones S, Zhang X, et al. An integrated genomic analysis of human glioblastoma multiforme. Science (80-). 2008;321(5897):1807–12. https://doi.org/10.1126/science.1164382.

6. McLendon R, Friedman A, Bigner D, et al. Comprehensive genomic characterization defines human glioblastoma genes and core pathways. Nature. 2008;455(7216):1061–8. https://doi.org/10.1038/nature07385.

7. Ohgaki H, Dessen P, Jourde B, et al. Genetic pathways to glioblastoma: a population-based study. Cancer Res. 2004;64(19):6892–9. https://doi.org/10.1158/0008-5472.CAN-04-1337.

8. Körber V, Yang J, Barah P, et al. Evolutionary trajectories of IDH WT glioblastomas reveal a common path of early tumorigenesis instigated years ahead of initial diagnosis. Cancer Cell. 2019;35(4):692–704.e12. https://doi.org/10.1016/j.ccell.2019.02.007.

9. Watanabe K, Tachibana O, Sato K, Yonekawa Y, Kleihues P, Ohgaki H. Overexpression of the EGF receptor and p53 mutations are mutually exclusive in the evolution of primary and secondary glioblastomas. Brain Pathol. 1996;6(3):217–23. https://doi.org/10.1111/j.1750-3639.1996.tb00848.x.

10. Sugawa N, Ekstrand AJ, James CD, Collins VP. Identical splicing of aberrant epidermal growth factor receptor transcripts from amplified rearranged genes in human glioblastomas. Proc Natl Acad Sci U S A. 1990;87(21):8602–6. https://doi.org/10.1073/pnas.87.21.8602.

11. Brennan CW, Verhaak RGW, McKenna A, et al. The somatic genomic landscape of glioblastoma. Cell. 2013;155(2):462. https://doi.org/10.1016/j.cell.2013.09.034.

12. Narita Y, Nagane M, Mishima K, Su Huang HJ, Furnari FB, Cavenee WK. Mutant epidermal growth factor receptor signaling down-regulates p27 through activation of the phosphatidylinositol 3-kinase/Akt pathway in glioblastomas. Cancer Res. 2002;62(22):6764–9.

13. Verhaak RGW, Hoadley KA, Purdom E, et al. Integrated genomic analysis identifies clinically relevant subtypes of glioblastoma characterized by abnormalities in PDGFRA, IDH1, EGFR, and NF1. Cancer Cell. 2010;17(1):98–110. https://doi.org/10.1016/j.ccr.2009.12.020.

14. Tamura M, Gu J, Matsumoto K, Aota SI, Parsons R, Yamada KM. Inhibition of cell migration, spreading, and focal adhesions by tumor suppressor PTEN. Science (80-). 1998;280(5369):1614–7. https://doi.org/10.1126/science.280.5369.1614.

15. Li J, Yen C, Liaw D, et al. PTEN, a putative protein tyrosine phosphatase gene mutated in human brain, breast, and prostate cancer. Science (80-). 1997;275(5308):1943–7. https://doi.org/10.1126/science.275.5308.1943.

16. Reifenberger G, Reifenberger J, Ichimura K, Meltzer PS, Collins VP. Amplification of multiple genes from chromosomal region 12q13-14 in human malignant gliomas: preliminary mapping of the amplicons shows preferential involvement of CDK4, SAS, and MDM2. Cancer Res. 1994;54(16):4299–303.

17. Dimitriadi M, Poulogiannis G, Liu L, et al. p53-independent mechanisms regulate the P2-MDM2 promoter in adult astrocytic tumours. Br J Cancer. 2008;99(7):1144–52. https://doi.org/10.1038/sj.bjc.6604643.

18. Biernat W, Kleihues P, Yonekawa Y, Ohgaki H. Amplification and overexpression of MDM2 in primary (de novo) glioblastomas. J Neuropathol Exp Neurol. 1997;56(2):180–5. https://doi.org/10.1097/00005072-199702000-00009.

19. Ghimenti C, Fiano V, Chiadò-Piat L, Chiò A, Cavalla P, Schiffer D. Deregulation of the p14ARF/Mdm2/p53 pathway and G1/S transition in two glioblastoma sets. J Neuro-Oncol. 2003;61(2):95–102. https://doi.org/10.1023/A:1022127302008.

20. Wang C-L, Wang J-Y, Liu Z-Y, et al. Ubiquitin-specific protease 2a stabilizes MDM4 and facilitates the p53-mediated intrinsic apoptotic pathway in glioblastoma. Carcinogenesis. 2014;35(7):1500–9. https://doi.org/10.1093/carcin/bgu015.

21. Serrano M, Hannon GJ, Beach D. A new regulatory motif in cell-cycle control causing specific inhibition of cyclin D/CDK4. Nature. 1993;366(6456):704–7. https://doi.org/10.1038/366704a0.

22. Ueki K, Ono Y, Henson JW, Efird JT, Von Deimling A, Louis DN. CDKN2/p16 or RB alterations occur in the majority of glioblastomas and are inversely correlated. Cancer Res. 1996;56(1):150–3.

23. Biernat W, Tohma Y, Yonekawa Y, Kleihues P, Ohgaki H. Alterations of cell cycle regulatory genes in primary (de novo) and secondary glioblastomas. Acta Neuropathol. 1997;94(4):303–9. https://doi.org/10.1007/s004010050711.

24. Shampay J, Szostak JW, Blackburn EH. DNA sequences of telomeres maintained in yeast. Nature. 1984;310(5973):154–7. https://doi.org/10.1038/310154a0.
25. Counter CM, Avilion AA, LeFeuvre CE, et al. Telomere shortening associated with chromosome instability is arrested in immortal cells which express telomerase activity. EMBO J. 1992;11(5):1921–9. https://doi.org/10.1002/j.1460-2075.1992.tb05245.x.
26. Harley CB, Futcher AB, Greider CW. Telomeres shorten during ageing of human fibroblasts. Nature. 1990;345(6274):458–60. https://doi.org/10.1038/345458a0.
27. Killela PJ, Reitman ZJ, Jiao Y, et al. TERT promoter mutations occur frequently in gliomas and a subset of tumors derived from cells with low rates of self-renewal. Proc Natl Acad Sci U S A. 2013;110(15):6021–6. https://doi.org/10.1073/pnas.1303607110.
28. Greider CW, Blackburn EH. The telomere terminal transferase of tetrahymena is a ribonucleoprotein enzyme with two kinds of primer specificity. 1987;51. https://www.cell.com/cell/pdf/0092-8674(87)90576-9.pdf. Accessed 22 Aug 2020.
29. Greider CW, Blackburn EH. Identification of a specific telomere terminal transferase activity in tetrahymena extracts. 1985;43. https://www.cell.com/pb/assets/raw/journals/research/cell/libraries/annotated-classics/ACGreider.pdf. Accessed 22 Aug 2020.
30. Greider CW, Blackburn EH. A telomeric sequence in the RNA of Tetrahymena telomerase required for telomere repeat synthesis. Nature. 1989;337(6205):331–7. https://doi.org/10.1038/337331a0.
31. Bell RJA, Rube HT, Kreig A, et al. The transcription factor GABP selectively binds and activates the mutant TERT promoter in cancer. Science (80-). 2015;348(6238):1036–9. https://doi.org/10.1126/science.aab0015.
32. Diplas BH, He X, Brosnan-Cashman JA, et al. The genomic landscape of TERT promoter wildtype-IDH wildtype glioblastoma. Nat Commun. 2018;9(1). https://doi.org/10.1038/s41467-018-04448-6.
33. Bryan TM, Englezou A, Dalla-Pozza L, Dunham MA, Reddel RR. Evidence for an alternative mechanism for maintaining telomere length in human tumors and tumor-derived cell lines. Nat Med. 1997;3(11):1271–4. https://doi.org/10.1038/nm1197-1271.
34. Bryan TM, Englezou A, Gupta J, Bacchetti S, Reddel RR. Telomere elongation in immortal human cells without detectable telomerase activity. EMBO J. 1995;14(17):4240–8. https://doi.org/10.1002/j.1460-2075.1995.tb00098.x.
35. Geisenberger C, Mock A, Warta R, et al. Molecular profiling of long-term survivors identifies a subgroup of glioblastoma characterized by chromosome 19/20 co-gain. Acta Neuropathol. 2015;130(3):419–34. https://doi.org/10.1007/s00401-015-1427-y.
36. Nakamura M, Watanabe T, Yonekawa Y, Kleihues P, Ohgaki H. Promoter methylation of the DNA repair gene MGMT in astrocytomas is frequently associated with G:C → A:T mutations of the TP53 tumor suppressor gene. 2001 undefined. academic.oup.com. https://academic.oup.com/carcin/article-abstract/22/10/1715/2733732. Accessed 22 May 2020.
37. Yang P, Zhang W, Wang Y, et al. IDH mutation and MGMT promoter methylation in glioblastoma: results of a prospective registry. Oncotarget. 2015;6(38):40896–906. https://doi.org/10.18632/oncotarget.5683.
38. Kleinschmidt-Demasters BK, Aisner DL, Birks DK, Foreman NK. Epithelioid GBMs show a high percentage of BRAF V600E mutation. Am J Surg Pathol. 2013;37(5):685–98. https://doi.org/10.1097/PAS.0b013e31827f9c5e.
39. Alexandrescu S, Korshunov A, Lai SH, et al. Epithelioid glioblastomas and anaplastic epithelioid pleomorphic xanthoastrocytomas-same entity or first cousins? Brain Pathol. 2016;26(2):215–23. https://doi.org/10.1111/bpa.12295.
40. Korshunov A, Chavez L, Sharma T, et al. Epithelioid glioblastomas stratify into established diagnostic subsets upon integrated molecular analysis. Brain Pathol. 2018;28(5):656–62. https://doi.org/10.1111/bpa.12566.
41. Nakajima N, Nobusawa S, Nakata S, et al. BRAF V600E, TERT promoter mutations and CDKN2A/B homozygous deletions are frequent in epithelioid glioblastomas: a histological and molecular analysis focusing on intratumoral heterogeneity. Brain Pathol. 2018;28(5):663–73. https://doi.org/10.1111/bpa.12572.

42. Oh JE, Ohta T, Nonoguchi N, et al. Genetic alterations in gliosarcoma and giant cell glioblastoma. Brain Pathol. 2016;26(4):517–22. https://doi.org/10.1111/bpa.12328.
43. Kozak KR, Moody JS. Giant cell glioblastoma: a glioblastoma subtype with distinct epidemiology and superior prognosis. Neuro-Oncology. 2009;11(6):833–41. https://doi.org/10.1215/15228517-2008-123.
44. Ogawa K, Kurose A, Kamataki A, Asano K, Katayama K, Kurotaki H. Giant cell glioblastoma is a distinctive subtype of glioma characterized by vulnerability to DNA damage. Brain Tumor Pathol. 2020;37(1):5–13. https://doi.org/10.1007/s10014-019-00355-w.
45. Shi Z, Li KK, Kwan JSH, et al. Whole-exome sequencing revealed mutational profiles of giant cell glioblastomas. Brain Pathol. 2019;29(6):782–92. https://doi.org/10.1111/bpa.12720.
46. Freije WA, Castro-Vargas FE, Fang Z, et al. Gene expression profiling of gliomas strongly predicts survival. Cancer Res. 2004;64(18):6503–10. https://doi.org/10.1158/0008-5472.CAN-04-0452.
47. Liang Y, Diehn M, Watson N, et al. Gene expression profiling reveals molecularly and clinically distinct subtypes of glioblastoma multiforme. Proc Natl Acad Sci U S A. 2005;102(16):5814–9. https://doi.org/10.1073/pnas.0402870102.
48. Mischel PS, Shai R, Shi T, et al. Identification of molecular subtypes of glioblastoma by gene expression profiling. Oncogene. 2003;22(15):2361–73. https://doi.org/10.1038/sj.onc.1206344.
49. Nutt CL, Mani DR, Betensky RA, et al. Gene expression-based classification of malignant gliomas correlates better with survival than histological classification. Cancer Res. 2003;63(7):1602–7.
50. Patel AP, Tirosh I, Trombetta JJ, et al. Single-cell RNA-seq highlights intratumoral heterogeneity in primary glioblastoma. Science (80-). 2014;344(6190):1396–401. https://doi.org/10.1126/science.1254257.
51. Klughammer J, Kiesel B, Roetzer T, et al. The DNA methylation landscape of glioblastoma disease progression shows extensive heterogeneity in time and space. Nat Med. 2018;24(10):1611–24. https://doi.org/10.1038/s41591-018-0156-x.
52. Wenger A, Vega SF, Kling T, Bontell TO, Jakola AS, Carén H. Intratumor DNA methylation heterogeneity in glioblastoma: implications for DNA methylation-based classification. Neuro-Oncology. 2019;21(5):616–27. https://doi.org/10.1093/neuonc/noz011.
53. Louis DN, et al. cIMPACT-NOW update 6: new entity and diagnostic principle recommendations of the cIMPACT-Utrecht meeting on future CNS tumor classification and grading. Brain Pathol. 2020;30(4):844–56. https://doi.org/10.1111/bpa.12832. Epub 2020 Apr 19. PMID: 32307792
54. Brat DJ, Aldape K, Colman H, et al. cIMPACT-NOW update 5: recommended grading criteria and terminologies for IDH-mutant astrocytomas. Acta Neuropathol. 2020;139(3):603–8. https://doi.org/10.1007/s00401-020-02127-9.
55. Sanson M, Marie Y, Paris S, et al. Isocitrate dehydrogenase 1 codon 132 mutation is an important prognostic biomarker in gliomas. J Clin Oncol. 2009;27(25):4150–4. https://doi.org/10.1200/JCO.2009.21.9832.
56. Songtao Q, Lei Y, Si G, et al. IDH mutations predict longer survival and response to temozolomide in secondary glioblastoma. Cancer Sci. 2012;103(2):269–73. https://doi.org/10.1111/j.1349-7006.2011.02134.x.
57. Lai A, Kharbanda S, Pope WB, et al. Evidence for sequenced molecular evolution of IDH1 mutant glioblastoma from a distinct cell of origin. J Clin Oncol. 2011;29(34):4482–90. https://doi.org/10.1200/JCO.2010.33.8715.
58. Balss J, Meyer J, Mueller W, Korshunov A, Hartmann C, von Deimling A. Analysis of the IDH1 codon 132 mutation in brain tumors. Acta Neuropathol. 2008;116(6):597–602. https://doi.org/10.1007/s00401-008-0455-2.
59. Watanabe T, Nobusawa S, Kleihues P, Ohgaki H. IDH1 mutations are early events in the development of astrocytomas and oligodendrogliomas. Am J Pathol. 2009;174(4):1149–53. https://doi.org/10.2353/ajpath.2009.080958.

60. Turcan S, Rohle D, Goenka A, et al. IDH1 mutation is sufficient to establish the glioma hypermethylator phenotype. Nature. 2012;483(7390):479–83. https://doi.org/10.1038/nature10866.

61. Dang L, White DW, Gross S, et al. Cancer-associated IDH1 mutations produce 2-hydroxyglutarate. Nature. 2009;462(7274):739–44. https://doi.org/10.1038/nature08617.

62. Noushmehr H, Weisenberger DJ, Diefes K, et al. Identification of a CpG island methylator phenotype that defines a distinct subgroup of glioma. Cancer Cell. 2010;17(5):510–22. https://doi.org/10.1016/j.ccr.2010.03.017.

63. Xu W, Yang H, Liu Y, et al. Oncometabolite 2-hydroxyglutarate is a competitive inhibitor of α-ketoglutarate-dependent dioxygenases. Cancer Cell. 2011;19(1):17–30. https://doi.org/10.1016/j.ccr.2010.12.014.

64. Flavahan WA, Drier Y, Liau BB, et al. Insulator dysfunction and oncogene activation in IDH mutant gliomas. Nature. 2016;529(7584):110–4. https://doi.org/10.1038/nature16490.

65. Bai H, Harmanci AS, Erson-Omay EZ, et al. Integrated genomic characterization of IDH1-mutant glioma malignant progression. Nat Genet. 2015;48(1):59–66. https://doi.org/10.1038/ng.3457.

66. Bunse L, Pusch S, Bunse T, et al. Suppression of antitumor T cell immunity by the onco-metabolite (R)-2-hydroxyglutarate. Nat Med. 2018;24(8):1192–203. https://doi.org/10.1038/s41591-018-0095-6.

67. Jiao Y, Killela PJ, Reitman ZJ, et al. Frequent ATRX, CIC, FUBP1 and IDH1 mutations refine the classification of malignant gliomas. Oncotarget. 2012;3(7):709–22. https://doi.org/10.18632/oncotarget.588.

68. Liu X-Y, Gerges N, Korshunov A, et al. Frequent ATRX mutations and loss of expression in adult diffuse astrocytic tumors carrying IDH1/IDH2 and TP53 mutations. Acta Neuropathol. 2012;124(5):615–25. https://doi.org/10.1007/s00401-012-1031-3.

69. Wiestler B, Capper D, Holland-Letz T, et al. ATRX loss refines the classification of anaplastic gliomas and identifies a subgroup of IDH mutant astrocytic tumors with better prognosis. Acta Neuropathol. 2013;3:443–51. https://doi.org/10.1007/s00401-013-1156-z.

70. Ceccarelli M, Barthel FP, Malta TM, et al. Molecular profiling reveals biologically discrete subsets and pathways of progression in diffuse glioma. Cell. 2016;164(3):550–63. https://doi.org/10.1016/j.cell.2015.12.028.

71. Brosnan-Cashman JA, Yuan M, Graham MK, et al. ATRX loss induces multiple hallmarks of the alternative lengthening of telomeres (ALT) phenotype in human glioma cell lines in a cell line-specific manner. Ouellette MM, ed. PLoS One. 2018;13(9):e0204159. https://doi.org/10.1371/journal.pone.0204159.

72. Mukherjee J, Johannessen TC, Ohba S, et al. Mutant IDH1 cooperates with ATRX loss to drive the alternative lengthening of telomere phenotype in glioma. Cancer Res. 2018;78(11):2966–77. https://doi.org/10.1158/0008-5472.CAN-17-2269.

73. Korshunov A, Casalini B, Chavez L, et al. Integrated molecular characterization of IDH-mutant glioblastomas. Neuropathol Appl Neurobiol. 2019;45(2):108–18. https://doi.org/10.1111/nan.12523.

74. Shirahata M, Ono T, Stichel D, et al. Novel, improved grading system(S) for IDH-mutant astrocytic gliomas. Acta Neuropathol. 2018;136(1):153–66. https://doi.org/10.1007/s00401-018-1849-4.

75. Aoki K, Nakamura H, Suzuki H, et al. Prognostic relevance of genetic alterations in diffuse lower-grade gliomas. Neuro-Oncology. 2018;20(1):66–77. https://doi.org/10.1093/neuonc/nox132.

76. Appay R, Dehais C, Maurage C-A, et al. CDKN2A homozygous deletion is a strong adverse prognosis factor in diffuse malignant IDH-mutant gliomas. Neuro-Oncology. 2019;21(12):1519–28. https://doi.org/10.1093/neuonc/noz124.

77. Phillips HS, Kharbanda S, Chen R, et al. Molecular subclasses of high-grade glioma predict prognosis, delineate a pattern of disease progression, and resemble stages in neurogenesis. Cancer Cell. 2006;9(3):157–73. https://doi.org/10.1016/j.ccr.2006.02.019.

78. Albright AL, Packer RJ, Zimmerman R, Rorke LB, Boyett J, Hammond GD. Magnetic resonance scans should replace biopsies for the diagnosis of diffuse brain stem gliomas. Neurosurgery. 1993;33(6):1026–30. https://doi.org/10.1097/00006123-199312000-00010.

79. Roujeau T, Machado G, Garnett MR, et al. Stereotactic biopsy of diffuse pontine lesions in children. J Neurosurg. 2007;107(1 Suppl):1–4. https://doi.org/10.3171/PED-07/07/001.

80. Khuong-Quang D-A, Buczkowicz P, Rakopoulos P, et al. K27M mutation in histone H3.3 defines clinically and biologically distinct subgroups of pediatric diffuse intrinsic pontine gliomas. Acta Neuropathol. 2012;124(3):439–47. https://doi.org/10.1007/s00401-012-0998-0.

81. Schwartzentruber J, Korshunov A, Liu XY, et al. Driver mutations in histone H3.3 and chromatin remodelling genes in paediatric glioblastoma. Nature. 2012;482(7384):226–31. https://doi.org/10.1038/nature10833.

82. Wu G, Broniscer A, McEachron TA, et al. Somatic histone H3 alterations in pediatric diffuse intrinsic pontine gliomas and non-brainstem glioblastomas. Nat Genet. 2012;44(3):251–3. https://doi.org/10.1038/ng.1102.

83. Buczkowicz P, Hoeman C, Rakopoulos P, et al. Genomic analysis of diffuse intrinsic pontine gliomas identifies three molecular subgroups and recurrent activating ACVR1 mutations. Nat Genet. 2014;46(5):451–6. https://doi.org/10.1038/ng.2936.

84. Wu G, Diaz AK, Paugh BS, et al. The genomic landscape of diffuse intrinsic pontine glioma and pediatric non-brainstem high-grade glioma. Nat Genet. 2014;46(5):444–50. https://doi.org/10.1038/ng.2938.

85. Sloan EA, Cooney T, Oberheim Bush NA, et al. Recurrent non-canonical histone H3 mutations in spinal cord diffuse gliomas. Acta Neuropathol. 2019;138(5):877–81. https://doi.org/10.1007/s00401-019-02072-2.

86. Yi S, Choi S, Ah Shin D, et al. Impact of H3.3 K27M mutation on prognosis and survival of grade IV spinal cord Glioma on the basis of new 2016 world health organization classification of the central nervous system. Neurosurgery. 2019;84(5):1072–81. https://doi.org/10.1093/neuros/nyy150.

87. Wang L, Li Z, Zhang M, et al. H3 K27M–mutant diffuse midline gliomas in different anatomical locations. Hum Pathol. 2018;78:89–96. https://doi.org/10.1016/j.humpath.2018.04.015.

88. Aboian MS, Solomon DA, Felton E, et al. Imaging characteristics of pediatric diffuse midline gliomas with histone H3 K27M mutation. Am J Neuroradiol. 2017;38(4):795–800. https://doi.org/10.3174/ajnr.A5076.

89. Karremann M, Gielen GH, Hoffmann M, et al. Diffuse high-grade gliomas with H3 K27M mutations carry a dismal prognosis independent of tumor location. Neuro-Oncology. 2018;20(1):123–31. https://doi.org/10.1093/neuonc/nox149.

90. Jiang H, Yang K, Ren X, et al. Diffuse midline glioma with H3 K27M mutation: a comparison integrating the clinical, radiological, and molecular features between adult and pediatric patients. Neuro-Oncology. 2019;1(August):1–9. https://doi.org/10.1093/neuonc/noz152.

91. Gessi M, Gielen GH, Dreschmann V, Waha A, Pietsch T. High frequency of H3F3A K27M mutations characterizes pediatric and adult high-grade gliomas of the spinal cord. Acta Neuropathol. 2015;130(3):435–7. https://doi.org/10.1007/s00401-015-1463-7.

92. Kleinschmidt-DeMasters BK, Levy JMM. H3 K27M-mutant gliomas in adults vs. children share similar histological features and adverse prognosis. Clin Neuropathol. 2018;37(2):53–63. https://doi.org/10.5414/NP301085.

93. Meyronet D, Esteban-Mader M, Bonnet C, et al. Characteristics of H3 K27M-mutant gliomas in adults. Neuro-Oncology. 2017;19(8):1127–34. https://doi.org/10.1093/neuonc/now274.

94. Louis DN, Giannini C, Capper D, et al. cIMPACT-NOW update 2: diagnostic clarifications for diffuse midline glioma, H3 K27M-mutant and diffuse astrocytoma/anaplastic astrocytoma, IDH-mutant. Acta Neuropathol. 2018;135(4):639–42. https://doi.org/10.1007/s00401-018-1826-y.

95. Buczkowicz P, Bartels U, Bouffet E, Becher O, Hawkins C. Histopathological spectrum of paediatric diffuse intrinsic pontine glioma: diagnostic and therapeutic implications. Acta Neuropathol. 2014;128(4):573–81. https://doi.org/10.1007/s00401-014-1319-6.

96. Lu VM, Alvi MA, McDonald KL, Daniels DJ. Impact of the H3K27M mutation on survival in pediatric high-grade glioma: a systematic review and meta-analysis. J Neurosurg Pediatr. 2019;23(3):308–16. https://doi.org/10.3171/2018.9.PEDS18419.

97. Venneti S, Garimella MT, Sullivan LM, et al. Evaluation of histone 3 lysine 27 trimethylation (H3K27me3) and enhancer of zest 2 (EZH2) in pediatric glial and glioneuronal tumors shows decreased H3K27me3 in H3F3A K27M mutant glioblastomas. Brain Pathol. 2013;23(5):558–64. https://doi.org/10.1111/bpa.12042.

98. Justin N, Zhang Y, Tarricone C, et al. Structural basis of oncogenic histone H3K27M inhibition of human polycomb repressive complex 2. Nat Commun. 2016;7:11316. https://doi.org/10.1038/ncomms11316.

99. Chan KM, Fang D, Gan H, et al. The histone H3.3K27M mutation in pediatric glioma reprograms H3K27 methylation and gene expression. Genes Dev. 2013;27(9):985–90. https://doi.org/10.1101/gad.217778.113.

100. Bender S, Tang Y, Lindroth AM, et al. Reduced H3K27me3 and DNA hypomethylation are major drivers of gene expression in K27M mutant pediatric high-grade gliomas. Cancer Cell. 2013;24(5):660–72. https://doi.org/10.1016/j.ccr.2013.10.006.

101. Lewis PW, Müller MM, Koletsky MS, et al. Inhibition of PRC2 activity by a gain-of-function H3 mutation found in pediatric glioblastoma. Science (80-). 2013;340(6134):857–61. https://doi.org/10.1126/science.1232245.

102. Harutyunyan AS, Krug B, Chen H, et al. H3K27M induces defective chromatin spread of PRC2-mediated repressive H3K27me2/me3 and is essential for glioma tumorigenesis. Nat Commun. 2019;10(1). https://doi.org/10.1038/s41467-019-09140-x.

103. Reddington JP, Perricone SM, Nestor CE, et al. Redistribution of H3K27me3 upon DNA hypomethylation results in de-repression of Polycomb target genes. Genome Biol. 2013;14(3):R25. https://doi.org/10.1186/gb-2013-14-3-r25.

104. Mackay A, Burford A, Carvalho D, et al. Integrated molecular meta-analysis of 1,000 pediatric high-grade and diffuse intrinsic pontine glioma. Cancer Cell. 2017;32(4):520–537.e5. https://doi.org/10.1016/j.ccell.2017.08.017.

105. Fontebasso AM, Papillon-Cavanagh S, Schwartzentruber J, et al. Recurrent somatic mutations in ACVR1 in pediatric midline high-grade astrocytoma. Nat Genet. 2014;46(5):462–6. https://doi.org/10.1038/ng.2950.

106. Taylor KR, Mackay A, Truffaux N, et al. Recurrent activating ACVR1 mutations in diffuse intrinsic pontine glioma. Nat Genet. 2014;46(5):457–61. https://doi.org/10.1038/ng.2925.

107. Fortin J, Tian R, Zarrabi I, et al. Mutant ACVR1 arrests glial cell differentiation to drive tumorigenesis in pediatric gliomas. Cancer Cell. 2020;37(3):308–323.e12. https://doi.org/10.1016/j.ccell.2020.02.002.

108. Carvalho D, Taylor KR, Olaciregui NG, et al. ALK2 inhibitors display beneficial effects in preclinical models of ACVR1 mutant diffuse intrinsic pontine glioma. Commun Biol. 2019;2(1):156. https://doi.org/10.1038/s42003-019-0420-8.

109. Zhang L, Chen LH, Wan H, et al. Exome sequencing identifies somatic gain-of-function PPM1D mutations in brainstem gliomas. Nat Genet. 2014;46(7):726–30. https://doi.org/10.1038/ng.2995.

110. Paugh BS, Qu C, Jones C, et al. Integrated molecular genetic profiling of pediatric high-grade gliomas reveals key differences with the adult disease. J Clin Oncol. 2010;28(18):3061–8. https://doi.org/10.1200/JCO.2009.26.7252.

111. Paugh BS, Zhu X, Qu C, et al. Novel oncogenic PDGFRA mutations in pediatric high-grade gliomas. Cancer Res. 2013;73(20):6219–29. https://doi.org/10.1158/0008-5472.CAN-13-1491.

112. Paugh BS, Broniscer A, Qu C, et al. Genome-wide analyses identify recurrent amplifications of receptor tyrosine kinases and cell-cycle regulatory genes in diffuse intrinsic pontine glioma. J Clin Oncol. 2011;29(30):3999–4006. https://doi.org/10.1200/JCO.2011.35.5677.

113. Carvalho D, Mackay A, Bjerke L, et al. The prognostic role of intragenic copy number breakpoints and identification of novel fusion genes in paediatric high grade glioma. Acta Neuropathol Commun. 2014;2(1):23. https://doi.org/10.1186/2051-5960-2-23.

114. Ebrahimi A, Skardelly M, Schuhmann MU, et al. High frequency of H3 K27M mutations in adult midline gliomas. J Cancer Res Clin Oncol. 2019;145(4):839–50. https://doi.org/10.1007/s00432-018-02836-5.

115. Gessi M, Capper D, Sahm F, et al. Evidence of H3 K27M mutations in posterior fossa ependymomas. Acta Neuropathol. 2016;132(4):635–7. https://doi.org/10.1007/s00401-016-1608-3.

116. Ryall S, Guzman M, Elbabaa SK, et al. H3 K27M mutations are extremely rare in posterior fossa group A ependymoma. Childs Nerv Syst. 2017;33(7):1047–51. https://doi.org/10.1007/s00381-017-3481-3.

117. Rodriguez FJ, Brosnan-Cashman JA, Allen SJ, et al. Alternative lengthening of telomeres, ATRX loss and H3-K27M mutations in histologically defined pilocytic astrocytoma with anaplasia. Brain Pathol. 2019;29(1):126–40. https://doi.org/10.1111/bpa.12646.

118. Hochart A, Escande F, Rocourt N, et al. Long survival in a child with a mutated K27M-H3.3 pilocytic astrocytoma. Ann Clin Transl Neurol. 2015;2(4):439–43. https://doi.org/10.1002/acn3.184.

119. Morita S, Nitta M, Muragaki Y, et al. Brainstem pilocytic astrocytoma with H3 K27M mutation: case report. J Neurosurg. 2018;129(3):593–7. https://doi.org/10.3171/2017.4.JNS162443.

120. Orillac C, Thomas C, Dastagirzada Y, et al. Pilocytic astrocytoma and glioneuronal tumor with histone H3 K27M mutation. Acta Neuropathol Commun. 2016;4(1):84. https://doi.org/10.1186/s40478-016-0361-0.

121. Pagès M, Beccaria K, Boddaert N, et al. Co-occurrence of histone H3 K27M and BRAF V600E mutations in paediatric midline grade I ganglioglioma. Brain Pathol. 2018;28(1):103–11. https://doi.org/10.1111/bpa.12473.

122. Kleinschmidt-DeMasters BK, Donson A, Foreman NK, Dorris K. H3 K27M mutation in gangliogliomas can be associated with poor prognosis. Brain Pathol. 2017;27(6):846–50. https://doi.org/10.1111/bpa.12455.

123. Pratt D, Natarajan SK, Banda A, et al. Circumscribed/non-diffuse histology confers a better prognosis in H3K27M-mutant gliomas. Acta Neuropathol. 2018;135(2):299–301. https://doi.org/10.1007/s00401-018-1805-3.

124. Sturm D, Witt H, Hovestadt V, et al. Hotspot mutations in H3F3A and IDH1 define distinct epigenetic and biological subgroups of glioblastoma. Cancer Cell. 2012;22(4):425–37. https://doi.org/10.1016/j.ccr.2012.08.024.

125. López G, Oberheim Bush NA, Berger MS, Perry A, Solomon DA. Diffuse non-midline glioma with H3F3A K27M mutation: a prognostic and treatment dilemma. Acta Neuropathol Commun. 2017;5(1):38. https://doi.org/10.1186/s40478-017-0440-x.

126. Linabery AM, Ross JA. Trends in childhood cancer incidence in the U.S. (1992–2004). Cancer. 2008;112(2):416–32. https://doi.org/10.1002/cncr.23169.

127. Heideman RL, Kuttesch J, Gajjar AJ, et al. Supratentorial malignant gliomas in childhood: a single institution perspective. Cancer. 1997;80(3):497–504. https://doi.org/10.1002/(SICI)1097-0142(19970801)80:3<497::AID-CNCR18>3.0.CO;2-S.

128. Fontebasso AM, Schwartzentruber J, Khuong-Quang DA, et al. Mutations in SETD2 and genes affecting histone H3K36 methylation target hemispheric high-grade gliomas. Acta Neuropathol. 2013;125(5):659–69. https://doi.org/10.1007/s00401-013-1095-8.

129. Bjerke L, Mackay A, Nandhabalan M, et al. Histone H3.3 mutations drive pediatric glioblastoma through upregulation of MYCN. Cancer Discov. 2013;3(5):512–9. https://doi.org/10.1158/2159-8290.CD-12-0426.

130. Heaphy CM, De Wilde RF, Jiao Y, et al. Altered telomeres in tumors with ATRX and DAXX mutations. Science (80-). 2011;333(6041):425. https://doi.org/10.1126/science.1207313.

131. Wong LH, McGhie JD, Sim M, et al. ATRX interacts with H3.3 in maintaining telomere structural integrity in pluripotent embryonic stem cells. Genome Res. 2010;20(3):351–60. https://doi.org/10.1101/gr.101477.109.

132. Sung T, Miller DC, Hayes RL, Alonso M, Yee H, Newcomb EW. Preferential inactivation of the p53 tumor suppressor pathway and lack of EGFR amplification distinguish de

novo high grade pediatric astrocytomas from de novo adult astrocytomas. Brain Pathol. 2000;10(2):249–59. https://doi.org/10.1111/j.1750-3639.2000.tb00258.x.

133. Korshunov A, Schrimpf D, Ryzhova M, et al. H3-/IDH-wild type pediatric glioblastoma is comprised of molecularly and prognostically distinct subtypes with associated oncogenic drivers. Acta Neuropathol. 2017;134(3):507–16. https://doi.org/10.1007/s00401-017-1710-1.

134. Bax DA, Mackay A, Little SE, et al. A distinct spectrum of copy number aberrations in pediatric high-grade gliomas. Clin Cancer Res. 2010;16(13):3368–77. https://doi.org/10.1158/1078-0432.CCR-10-0438.

135. Zarghooni M, Bartels U, Lee E, et al. Whole-genome profiling of pediatric diffuse intrinsic pontine gliomas highlights platelet-derived growth factor receptor α and poly (ADP-ribose) polymerase as potential therapeutic targets. J Clin Oncol. 2010;28(8):1337–44. https://doi.org/10.1200/JCO.2009.25.5463.

136. Koschmann C, Zamler D, MacKay A, et al. Characterizing and targeting PDGFRA alterations in pediatric high-grade glioma. Oncotarget. 2016;7(40):65696–706. https://doi.org/10.18632/oncotarget.11602.

137. Tauziède-Espariat A, Debily MA, Castel D, et al. The pediatric supratentorial MYCN-amplified high-grade gliomas methylation class presents the same radiological, histopathological and molecular features as their pontine counterparts. Acta Neuropathol Commun. 2020;8(1):104. https://doi.org/10.1186/s40478-020-00974-x.

138. Tauziède-Espariat A, Debily MA, Castel D, et al. An integrative radiological, histopathological and molecular analysis of pediatric pontine histone-wildtype glioma with MYCN amplification (HGG-MYCN). Acta Neuropathol Commun. 2019;7(1):10. https://doi.org/10.1186/s40478-019-0738-y.

139. Suri V, Das P, Jain A, et al. Pediatric glioblastomas: a histopathological and molecular genetic study. Neuro-Oncology. 2009;11(3):274–80. https://doi.org/10.1215/15228517-2008-092.

140. Bredel M, Pollack IF, Hamilton RL, James CD. Epidermal growth factor receptor expression and gene amplification in high-grade non-brainstem gliomas of childhood. Clin Cancer Res. 1999;5(7):1786–92.

141. Pollack IF, Hamilton RL, James CD, et al. Rarity of PTEN deletions and EGFR amplification in malignant gliomas of childhood: results from the Children's Cancer Group 945 cohort. J Neurosurg Pediatr. 2006;105(5):418–24. https://doi.org/10.3171/ped.2006.105.5.418.

142. Li G, Mitra SS, Monje M, et al. Expression of epidermal growth factor variant III (EGFRvIII) in pediatric diffuse intrinsic pontine gliomas. J Neuro-Oncol. 2012;108(3):395–402. https://doi.org/10.1007/s11060-012-0842-3.

143. Guerreiro Stucklin AS, Ryall S, Fukuoka K, et al. Alterations in ALK/ROS1/NTRK/MET drive a group of infantile hemispheric gliomas. Nat Commun. 2019;10(1). https://doi.org/10.1038/s41467-019-12187-5.

144. Reyes D, Prayson R. Glioblastoma in the setting of tuberous sclerosis. J Clin Neurosci. 2015;22(5):907–8. https://doi.org/10.1016/j.jocn.2014.12.001.

145. Vignoli A, Lesma E, Alfano RM, et al. Glioblastoma multiforme in a child with tuberous sclerosis complex. Am J Med Genet A. 2015;167(10):2388–93. https://doi.org/10.1002/ajmg.a.37158.

146. Azriel A, Gogos A, Rogers TW, Moscovici S, Lo P, Drummond K. Glioblastoma in a patient with tuberous sclerosis. J Clin Neurosci. 2019;60:153–5. https://doi.org/10.1016/j.jocn.2018.10.083.

147. Kendroud S, Groepper D, Choi YJ. Apparent germline IDH1 mutation in a patient with ollier disease and glioblastomas: a case report. Neurology. 2019;92 (15 Supplement):1.9–042.

148. Gajavelli S, Nakhla J, Nasser R, Yassari R, Weidenheim KM, Graber J. Ollier disease with anaplastic astrocytoma: a review of the literature and a unique case. Surg Neurol Int. 2016;7(24):S607–11. https://doi.org/10.4103/2152-7806.189731.

149. Patay Z, Orr BA, Shulkin BL, et al. Successive distinct high-grade gliomas in L-2-hydroxyglutaric aciduria. J Inherit Metab Dis. 2015;38(2):273–7. https://doi.org/10.1007/s10545-014-9782-8.

150. Tan AP, Mankad K. Intraventricular glioblastoma multiforme in a child with L2-hydroxyglutaric aciduria. World Neurosurg. 2018;110:288–90. https://doi.org/10.1016/j.wneu.2017.11.106.
151. Ars E, Kruyer H, Morell M, et al. Recurrent mutations in the NF1 gene are common among neurofibromatosis type 1 patients. J Med Genet. 2003;40(6):e82. https://doi.org/10.1136/jmg.40.6.e82.
152. Huttner AJ, Kieran MW, Yao X, et al. Clinicopathologic study of glioblastoma in children with neurofibromatosis type 1. Pediatr Blood Cancer. 2010;54(7):n/a-n/a. https://doi.org/10.1002/pbc.22462.
153. D'Angelo F, Ceccarelli M, Tala, et al. The molecular landscape of glioma in patients with neurofibromatosis 1. Nat Med. 2019;25(1):176–87. https://doi.org/10.1038/s41591-018-0263-8.
154. Li FP, Fraumeni JF. Soft-tissue sarcomas, breast cancer, and other neoplasms. A familial syndrome? Ann Intern Med. 1969;71(4):747–52. https://doi.org/10.7326/0003-4819-71-4-747.
155. Birch JM, Hartley AL, Tricker KJ, et al. Prevalence and diversity of constitutional mutations in the p53 gene among 21 Li-Fraumeni families. Cancer Res. 1994;54(5):1298–304.
156. Nichols KE, Malkin D, Garber JE, Fraumeni JFJ, Li FP. Germ-line p53 mutations predispose to a wide spectrum of early-onset cancers. Cancer Epidemiol Biomarkers Prev. 2001;10(2):83–7.
157. Zapotocky M, Misove A, Vlckova M, et al. Gene-14. Unique molecular and clinical features of Li-Fraumeni syndrome associated brain tumours. Neuro-Oncology. 2019;21(Suppl_2):ii84. https://doi.org/10.1093/neuonc/noz036.085.
158. Watanabe T, Anne AE, Ae V, et al. Selective acquisition of IDH1 R132C mutations in astrocytomas associated with Li-Fraumeni syndrome. https://doi.org/10.1007/s00401-009-0528-x.
159. Sloan EA, Hilz S, Gupta R, et al. Gliomas arising in the setting of Li-Fraumeni syndrome stratify into two molecular subgroups with divergent clinicopathologic features. Acta Neuropathol. 2020;139:953–7. https://doi.org/10.1007/s00401-020-02144-8.
160. Turcot J, Després JP, St. Pierre F. Malignant tumors of the central nervous system associated with familial polyposis of the colon – report of two cases. Dis Colon Rectum. 1959;2(5):465–8. https://doi.org/10.1007/BF02616938.
161. Leung SY, Yuen ST, Chan TL, et al. Chromosomal instability and p53 inactivation are required for genesis of glioblastoma but not for colorectal cancer in patients with germline mismatch repair gene mutation. Oncogene. 2000;19(35):4079–83. https://doi.org/10.1038/sj.onc.1203740.
162. Galuppini F, Opocher E, Tabori U, et al. Concomitant IDH wild-type glioblastoma and IDH1 -mutant anaplastic astrocytoma in a patient with constitutional mismatch repair deficiency syndrome. Neuropathol Appl Neurobiol. 2018;44(2):233–9. https://doi.org/10.1111/nan.12450.
163. AlHarbi M, Ali Mobark N, AlMubarak L, et al. Durable response to nivolumab in a pediatric patient with refractory glioblastoma and constitutional biallelic mismatch repair deficiency. Oncologist. 2018;23(12):1401–6. https://doi.org/10.1634/theoncologist.2018-0163.
164. Larouche V, Atkinson J, Albrecht S, et al. Sustained complete response of recurrent glioblastoma to combined checkpoint inhibition in a young patient with constitutional mismatch repair deficiency. Pediatr Blood Cancer. 2018;65(12):e27389. https://doi.org/10.1002/pbc.27389.
165. Westdorp H, Kolders S, Hoogerbrugge N, de Vries IJM, Jongmans MCJ, Schreibelt G. Immunotherapy holds the key to cancer treatment and prevention in constitutional mismatch repair deficiency (CMMRD) syndrome. Cancer Lett. 2017;403:159–64. https://doi.org/10.1016/j.canlet.2017.06.018.
166. Pavelka Z, Zitterbart K, Nosková H, Bajčiová V, Slabý O, Štěrba J. Effective immunotherapy of glioblastoma in an adolescent with constitutional mismatch repair-deficiency syndrome. Klin Onkol. 2019;32(1):70–4. https://doi.org/10.14735/amko201970.

Additional Resources

Ellison D, Love S, Chimelli LMC, et al., editors. Neuropathology. 3rd ed. Mosby Ltd.; 2012.

Kleinschmidt-DeMasters BK, Tihan T, Rodriguez F, editors. Diagnostic pathology: neuropathology. 3rd ed. Elsevier; 2021.

Louis DN, Ohgaki H, Wiestler OD, et al., editors. WHO classification of tumours of the central nervous system. 4th ed. Lyon: International Agency for Research on Cancer; 2016.

Love S, Perry A, Ironside J, Budka H, editors. Greenfield's neuropathology. 9th ed. CRC Press; 2015.

Chapter 9
Genomic Heterogeneity of Aggressive Pediatric and Adult Diffuse Astrocytomas

Christopher R. Pierson and Diana L. Thomas

Introduction

Glioblastoma, formerly known as glioblastoma multiforme (GBM), is remarkable for its degree of both morphologic and genomic heterogeneity. In children and adults, as defined by the World Health Organization (WHO), GBM is a grade IV neoplasm with a diffusely infiltrative growth pattern populated by cells showing predominately astrocytic differentiation [1]. As discussed in previous chapters, GBM features prominent nuclear atypia and cellular pleomorphism, as well as high tumor cell mitotic activity accompanied by microvascular proliferation and/or necrosis. As its former name indicates, GBM may include one or many morphologic patterns within a single tumor. In some tumors, this reflects underlying clonal evolution with newly acquired genetic changes in tumor cell subpopulations [2–5]. Even more variable than GBM morphology is the range of genomic heterogeneity, creating multiple molecular signatures that define tumor behavior, prognosis and treatment response independent of tumor histopathology. Furthermore, while pediatric and adult glioblastoma share many histopathologic similarities, they are unequivocally biologically distinct neoplasms. In many pediatric and adult gliomas, the molecular subgroup is a better predictor of tumor behavior than histologic grade. In particular, WHO grade II or III diffuse astrocytomas lacking morphologic features associated with GBM (microvascular proliferation and necrosis), but with

C. R. Pierson
Department of Pathology, Nationwide Children's Hospital, Columbus, OH, USA
e-mail: christopher.pierson@nationwidechildrens.org

D. L. Thomas (✉)
Department of Pathology, The Ohio State University and Nationwide Children's Hospital, Columbus, OH, USA
e-mail: diana.thomas@nationwidechildrens.org

© The Author(s), under exclusive license to Springer Nature Switzerland AG 2021
J. J. Otero, A. P. Becker (eds.), *Precision Molecular Pathology of Glioblastoma*, Molecular Pathology Library, https://doi.org/10.1007/978-3-030-69170-7_9

certain defined molecular alterations, should be considered GBM for prognostic and therapeutic purposes due to their expected WHO grade IV-like behavior. The focus of this chapter centers on the genomic heterogeneity and pathobiology of aggressive pediatric and adult diffuse astrocytomas with WHO grade IV behavior independent of morphologic features.

Pediatric GBM is traditionally grouped with anaplastic astrocytoma and diffuse intrinsic pontine glioma (DIPG) as the high-grade gliomas (HGG). HGG are common in adults, whereas in children low-grade gliomas are more common; nonetheless, HGG are estimated to occur in slightly less than 1 per 100,000 children each year [6]. In adults, HGG commonly arise in the supratentorial structures, while in children GBMs tend to be located in midline structures such as the thalamus, spinal cord and pons. DIPGs are diffusely infiltrative astrocytomas of the pons and many, but not all, fulfill WHO histological criteria for HGG. DIPGs occur nearly exclusively in children with a peak age incidence of 6–8 years, while HGG located in supratentorial structures occur in older children with a peak incidence in adolescence. Overall, pediatric HGG patients have a grim prognosis with less than 5% of GBM patients surviving 5 years after diagnosis while DIPG patients have a median survival that is less than 1 year after diagnosis [7]. Curiously, infants with histologic HGG tend to show better clinical outcomes than older children do and can have a more favorable clinical course than infants with low-grade gliomas, suggesting that infant HGG has unique biological properties [8, 9]. Clearly, there is a pressing need to better understand the biology of these tumors and for effective therapeutic approaches for pediatric GBM.

The diversity of pediatric GBM biology was recognized relatively recently when advanced molecular testing techniques were applied in collaborative studies that amassed large cohorts of GBM. The data generated from these studies has clearly shown that childhood GBM is a distinct disease from adult GBM. Furthermore, these studies conclusively demonstrate that pediatric GBMs develop following unique molecular pathogenetic events, which are different from those that underlie the pathogenesis of their adult counterparts. The advances in genomic and epigenetic profiling have further permitted the characterization of these molecular and cellular differences with precision, expanding our understanding of GBM biology, and resolving distinct subgroups of GBM that arise in children and adults.

The application of molecular profiling to large cohorts of tumor samples from pediatric and adult GBM patients has identified a number of recurrent genomic and epigenetic alterations that subdivide GBM into discrete subgroups, which correlate with various clinical parameters including patient age and tumor location [10, 11]. Moving away from traditional histologic classification of GBM, this chapter will provide an overview of the key features of adult and pediatric GBM based on gene expression profiling, genomic structural variations, copy number alterations (CNA), DNA methylation profiling, and the mutational landscape of single nucleotide variants (SNV). This will be followed by a description of adult and pediatric GBM subgroups that have emerged from these studies.

Gene Expression Profiling

Genome wide gene expression profiling microarray studies analyzing large cohorts of adult and pediatric GBM have been used to characterize differentially expressed genes that successfully identified subgroups within GBM that were not discernable histopathologically. The gene expression profiling studies were initially performed using cohorts of adult GBMs and subsequently the gene expression subgroups were identified in pediatric GBM (Table 9.1). The first gene expression profiling study in GBM identified three subgroups according to the functions of signature genes: proneural, mesenchymal and proliferative, with different patient outcomes including longer survival of patients with proneural tumors [12]. Subsequent gene expression profiling performed on the Cancer Genome Atlas (TCGA) tumor cohort characterized four different groups of GBM in adults: proneural, neural, classical and

Table 9.1 Molecular features and subgroups of pediatric and adult HGG

	Pediatric	Adult
Gene expression profiling	*PDGFRA* Proneural (G-CIMP+ and G-CIMP-) (very rare) Neural (very rare) Classical (very rare)	Proneural (G-CIMP+ and G-CIMP-) Neural Classical Mesenchymal
Structural variants	*ALK, ROS1, NTRK1/2/3, MET* fusions *BCOR* fusions Deletion in *PTEN, RB1, CDKN2C, NF1, TP53* Amplification in *CDK4, CDK6, PDGFRA, MET, MDM2* *EGFR* exon 20 insertions (bithalamic glioma)	*EGFRvIII* Deletions in *PTEN, RB1, CDKN2C, NF1, TP53* Amplification in *CDK4, CDK6, PDGFRA, MET, MDM2* *FGFR-TACC* fusions
Copy number alterations	Chromosome 1q gain *PDGFRA* amplification MYC and MYCN amplification *CDK4, CDK6* amplification *CCND1, CCND2* or *CCDN3* amplification EGFR amplification (very rare)	*EGFR* amplification *CDKN2A/B* homozygous loss Chromosome +7/−10 *PDGFRA* amplification
DNA methylation profiling clusters	RTK I K27 G34 *MYCN* amplified	IDH Mesenchymal RTK II
Single nucleotide variants	*PDGFRA* *FGFR1* *BRAF V600E* *PIK3CA/PIK3R1* *TP53* *H3F3A* mutations (H3 K27M, H3 G34R/V) *HIST1H3B* K27M	*IDH1/IDH2* *ATRX* *EGFR* *TERT* promoter *BRAF* V600E *PTEN* *TP53* H3 K27M, H3 G34R/V (very rare)

mesenchymal [13, 14]. The identified gene expression subtypes showed additional correlative molecular features. For instance, the proneural subtype had alterations in *PDGFRA* or *IDH*, while *NF1* mutations occurred in mesenchymal tumors and *EGFR* mutations appeared in the classical subgroup. In time, proneural GBMs were distinguished as glioma-CpG island methylator phenotype (G-CIMP)-positive and G-CIMP-negative subtypes based on *IDH1* mutation status and DNA methylation pattern. The favorable prognosis of proneural GBM was discovered to apply to the G-CIMP-positive subset, while C-CIMP-negative and mesenchymal tumors have a less favorable prognosis [13].

Gene expression profiling studies of pediatric GBM demonstrated significant differences from adult GBM, suggesting distinct pathogenetic mechanisms are responsible (Table 9.1) [15, 16]. A prominent proportion of pediatric GBMs show enhanced *PDGFRA*-driven gene expression, which is not surprising given the high frequency of *PDGFRA* gene amplification in pediatric tumors [10, 16–19]. Gene expression profiling studies demonstrated similarities between some midline GBMs and DIPG, foreshadowing their common pathogenesis prior to sequencing studies that later showed these tumor types share *H3F3A* K27M mutations [10, 20, 21].

Genomic Structural Changes and Copy Number Alterations

The genome of pediatric GBM may contain a number of DNA copy number alterations (CNA) and structural alterations, although these changes tend to occur less frequently in childhood than in adult GBM (Table 9.1) [18, 19, 22, 23]. These alterations are variable in degree and range from simple rearrangements to complicated structural anomalies due to chromothripsis [20, 22]. Most pediatric GBM have about five large CNAs along with amplifications and focal deletions, although some cases have fewer and some lack detectable CNAs altogether [16, 19]. Chromosome 1q gain occurs at a higher rate than it does in adult GBM and may be enriched in *H3F3A* G34-mutated tumors [16]. As more pediatric GBM are studied and technological advances continue, smaller CNAs can be resolved and more complex structural rearrangements and gene fusion events can be identified.

A number of CNA including gain and losses of chromosomes as well as chromothripsis have been described in adult GBM [13, 24, 25]. Total CNAs are associated with overall prognosis in a number of diffuse glioma subsets [26, 27]. *IDH*-wildtype GBM have uniformly high total CNA and poor outcomes [27]. Increased numbers of total CNAs in addition to *CDK4* amplification and *CDKN2A/B* homozygous deletion are found in *IDH*-mutant low grade gliomas that show rapid progression and outcomes similar to *IDH*-wildtype GBM [26].

EGFR amplification is an important copy number alteration occurring in approximately 40–50% of adult glioblastomas, mostly primary glioblastomas arising in the fourth decade of life and beyond, and the level of amplification may correlate with patient outcomes [28]. *EGFR* is positioned on the short arm of chromosome 7 (7p12) and encodes a cell surface receptor tyrosine kinase (EGFR/Erb-1). EGFR is activated following binding of its growth factor ligand to the extracellular domain of

EGFR with subsequent phosphorylation of its intracellular tyrosine kinase domain. Activation of EGFR initiates signal transduction of the Ras/MAPK and PI3K/Akt pathways resulting in increased DNA transcription, cellular proliferation, angiogenesis and resistance to apoptosis (Fig. 9.1) [29]. Importantly, *EGFR* amplification is defined as high level gains of the *EGFR* gene by validated molecular techniques including fluorescence in-situ hybridization (FISH), next generation sequencing (NGS) and array comparative genomic hybridization (aCGH). Low level gains such as trisomy of chromosome 7 are insufficient for designation as an EGFR amplified tumor. Currently immunohistochemistry for EGFR protein expression is not considered a reproducible test for detection of *EGFR* amplification.

Gain of chromosome 7 (+7) and loss of chromosome 10 (−10) are the most common chromosomal aberrations and occur in about 80% of GBMs arising in adults and especially older adults however, these chromosomal changes are far less common in pediatric GBM [13, 24]. As such, GBMs in the receptor tyrosine kinase (RTK) II or classical methylation cluster are significantly more likely to harbor +7+ and −10, while they are distinctly uncommon in proneural GBM and GBM bearing *IDH* or *H3F3A* mutations.

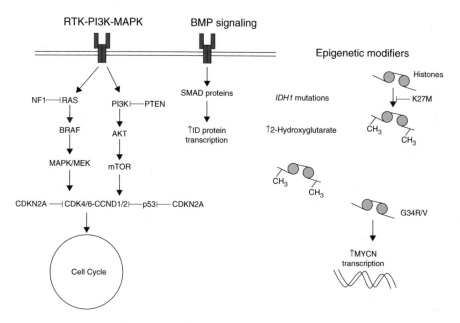

Fig. 9.1 Summary of key signaling pathways and epigenetic modifiers involved in the pathogenesis of glioblastoma. Multiple genes encoding proteins in the RTK-PI3K-MAPK signaling axis, which are involved in cell growth, proliferation and survival, are affected in GBM. The involved proteins include RTK on the cell membrane and its downstream mediators such as PI3K, RAS and BRAF. The function of negative regulators of this axis such as NF1 and PTEN may be ablated due to gene mutations. BMP signaling is upregulated in a subset of DIPGs. Diverse epigenetic modifiers are important to the pathogenesis of GBM and include direct mutations of histone 3 proteins (K27M, G34R/V) and indirect alterations such as *IDH* mutations that generate the oncometabolite, 2-hydroxyglutarate, which alters methylation marks on chromatic and in turn, gene expression

Grade II or III *IDH*-wildtype diffuse astrocytomas with combined loss of whole chromosome 10 and gain of whole chromosome 7 typically exhibit WHO grade IV behavior and overall poor survival. Some studies suggest that partial gains (e.g. +7q or +7p) or partial losses (e.g. -10q or -10p) in diffuse astrocytomas can also predict aggressive clinical behavior, but larger studies are needed to confirm [30–34]. The −10/+7 molecular profile has also been reported, together with *BRAF* V600E and homozygous loss of *CDKN2A/B* in pleomorphic xanthroastrocytoma, a potential morphologic mimic of GBM on small biopies, and therefore caution should be used in diagnostically challenging cases [31, 35].

Interchromosomal and intrachromosomal rearrangements are present in most GBMs [36]. In adult GBM certain rearrangements result in the upregulation of growth factor signaling pathways, including *EGFR*, resulting in the activation of TRK-PI3K-MAPK signaling. The well-known *EGFR* variant III (*EGFRvIII*) of adult RTK II GBM occurs following an intrachromosomal deletion that removes exons 2–7 leading to the constitutive activation of *EGFR* signaling [37]. In adults, intragenic deletions or missense mutations involve exons that encode the extracellular domains of EGFR that are often present on the amplified *EGFR* allele [13, 38]. EGFR alterations are far less common in pediatric GBM (about 4%) but they seem to characterize an emerging and possible new subtype [9, 39]. This new subtype consists of bithalamic gliomas that characteristically show small in-frame insertions involving exon 20 of *EGFR*, which encodes the intracellular tyrosine kinase domain, as well as *TP53* mutations and unlike unilateral thalamic GBMs, only rare histone H3 mutations [39]. These bithalamic GBM also have a distinct genome methylation profile that shows some overlap with the RTK III methylation subclass of IDH wild-type GBM, a poorly defined group of cerebral pediatric GBMs with EGFR amplification. Nonetheless this suggests that bithalamic tumors may arise due epigenetic mechanisms distinct from other pediatric GBM [39]. Other commonly altered RTKs include a subset of *PDGFRA* amplified GBMs in adults and children, which show intrachromosomal deletions that generate constitutively active PDGFRA [19, 36, 40–42].

Intrachromosomal CNA can be identified in the majority of pediatric HGG and when present in high number, are associated with shorter overall survival, while their absence is associated with a longer overall survival. These data are likely driven by the infant age group, which is known to have a better clinical outcome relative to older children [23, 43–45]. GBMs bearing *H3F3A* K27M have increased numbers of intrachromosomal CNA [23]. The DNA breakpoints of most intrachromosomal structural alterations disrupt the involved gene, leading to a loss of function, which provides a mechanism by which tumor cells can obviate the effects of tumor suppressor genes such as *RB1* and *NF1*, among others [23].

Most chromosomal structural alterations are damaging; however, others may result in a gain of function that promotes gliomagenesis. If the breakpoints come together and align in a single reading frame a novel protein with new function may result and promote gliomagenesis. These so-called gene fusions can be detected using RNA sequencing and are seen in about 50% of childhood GBMs and they are particularly prominent in infant GBMs [22]. A high proportion of fusion genes are potentially targetable therapeutically [8, 22, 23, 45, 46]. It should be noted that many of the discovered gene fusions are not unique to GBM or even limited to HGG [8, 47, 48].

A large international cohort study defined three subgroups of infant GBM and Group 1 was primarily made up of HGG hemispheric tumors bearing fusions of the receptor tyrosine kinase genes *ALK, ROS1, NTRK1/2/3* or *MET* [8]. Rearrangements involving any one of the three *NTRK* genes may generate fusions with a variety of partner genes in pediatric HGG and are believed to constitutively activate MAPK, PI3K and PKC signaling pathways potentiating cell growth and proliferation and aiding cell survival [22, 47]. *MET* fusions are less common than *NTRK* fusions and they also activate MAPK signaling [46].

Gene fusions can also occur in adult gliomas although they are much less common. In frame *FGFR3-TACC3* fusions are found in WHO grade II to IV diffuse astrocytomas and these patients may benefit from targeted therapy with *FGFR* inhibitors [49–51]. The *FGFR3-TACC3* fusion protein results in a constitutively active tyrosine kinase domain and promotes aneuploidy [52]. These tumors share morphologic similarities including monomorphous ovoid nuclei, nuclear palisading, and thin capillary networks [50]. Identification of these tumors can be challenging without a full molecular panel or directed sequencing; however, immunoreactivity with an FGFR3 antibody shows promise as a robust screening method [50, 53]. The *FGFR3-TACC3* fusion gene appears to be mutually exclusive with *IDH* mutations and *EGFR, PDGFR* and *MET* amplification in adult GBM [49, 54].

Not all of the identified gene fusions involve receptor tyrosine kinase genes. BCL6 corepressor protein is encoded by *BCOR* and mediates transcriptional silencing of genes epigenetically via its interactions with histone deacetylases and the polycomb repressive complex [55, 56]. *BCOR* alterations are known to occur in other types of brain tumors and in some tumor types arising outside of the central nervous system (CNS) [57, 58]. *BCOR* fusions are uncommon and not unique to HGG, but are associated with aggressive clinical behavior [59, 60]. While most reported fusions result in a gain-of-function such as enhanced kinase activity, *BCOR* fusions may drive gliomagenesis by leading to a loss of function in BCOR and its fusion partner [59, 60]. This would be consistent with a tumor suppressor effect as described with *BCOR* nonsense, frameshift, deletions and splice site mutations encountered in histone *H3*-mutated gliomas [9, 22, 56].

Focal copy number alterations in pediatric GBM overlap with those occurring in adult GBM and include deletions in *PTEN, RB1, CDKN2C, NF1* and *TP53* as well as amplifications of *CDK4, CDK6, PDGFRA, MET* and *MDM2* among others [61]. *PDGFRA* and either *MYC* or *MYCN* amplifications are more frequent in pediatric than adult GBMs [10, 19, 62]. *PDGFRA* amplifications are prominent in DIPG, particularly in DIPG with H3 mutations and are enriched in radiation-induced gliomas [10, 17, 18, 63]. The H3 K27-mutant midline gliomas show a high frequency of *PDGFRA* amplifications and are enriched for proneural gene expression signature [10]. In DIPG *PDGFRA* amplifications are associated with a dismal prognosis and resistance to therapy [17, 62]. *MYCN* amplifications are seen in a subgroup of DIPGs that have hypermethylated genomes [64].

DNA Methylation Profiling

Hypermethylation of gene promoter regions is an epigenetic mechanism of gene silencing that impacts the expression of many types of genes including tumor suppressors and others that are important in cell cycle regulation and additional key functions of neoplastic cells. The most widely used application of DNA methylation testing concerns assessing the methylation status of the *MGMT* promoter, which regulates the expression of O^6-methylguanine methyltransferase. *MGMT* promoter methylation silences gene expression and limits the ability of the cell to repair DNA damage induced by alkylating agent chemotherapy, particularly temozolomide. *MGMT* promoter methylation is a useful biomarker in adult GBM patients and is responsible in part to the improved outcome in *IDH*-mutant tumors, but its predictive capacity in pediatric patients is unclear [65–67].

DNA microarray technology facilitated the evaluation of the pediatric GBM methylome in an unbiased, genome-wide fashion and led to the delineation of tumor subgroups that differed from those identified in adult GBM patients. Early studies of the GBM methylome in adults discerned a group in the proneural gene expression class with hypermethylation at many loci and coexisting *IDH1* alterations, i.e. the so-called G-CIMP-positive tumors [68]. A more comprehensive genome-wide DNA methylation analysis of a large cohort of pediatric and adult GBMs demonstrated that, when correlated with gene expression profiles, mutational status, and DNA copy number alterations, GBMs cluster into six distinct groups known as IDH, K27, G34, receptor tyrosine kinase (RTK) I and II, and mesenchymal that also align with clinicopathologic parameters including patient age and tumor location (Table 9.1) [10]. These GBM methylation groups correlated relatively well with the groups identified by expression profiling, underscoring the importance of epigenetic mechanisms in the pathogenesis of GBM [14].

A subset of GBM in the RTK I cluster arose in some pediatric patients and included *PDGFRA* amplified, G-CIMP-negative, proneural GBMs [10, 14]. Tumors in the IDH cluster were G-CIMP-positive, proneural gliomas that primarily arose in young adults; however, some adolescents were also affected (median age 40 years; range 13–71 years). GBMs clustering in the mesenchymal methylation group arose in patients with a wide range of ages that included elderly patients and showed a mesenchymal pattern of gene expression as well as *PTEN* and *NF1* mutations. The RTK II cluster showed classical gene expression profile, chromosome 7 loss and chromosome 10 gain as well as *EGFR* alterations and had a median age 58 years with no pediatric GBM patients.

Two of the methylation clusters, K27 and G34, preferentially occurred in the pediatric population and were tightly correlated with the presence of *H3F3A* mutations at positions K27 and G34 [10]. *H3F3A* encodes the replication-independent histone, H3.3, which primarily binds transcriptionally activated genes and telomeres. H3.3 is often methylated at or near the mutated residues, which affects DNA methylation likely by altering DNA accessibility, so *H3F3A* mutations can account for the global changes in methylation noted in these GBM subgroups. The two main recurrent *H3F3A* mutations are only seven amino acid residues apart in the H3.3 protein, yet they result in significant differences in terms of methylation profile, tumor location in the central nervous system and clinical setting. Tumors in the K27 cluster predominately arise in the midline central nervous system structures including the thalami and pons of children with a median age of about 10 years, while G34 tumors tend to occur in the cerebral hemispheres of adolescents with a median age of 18 years [10, 20, 69]. *IDH1* and *H3F3A* mutations are mutually exclusive between individual GBMs, yet it seems that each favors tumor development by impairing the normal differentiation program of progenitor cells using a pathogenetic mechanism with some overlapping features [70]. Mutant IDH1 protein produces 2-hydroxyglutarate, an oncometabolite, which is responsible for the increased global methylation pattern of CIMP-positive, proneural GBM. Increased intracellular 2-hydroxyglutarate concentrations increases H3 K27 methylation, inhibiting progenitor cell differentiation by increasing the expression of stem cell markers while decreasing the expression of differentiation-related markers. In a related fashion, H3.3 bearing mutations at G34 favors tumor formation in part, by reducing the expression of the important developmental transcription factor, OLIG2, due to hypermethylation of its gene locus [10].

The K27 and G34 mutations are associated with different methylation patterns [10]. Despite the increased methylation of the *OLIG2* locus, tumors in the G34 subgroup show global hypomethylation across the genome, which is prominent in non-promoter regions, including subtelomeric zones near the ends of chromosomes, suggesting that the loss of methylation in subtelomeric areas may have a role in the alternative lengthening of telomeres observed in tumors with *H3F3A* G34 mutations [10, 20]. The marked differences in methylation signatures correlate with tumor location and clinical course, suggesting that the mechanisms by which these epigenetic alterations lead to tumor formation are critical to understand and will likely be a focus of intense study for years to come.

Approximately half of pediatric GBMs have recurrent somatic mutations in histone H3 genes or in *IDH1/2*. The remaining GBMs are a diverse group; however, genome-wide molecular profiling studies are starting to delineate new subgroups, identify potential previously unrecognized therapeutic targets, and also reveal prognostic information in these tumors [67, 71]. A cohort of H3-/*IDH*-wild type pediatric GBM was comprehensively studied using an integrated approach that included genome-wide DNA methylation, targeted mutation detection and CNA and identified three molecular subtypes with different genomic and epigenetic signatures and clinical behavior. These were designated as MYCN, enriched for *MYCN* amplification, RTK 1, enriched for *PDGFRA* amplification and RTK 2, enriched for *EGFR* amplification [67]. The MYCN subtype of H3-/*IDH*- wild type tumors is the most aggressive with a survival period that is similar to that of H3 K27M mutant tumors [10, 67, 69]. These tumors tend to arise outside of the brainstem, have high level *MYCN* amplification, which often co-exist with amplification of Inhibitor of DNA Binding 2 (*ID2*) and recurrent *TP53* mutations [67, 72]. The RTK 1 subtype of H3-/*IDH*- wild type tumors frequently bear *PDGRFA* amplification and a paucity of other typical GBM cytogenetic alterations [67]. The RTK I tumors have an intermediate prognosis. H3-/*IDH*- wild type tumors of the RTK 2 subtype differed from adult GBM despite having *EGFR* amplification in common. Tumors in this subtype showed an overall 5 year survival at close to 50% and the methylation profile differed from all adult GBM variants [67].

Korshunov et al. studied a large cohort of pediatric GBMs using genome wide DNA methylation and candidate gene screening, which revealed that a subset of histologically high-grade tumors showed a methylation profile similar to low-grade glioma or pleomorphic xanthoastrocytoma [71]. These tumors had a favorable prognosis and often had *BRAF* V600E mutations with chromosome 9p21 loss leading to homozygous deletion of the *CDKN2A* tumor suppressor locus [71]. *BRAF* V600E is common in PXA, but its frequency is unknown in genuine GBM and the histologic features of PXA, especially anaplastic PXA, overlap with GBM, so molecular testing will likely be required to distinguish these entities with confidence [73, 74].

Single Nucleotide Variants and Deregulated Cancer Cell Signaling Pathways

The 2016 update of the WHO Classification of CNS tumors subclassifies diffuse astrocytomas including GBM by *IDH* mutation status. This distinction principally pertains to adults and a subset of older adolescents as pediatric gliomas are very rarely *IDH*-driven [61, 75, 76]. As with essentially all GBM, *IDH*-wildtype and *IDH*-mutant tumors are not distinguishable on morphology despite their distinct biologic differences. *IDH*-wildtype GBM are significantly more common with poorer overall survival [77–79]. *IDH*-mutant glioblastomas account for 10% or fewer of all GBM [1, 80]. *IDH1* and *IDH2*-mutant GBM are associated with younger age at presentation, DNA hypermethylation phenotype, and overall better outcome compared to *IDH*-wildtype GBM [78, 80]. Despite a better overall prognosis, *IDH*-mutant GBM are designated WHO grade IV as most patients develop tumor progression and die of their disease.

Patient outcomes are highly variable among *IDH*-mutant GBM suggesting genomic heterogeneity among *IDH*-mutant tumors [81]. Furthermore, histologic grading of *IDH*-mutant tumors and assessment of mitotic activity are not good predictors of overall patient outcomes [80, 82]. Analysis of large cohorts of *IDH*-mutant GBM has revealed a strong association between patient outcome and distinct copy number alterations, particularly homozygous deletion of *CDKN2A/B* [30, 80, 83–85]. As a result, the Consortium to Inform Molecular and Practical Approaches to CNS Tumor Taxonomy (cIMPACT-NOW) issued recommendations to reflect the current understanding of *IDH*-mutant tumors. The recommended integrated diagnosis for *IDH*-mutant diffuse astrocytomas with either necrosis, microvascular proliferation, or *CDKN2A/B* homozygous deletion is "astrocytoma, IDH-mutant, grade 4" [86, 87]. *CDKN2A/B* homozygous deletions are also found in approximately 60% of *IDH*-wildtype GBM but do not carry the same prognostic significance.

Sequencing technology has evolved and an ever-increasing number of recurrent somatic SNV have been identified, sometimes at low frequency, and occasionally in genes that were not expected to be involved in gliomagenesis or even in neoplasia. Adult and pediatric GBM share common SNV in a number of genes, although some are unique to one patient population or the other [61]. Nonetheless, the gene mutations encountered in pediatric GBM perturb many of the same cancer cell pathways

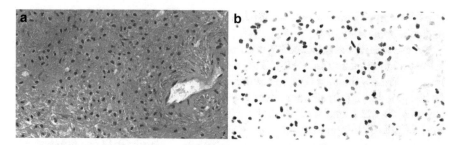

Fig. 9.2 Brainstem glioma in a 65 year old. (**a**) H&E stained section showing a diffusely infiltrative astrocytoma without mitoses, microvascular proliferation or necrosis. (**b**) Immunostaining for H3 K27M is consistent with mutation status that was later confirmed by NGS

and functions that are altered in adult GBM, which include RTK-RAS-PI3K pathway, p53 function, cell cycle control and epigenetic regulation [10, 20, 88].

The genetic hallmarks of adult *IDH*-wildtype and *IDH*-mutant tumors are described in previous chapters and will only be briefly mentioned here. Common somatic mutations in adult *IDH*-wildtype GBM include *TERT, PTEN, EGFR, TP53, NF1, PIC3CA*, and *RB1*, while ATRX mutations are very rare [1, 89, 90]. *TP53* and *ATRX* mutations are found in 70–80% of *IDH*-mutant GBM while *EGFR and PTEN* mutations are exceedingly rare [89, 90]. *H3F3A* K27M mutations are uncommon in adults but do occur in older patients over, and immunohistochemistry or other testing should be considered in diffusely infiltrating midline gliomas presenting at any age (Fig. 9.2) [91, 92].

Mutations in the promoter region of *telomerase reverse transcriptase (TERT)* gene are frequent in *IDH*-wildtype GBM and less frequent among *IDH*-mutant GBM but do occur [89, 90]. Telomerase, a reverse transcriptase that maintains telomere length, is inactive in mature somatic cells in adulthood but activated in glioma cells via defined *TERT* promoter mutations. Mutations in the *TERT* promoter result in upregulation of telomerase complex activity and elongation of telomere length leading to uncontrolled cell proliferation. The most common mutations in the *TERT* promoter, C228T and C250T are located upstream of the *TERT* start site. Recent studies have elucidated the prognostic significance of *TERT* promoter mutations by demonstrating patients with WHO grade II and III *IDH*-wildtype gliomas often follow a similar clinical course as *IDH*-wildtype WHO grade IV GBM [93]. As such, the cIMPACT-NOW working group has recommended an integrated diagnosis of "diffuse glioma, WHO grade II or III, with molecular features of glioblastoma". This recommended terminology refers to diffuse astrocytomas of any grade with *TERT* promoter mutations, *EGFR* amplification, and/ or chromosome +7/−10. Long-term follow-up studies have subsequently validated this recommendation and conclude diffuse astrocytomas with *TERT* promoter mutations are as clinically aggressive as WHO grade IV tumors [93]. It is important to note that *TERT* promoter mutations are not limited to *IDH*-wildtype or *IDH*-mutant GBM. *TERT* promoter mutations are very common in adult oligodendrogliomas and occasionally found in pleomorphic xanthoastrocytoma, ependymoma, and low-grade glioneuronal tumors [94, 95]. *TERT* promoter mutations frequently occur together with *EGFR* amplification or chromosome −10/+7. TERT promoter mutations are rare in the pediatric population [96].

As mentioned, the RTK *EGFR*, commonly mutated to potentiate cell growth and proliferation signaling in adult GBM is rare in childhood GBM. *PDGFRA* is the most commonly mutated RTK in children and is seen in about 30% of all childhood HGGs [16, 42, 63]. In addition, pediatric GBMs may activate the RTK-RAS-PI3K pathway via *MET* amplification or by activating mutations in other RTKs, such as *FGFR1* [22, 97]. Inhibiting RTK is an attractive treatment strategy; however, the degree of intratumoral heterogeneity within a given pediatric GBM can be considerable, suggesting that a given tumor would have a population of drug resistant cells prior to initiating therapy, since not all of the cells in the tumor may contain the therapeutic target [18].

GBM cells can also activate RTK-RAS-PI3K signaling downstream of RTK. BRAF binds RAS, transducing the cell growth signal of the RTK-RAS-PI3K pathway. Amino acid position 600 of *BRAF* is a hotspot where the amino acid, valine is substituted for a glutamic acid, due to a point mutation in the *BRAF* gene. *BRAF* V600E mutations are present in a subset of pediatric and adult HGG [20, 73, 98]. PI3K is activated in pediatric GBM by either gain of function mutations in *PIK3CA*, which encodes the catalytic subunit of PI3K or by deregulating mutations in *PIK3R1*, which encodes the regulatory subunit of PI3K [97]. In adults, PI3K activity may be upregulated following biallelic inactivation of the tumor suppressor, *PTEN* but this is uncommon in pediatric HGG [24, 88].

Loss of cell cycle control is a key event in pediatric GBM pathogenesis. Approximately half of all pediatric HGGs bear mutations in *TP53*, which encodes p53, a critical tumor suppressor that regulates cell division and survival (apoptosis) as well as senescence [20, 22]. Proteins of the cyclin-CDK complex phosphorylate RB at the G1 checkpoint, which is a key cell cycle regulatory step that commits a cell to synthesize DNA and divide. Amplifications of *CDK4*, *CDK6* or the cyclin genes, *CCND1*, *CCND2* or *CCDN3* have been identified in pediatric HGG and have potential to allow a tumor cell to divide by overcoming the checkpoint [18]. Homozygous deletion of *CDKN2A*, which encodes the tumor suppressor proteins, p14 and p16, occurs in about a quarter of non-brainstem HGGs [61]. CDK4 and CDK6 normally induce the cell to divide by promoting the completion of the cell cycle. The p16 protein normally binds CDK4 and CDK6, blocking their ability to stimulate cell proliferation. The p14 protein normally binds p53, protecting it from degradation. Therefore, *CDKN2A* deletions can profoundly deregulate the cell cycle; losing the effect of p14 on p53 effectively removes a brake on the cell cycle, while losing the effect of p16 on CDK4 and CDK6 is akin to depressing a cell cycle accelerator. Curiously, unlike in adults, *RB1* biallelic loss of function mutations are uncommon childhood GBM, although about 30% of tumors show chromosome 13q loss, which contains the *RB1* locus [20, 22].

Perhaps the most unexpected finding to come from genome-wide sequencing studies of large cohorts of pediatric GBM and DIPG was the prominence of SNV in H3 histone family 3A (*H3F3A*) and histone cluster 1, H3b (*HIST1H3B*) genes, encoding H3.3 and H3.1, respectively [20, 22, 99]. *H3F3A* and *HIST1H3B* mutations are extremely rare adult GBM and likely contribute to the significant differences in HGG pathogenesis in adults and children and the previously discussed differences in the tumor methylome between these patients.

Histone H3 mutations in GBM occur at two amino acid positions resulting in the lysine at position 27 being replaced by methionine (K27M) or the glycine at position 34 being replaced by either arginine (G34R) or valine (G34V) [20, 22]. Ten identical genes encode histone 3.1, but *HIST1H3B* is most commonly mutated in GBM [20, 22]. Nucleosomes are disrupted during the cell cycle and the cell synthesizes H3.3 in all phases of the cell cycle to replace lost histones [100, 101]. The role of H3.1 and H3.2 is to package newly synthesized DNA and these histones are synthesized during S phase of the cell cycle [100, 101].

K27M mutations in *H3F3A* or *HIST1H3B* are both encountered in DIPG and other midline gliomas that arise in the spinal cord of thalamus [10, 20, 22, 69, 99]. H3.3 K27M bearing tumors have an age of onset at about 6 years and a median survival period of about 12 months [22, 64, 102–104]. H3.3 K27M can be identified in about two-thirds of DIPGs and in two-thirds of midline line HGGs arising outside of the brainstem [9]. Curiously, co-segregating alterations differ by tumor location with *PDGFRA* alterations tending to occur in the pons and *FGFR* alterations occurring in the thalamus [9, 102]. A meta-analysis showed H3.3 K27M tumors located in the pons are associated with *CCND2* amplification, while non-brainstem midline tumors have amplification of *CDK4* [9]. A complex rearrangement in H3.3 K27M tumors was found resulting in amplification at 17p11.2 increasing *TOP3A* copy number and expression and the loss of the distal aspect of 17p, which contains the *TP53* locus [9]. *TOP3A* is a topoisomerase with roles in homologous recombination and alternative lengthening of telomeres and in H3.3 K27M DIPG *TOP3A* alterations are mutually exclusive with *ATRX* mutations, providing another means gliomas can use to activate alternative lengthening of telomeres [105].

HIST1H3B K27M mutations are associated with a younger age of onset and a slightly longer survival period [22, 64, 102, 103]. H3.1 K27M tumors are restricted to the pons. DIPGs harboring a *HIST1H3B* mutation also often have coexisting somatic activating mutations in *ACVR1* suggesting that BMP signaling is important to their pathogenesis [22, 64, 102, 103]. *ACVR1* mutations are exclusive to DIPG, predominate in females and enriched in tumors bearing histone 3.1 gene mutations [22]. *ACVR1* mutations phosphorylate and activate SMAD proteins, increasing the expression of downstream effectors including the ID protein family members ID1 and ID2 [64, 102, 103]. Histone H3 and *ACVR1* mutations seem to work cooperatively to enhance the downstream effect on ID proteins [64]. H3.1 K27M tumors are enriched for mutations that activate the PI3K pathway, including *PIK3CA* and *PIK3R1* and are associated with *BCOR* mutations [9].

G34 mutations do not occur in *HIST1H3B* and GBMs bearing *H3F3A* G34 mutations have distinct clinical profiles. In contrast to tumors with K27M, G34 tumors arise in the peripheral aspect of the cerebral hemispheres and not in midline structures. In addition, G34 tumors tend to occur in older children with an onset at about 13 years and patients survive longer (about 24 months) [22, 64, 102–104]. The differences in the timing of diagnosis and the survival interval likely stem from the differences in tumor location with brainstem and midline tumors presenting earlier than hemispheric tumors and affording little opportunity for maximal safe surgical resection, which may be achieved in hemispheric tumors. G34R/V and K27M mutations predominate in children but can be identified in adult GBMs, with the latter seen in the majority of young adults with thalamic tumors [10, 106]. H3.3 G34R/V mutations co-segregate with *ATRX* and *TP53* mutations and are the only pediatric GBM subgroup to commonly show *MGMT* promoter methylation [71]. A meta-analysis showed frequent loss of chromosomal arms at 3q, 4q, 5q and 18q, with loss of 4q31.3 leading to loss of *FBXW7*, a candidate tumor suppressor [9, 107]. *FBXW7* is part of the SCF-like ubiquitin ligase complex that targets MYC and MYCN for proteasomal destruction, so the loss of *FBXW7* in H3.3 G34R/V tumors would enhance the life span of MYC proteins [108]. MYCN expression is also increased in H3.3 G34R/V tumors due to the effects of H3 K36me3, making MYNC a critically important driver of this subgroup [109].

K27M and G34R/V have structural consequences that impact histone function in gene transcription. These amino acids occur in the amino-terminal tail of the histone H3 protein and the post-translation modification of the tail region has regulatory roles on gene transcription and chromatin compaction and structure that are important in cell differentiation [101, 110, 111]. The post-translational modifications of the tail region are diverse and include acetylation, methylation and ubiquitylation of lysine residues, phosphorylation of serine of threonine residues and methylation of arginine residues. A wide scope of enzymes catalyze these changes and include writers which add and erasers which remove these moieties, while readers are effector proteins that bind to chromatin according to the pattern of moieties on the histone tail, thereby regulating the location of the transcriptional complexes to chromatin [101, 112]. These readers, writers and erasers are increasingly recognized as critical to the pathogenesis of many different types of cancer arising in diverse tissues [113, 114].

The role histone mutations play in gliomagenesis is not entirely understood. The lysine that is abrogated due to the K27M mutation is normally either methylated or acetylated. When K27 is trimethylated (K27me3) it interacts with the polycomb repressive complex 2 (PCR2) to selectively repress gene transcription. The K27M mutation effectively removes the ability of this key methylation site on the histone tail leading to general hypomethylation followed by an upregulation in gene expression with PRC2 target gene derepression, which together potentiate gliomagenesis [21, 101, 115]. The impact of the K27M mutation is likely enormous to tumor cell biology. Immunostaining shows that the H3 K27M mutant protein is often detectable in nearly 100% of tumor cells, which suggests that tumor cells bearing H3 K27M are favorably selected within the overall tumor cell population [69, 99]. Furthermore, H3 K27M protein expression makes up a small fraction of the total H3 protein in the tumor cell, yet these tumors essentially show a total loss of K27me3, indicating a trans-dominant-negative effect across all isoforms of wild type H3 occurs in the tumor cell [97, 116]. K27 seems to hold a critical place in pediatric gliomagenesis because mutations in the writers or erasers of each post-translationally modified lysine residue of the histone tail has been identified except for K27, which is only impacted by direct mutation [20, 22].

H3 bearing G34R/V mutations also impair epigenetic regulation of gene expression but the mechanism is different from that of K27M. The G34 residue does not undergo a direct post-translational modification it is, however, near the lysine residue at position 36 (K36), which is directly modified. In support of the importance of K36 methylation, *SETD2,* the methyltransferase that writes the methyl marks on K36, is mutated in about 10% of pediatric GBMs [22, 102, 104]. K36 trimethylation activates gene transcription, and also impacts alternative splicing and DNA repair [97]. G34R is associated with reduced K36 trimethylation on one mutant allele so the dominant effect over total cell histone H3 as seen in the presence of K27M, does not occur [97, 115]. Experiments show that histone 3 bearing G34V binds genes associated with stem cell maintenance and cortical development with the oncogene, *MYCN*, showing significant G34 binding and increased expression [97, 109]. The presence of *MYNC* amplification and G34R/V are mutually exclusive [109]. The differential impact of G34R and G34V substitution on gliomagenesis are not fully characterized, although the arginine in G34R has the potential to undergo post-translational modifications, suggesting that there may be differences [97, 117].

Mutations in other chromatin regulatory genes besides histone genes have been identified in pediatric GBM including members of the *MLL* (writers), *KDM* (erasers) and *CHD* (chromatin remodelers) gene families [20, 22]. *ATRX* and *DAXX* encode histone chaperones that load histone H3.3 to regions of heterochromatin located at telomeres and co-segregate with H3 G34R/and they are mutated in up to 20% of pediatric HGG [20, 22, 102]. Tumors with *H3F3A* and *ATRX* or *DAXX* mutations show telomerase independent alternative lengthening of telomeres [20]. *TERT* promoter mutations are rare in pediatric GBMs but are present in most adult GBMs and in adults they are mutually exclusive to *ATRX* mutations [22, 118].

Future Directions and Conclusion

The amount of information regarding the origin and drivers of GBM has vastly expanded in the past several years. It is now well understood that molecular features better predict tumor behavior and patient outcomes compared to traditional histologic classification, especially on small or non-representative tumor biopsies. Many of the recently recognized molecular subgroups will undoubtedly find their way into future revisions of the WHO classification. Despite our increasing understanding of distinct glioma molecular signatures, it is important to emphasize that a combined approach of morphologic evaluation and molecular characterization improves diagnostic classification for glioblastoma [119].

In this timeframe, we have also learned that pediatric and adult GBMs are significantly different biologically. Adult and pediatric GBM are truly a group of diseases that arise due to unique pathogenetic mechanisms, but how can this new information be applied in patient care to improve outcomes for this dreaded, essentially fatal disease? First, we cannot expect that data from clinical trials of adults GBM patients will properly inform trials in pediatric GBM patients. This approach was used in the past and as a result, trials were largely ineffective with only slight improvements in clinical outcome. Clearly, these biological differences in adult and pediatric disease cannot be overlooked. Second, we now realize that each pediatric GBM subgroup and some adult subgroups appear to have distinct cellular origins and oncogenic drivers, which may be therapeutically targetable [120, 121]. It is hoped that tumors targeted with such specificity would lead to more effective therapies and perhaps fewer treatment-related complications. We now realize that past clinical trials, which enrolled an unselected patient population and failed to take GBM subgroups into account, were underpowered to detect subgroup-specific efficacy [120]. Taking tumor subgroup into account when tailoring therapeutic approach is critical as clinical behavior is more accurately predicted by tumor biology, which is reflected in genetic and epigenetic alterations rather than tumor grade or various clinical parameters [120].

BRAF V600E mutations, while not unique to GBM, are known to activate MAPK signaling and BRAF inhibiting drugs such as the MEK-inhibitors and *BRAF* V600E-specific inhibitors have shown success [122]. RTK gene fusions are now recognized as key drivers of tumor biology in a significant subset of GBMs, particularly those arising in infants and these alterations are potential therapeutic targets [8, 123–125]. DIPG and midline GBM with histone 3 mutations may be treatable with drugs that are epigenetic modifiers with activity toward histone demethylases and deacetylases [126, 127]. *IDH* mutations are rare in pediatric GBM and likely represent the tail end of the peak incidence in adulthood. As such patients with these tumors may be better off enrolling on separate strata of adult clinical trials [120].

It is hoped that as our knowledge of the molecular alterations driving tumor biology grows, new molecular targets will continue to emerge and innovative agents can be designed to allow even more refined subgroup specific therapies and trials with the goal of improving patient outcome.

References

1. Louis DN, et al. WHO classification of tumours of the central nervous system. Revised 4th ed. Lyon: International Agency for Research on Cancer; 2016.
2. Fujisawa H, et al. Acquisition of the glioblastoma phenotype during astrocytoma progression is associated with loss of heterozygosity on 10q25-qter. Am J Pathol. 1999;155(2):387–94.
3. Georgescu M-M, Olar A. Genetic and histologic spatiotemporal evolution of recurrent, multifocal, multicentric and metastatic glioblastoma. Acta Neuropathol Commun. 2020;8(1):10.
4. Consortium TG. Glioma through the looking GLASS: molecular evolution of diffuse gliomas and the Glioma Longitudinal Analysis Consortium. Neuro Oncol. 2018;20(7):873–84.
5. Riehmer V, et al. Genomic profiling reveals distinctive molecular relapse patterns in IDH1/2 wild-type glioblastoma. Genes Chromosom Cancer. 2014;53(7):589–605.

6. Ostrom QT, et al. CBTRUS Statistical Report: Primary brain and other central nervous system tumors diagnosed in the United States in 2012–2016. Neuro Oncol. 2019;21(Supplement_5):v1–v100.
7. Stupp R, et al. Effects of radiotherapy with concomitant and adjuvant temozolomide versus radiotherapy alone on survival in glioblastoma in a randomised phase III study: 5-year analysis of the EORTC-NCIC trial. Lancet Oncol. 2009;10(5):459–66.
8. Guerreiro Stucklin AS, et al. Alterations in ALK/ROS1/NTRK/MET drive a group of infantile hemispheric gliomas. Nat Commun. 2019;10(1):4343.
9. Mackay A, et al. Integrated molecular meta-analysis of 1,000 pediatric high-grade and diffuse intrinsic pontine glioma. Cancer Cell. 2017;32(4):520–537 e5.
10. Sturm D, et al. Hotspot mutations in H3F3A and IDH1 define distinct epigenetic and biological subgroups of glioblastoma. Cancer Cell. 2012;22(4):425–37.
11. Jones DTW, et al. Molecular characteristics and therapeutic vulnerabilities across paediatric solid tumours. Nat Rev Cancer. 2019;19(8):420–38.
12. Phillips HS, et al. Molecular subclasses of high-grade glioma predict prognosis, delineate a pattern of disease progression, and resemble stages in neurogenesis. Cancer Cell. 2006;9(3):157–73.
13. Brennan CW, et al. The somatic genomic landscape of glioblastoma. Cell. 2013;155(2):462–77.
14. Verhaak RG, et al. Integrated genomic analysis identifies clinically relevant subtypes of glioblastoma characterized by abnormalities in PDGFRA, IDH1, EGFR, and NF1. Cancer Cell. 2010;17(1):98–110.
15. Faury D, et al. Molecular profiling identifies prognostic subgroups of pediatric glioblastoma and shows increased YB-1 expression in tumors. J Clin Oncol. 2007;25(10):1196–208.
16. Paugh BS, et al. Integrated molecular genetic profiling of pediatric high-grade gliomas reveals key differences with the adult disease. J Clin Oncol. 2010;28(18):3061–8.
17. Puget S, et al. Mesenchymal transition and PDGFRA amplification/mutation are key distinct oncogenic events in pediatric diffuse intrinsic pontine gliomas. PLoS One. 2012;7(2):e30313.
18. Paugh BS, et al. Genome-wide analyses identify recurrent amplifications of receptor tyrosine kinases and cell-cycle regulatory genes in diffuse intrinsic pontine glioma. J Clin Oncol. 2011;29(30):3999–4006.
19. Bax DA, et al. A distinct spectrum of copy number aberrations in pediatric high-grade gliomas. Clin Cancer Res. 2010;16(13):3368–77.
20. Schwartzentruber J, et al. Driver mutations in histone H3.3 and chromatin remodelling genes in paediatric glioblastoma. Nature. 2012;482(7384):226–31.
21. Bender S, et al. Reduced H3K27me3 and DNA hypomethylation are major drivers of gene expression in K27M mutant pediatric high-grade gliomas. Cancer Cell. 2013;24(5):660–72.
22. Wu G, et al. The genomic landscape of diffuse intrinsic pontine glioma and pediatric nonbrainstem high-grade glioma. Nat Genet. 2014;46(5):444–50.
23. Carvalho D, et al. The prognostic role of intragenic copy number breakpoints and identification of novel fusion genes in paediatric high grade glioma. Acta Neuropathol Commun. 2014;2:23.
24. Cancer Genome Atlas Research, N. Comprehensive genomic characterization defines human glioblastoma genes and core pathways. Nature. 2008;455(7216):1061–8.
25. Malhotra A, et al. Breakpoint profiling of 64 cancer genomes reveals numerous complex rearrangements spawned by homology-independent mechanisms. Genome Res. 2013;23(5):762–76.
26. Richardson TE, et al. Genetic and epigenetic features of rapidly progressing IDH-mutant astrocytomas. J Neuropathol Exp Neurol. 2018;77(7):542–8.
27. Mirchia K, et al. Total copy number variation as a prognostic factor in adult astrocytoma subtypes. Acta Neuropathol Commun. 2019;7(1):92.
28. Hobbs J, et al. Paradoxical relationship between the degree of EGFR amplification and outcome in glioblastomas. Am J Surg Pathol. 2012;36(8):1186–93.

29. An Z, et al. Epidermal growth factor receptor and EGFRvIII in glioblastoma: signaling pathways and targeted therapies. Oncogene. 2018;37(12):1561–75.
30. Aoki K, et al. Prognostic relevance of genetic alterations in diffuse lower-grade gliomas. Neuro Oncol. 2018;20:66–77.
31. Stichel D, et al. Distribution of EGFR amplification, combined chromosome 7 gain and chromosome 10 loss, and TERT promoter mutation in brain tumors and their potential for the reclassification of IDHwt astrocytoma to glioblastoma. Acta Neuropathol. 2018;136(5):793–803.
32. Tabouret E, et al. Prognostic impact of the 2016 WHO classification of diffuse gliomas in the French POLA cohort. Acta Neuropathol. 2016;132(4):625–34.
33. Weller M, et al. Molecular classification of diffuse cerebral WHO grade II/III gliomas using genome- and transcriptome-wide profiling improves stratification of prognostically distinct patient groups. Acta Neuropathol. 2015;129(5):679–93.
34. Wijnenga MMJ, et al. Molecular and clinical heterogeneity of adult diffuse low-grade IDH wild-type gliomas: assessment of TERT promoter mutation and chromosome 7 and 10 copy number status allows superior prognostic stratification. Acta Neuropathol. 2017;134(6):957–9.
35. Vaubel RA, et al. Recurrent copy number alterations in low-grade and anaplastic pleomorphic xanthoastrocytoma with and without BRAF V600E mutation. Brain Pathol. 2018;28(2):172–82.
36. Zheng S, et al. A survey of intragenic breakpoints in glioblastoma identifies a distinct subset associated with poor survival. Genes Dev. 2013;27(13):1462–72.
37. Biernat W, et al. Predominant expression of mutant EGFR (EGFRvIII) is rare in primary glioblastomas. Brain Pathol. 2004;14(2):131–6.
38. Wong AJ, et al. Structural alterations of the epidermal growth factor receptor gene in human gliomas. Proc Natl Acad Sci U S A. 1992;89(7):2965–9.
39. Mondal G, et al. Pediatric bithalamic gliomas have a distinct epigenetic signature and frequent EGFR exon 20 insertions resulting in potential sensitivity to targeted kinase inhibition. Acta Neuropathol. 2020;139(6):1071–88.
40. Cho J, et al. Glioblastoma-derived epidermal growth factor receptor carboxyl-terminal deletion mutants are transforming and are sensitive to EGFR-directed therapies. Cancer Res. 2011;71(24):7587–96.
41. Ozawa T, et al. PDGFRA gene rearrangements are frequent genetic events in PDGFRA-amplified glioblastomas. Genes Dev. 2010;24(19):2205–18.
42. Paugh BS, et al. Novel oncogenic PDGFRA mutations in pediatric high-grade gliomas. Cancer Res. 2013;73(20):6219–29.
43. Duffner PK, et al. Treatment of infants with malignant gliomas: the Pediatric Oncology Group experience. J Neuro-Oncol. 1996;28(2–3):245–56.
44. Wu W, et al. Joint NCCTG and NABTC prognostic factors analysis for high-grade recurrent glioma. Neuro Oncol. 2010;12(2):164–72.
45. Clarke M, et al. Infant high-grade gliomas comprise multiple subgroups characterized by novel targetable gene fusions and favorable outcomes. Cancer Discov. 2020;10(7):942 63.
46. International Cancer Genome Consortium PedBrain Tumor, P. Recurrent MET fusion genes represent a drug target in pediatric glioblastoma. Nat Med. 2016;22(11):1314–20.
47. Torre M, et al. Molecular and clinicopathologic features of gliomas harboring NTRK fusions. Acta Neuropathol Commun. 2020;8(1):107.
48. Jones DT, et al. Recurrent somatic alterations of FGFR1 and NTRK2 in pilocytic astrocytoma. Nat Genet. 2013;45(8):927–32.
49. Di Stefano AL, et al. Detection, characterization, and inhibition of FGFR-TACC fusions in IDH wild-type glioma. Clin Cancer Res. 2015;21(14):3307–17.
50. Bielle F, et al. Diffuse gliomas with FGFR3-TACC3 fusion have characteristic histopathological and molecular features. Brain Pathol. 2018;28(5):674–83.
51. Lasorella A, Sanson M, Iavarone A. FGFR-TACC gene fusions in human glioma. Neuro Oncol. 2017;19(4):475–83.

52. Costa R, et al. FGFR3-TACC3 fusion in solid tumors: mini review. Oncotarget. 2016;7(34):55924–38.
53. Granberg KJ, et al. Strong FGFR3 staining is a marker for FGFR3 fusions in diffuse gliomas. Neuro Oncol. 2017;19(9):1206–16.
54. Parker BC, et al. The tumorigenic FGFR3-TACC3 gene fusion escapes miR-99a regulation in glioblastoma. J Clin Invest. 2013;123(2):855–65.
55. Huynh KD, et al. BCoR, a novel corepressor involved in BCL-6 repression. Genes Dev. 2000;14(14):1810–23.
56. Astolfi A, et al. BCOR involvement in cancer. Epigenomics. 2019;11(7):835–55.
57. Sturm D, et al. New brain tumor entities emerge from molecular classification of CNS-PNETs. Cell. 2016;164(5):1060–72.
58. Roy A, et al. Recurrent internal tandem duplications of BCOR in clear cell sarcoma of the kidney. Nat Commun. 2015;6:8891.
59. Torre M, et al. Recurrent EP300-BCOR fusions in pediatric gliomas with distinct clinico-pathologic features. J Neuropathol Exp Neurol. 2019;78(4):305–14.
60. Pisapia DJ, et al. Fusions involving BCOR and CREBBP are rare events in infiltrating glioma. Acta Neuropathol Commun. 2020;8(1):80.
61. Sturm D, et al. Paediatric and adult glioblastoma: multiform (epi)genomic culprits emerge. Nat Rev Cancer. 2014;14(2):92–107.
62. Phillips JJ, et al. PDGFRA amplification is common in pediatric and adult high-grade astrocytomas and identifies a poor prognostic group in IDH1 mutant glioblastoma. Brain Pathol. 2013;23(5):565–73.
63. Zarghooni M, et al. Whole-genome profiling of pediatric diffuse intrinsic pontine gliomas highlights platelet-derived growth factor receptor alpha and poly (ADP-ribose) polymerase as potential therapeutic targets. J Clin Oncol. 2010;28(8):1337–44.
64. Buczkowicz P, et al. Genomic analysis of diffuse intrinsic pontine gliomas identifies three molecular subgroups and recurrent activating ACVR1 mutations. Nat Genet. 2014;46(5):451–6.
65. Donson AM, et al. MGMT promoter methylation correlates with survival benefit and sensitivity to temozolomide in pediatric glioblastoma. Pediatr Blood Cancer. 2007;48(4):403–7.
66. Lee JY, et al. MGMT promoter gene methylation in pediatric glioblastoma: analysis using MS-MLPA. Childs Nerv Syst. 2011;27(11):1877–83.
67. Korshunov A, et al. H3-/IDH-wild type pediatric glioblastoma is comprised of molecularly and prognostically distinct subtypes with associated oncogenic drivers. Acta Neuropathol. 2017;134(3):507–16.
68. Noushmehr H, et al. Identification of a CpG island methylator phenotype that defines a distinct subgroup of glioma. Cancer Cell. 2010;17(5):510–22.
69. Khuong-Quang DA, et al. K27M mutation in histone H3.3 defines clinically and biologically distinct subgroups of pediatric diffuse intrinsic pontine gliomas. Acta Neuropathol. 2012;124(3):439–47.
70. Lu C, et al. IDH mutation impairs histone demethylation and results in a block to cell differentiation. Nature. 2012;483(7390):474–8.
71. Korshunov A, et al. Integrated analysis of pediatric glioblastoma reveals a subset of biologically favorable tumors with associated molecular prognostic markers. Acta Neuropathol. 2015;129(5):669–78.
72. Tauziède-Espariat A, et al. The pediatric supratentorial MYCN-amplified high-grade gliomas methylation class presents the same radiological, histopathological and molecular features as their pontine counterparts. Acta Neuropathol Commun. 2020;8(1):104.
73. Schindler G, et al. Analysis of BRAF V600E mutation in 1,320 nervous system tumors reveals high mutation frequencies in pleomorphic xanthoastrocytoma, ganglioglioma and extra-cerebellar pilocytic astrocytoma. Acta Neuropathol. 2011;121(3):397–405.

74. Ida CM, et al. Pleomorphic xanthoastrocytoma: natural history and long-term follow-up. Brain Pathol. 2015;25(5):575–86.
75. Louis DN, et al. The 2016 World Health Organization Classification of tumors of the central nervous system: a summary. Acta Neuropathol. 2016;131:803.
76. Pollack IF, et al. IDH1 mutations are common in malignant gliomas arising in adolescents: a report from the Children's Oncology Group. Childs Nerv Syst. 2011;27(1):87–94.
77. Nobusawa S, et al. IDH1 mutations as molecular signature and predictive factor of secondary glioblastomas. Clin Cancer Res. 2009;15(19):6002–7.
78. Yan H, et al. IDH1 and IDH2 mutations in gliomas. N Engl J Med. 2009;360(8):765–73.
79. Hartmann C, et al. Long-term survival in primary glioblastoma with versus without isocitrate dehydrogenase mutations. Clin Cancer Res. 2013;19(18):5146–57.
80. Korshunov A, et al. Integrated molecular characterization of IDH-mutant glioblastomas. Neuropathol Appl Neurobiol. 2019;45:108–18.
81. Gerber NK, et al. Transcriptional diversity of long-term glioblastoma survivors. Neuro Oncol. 2014;16(9):1186–95.
82. Yoda RA, et al. Mitotic index thresholds do not predict clinical outcome for IDH-mutant astrocytoma. J Neuropathol Exp Neurol. 2019;78(11):1002–10.
83. Appay R, et al. CDKN2A homozygous deletion is a strong adverse prognosis factor in diffuse malignant IDH-mutant gliomas. Neuro Oncol. 2019;21:1519.
84. Cimino PJ, Holland EC. Targeted copy number analysis outperforms histological grading in predicting patient survival for WHO grade II/III IDH-mutant astrocytomas. Neuro Oncol. 2019;21(6):819.
85. Perry A, et al. CDKN2A loss is associated with shortened survival in infiltrating astrocytomas but not oligodendrogliomas or mixed oligoastrocytomas. Neuro Oncol. 2014;16(suppl_3):iii1–iii22.
86. Louis DN, et al. cIMPACT-NOW update 6: new entity and diagnostic principle recommendations of the cIMPACT-Utrecht meeting on future CNS tumor classification and grading. Brain Pathol. 2020;30(4):844–856. https://doi.org/10.1111/bpa.12832. Epub 2020 Apr 19. PMID: 32307792.
87. Brat DJ, et al. cIMPACT-NOW update 5: recommended grading criteria and terminologies for IDH-mutant astrocytomas. Acta Neuropathol. 2020;139(3):603–8.
88. Parsons DW, et al. An integrated genomic analysis of human glioblastoma multiforme. Science. 2008;321(5897):1807–12.
89. Nonoguchi N, et al. TERT promoter mutations in primary and secondary glioblastomas. Acta Neuropathol. 2013;126(6):931–7.
90. Liu XY, et al. Frequent ATRX mutations and loss of expression in adult diffuse astrocytic tumors carrying IDH1/IDH2 and TP53 mutations. Acta Neuropathol. 2012;124(5):615–25.
91. Solomon DA, et al. Diffuse midline gliomas with histone H3-K27M mutation: a series of 47 cases assessing the spectrum of morphologic variation and associated genetic alterations. Brain Pathol. 2016;26(5):569–80.
92. Meyronet D, et al. Characteristics of H3 K27M-mutant gliomas in adults. Neuro Oncol. 2017;19(8):1127–34.
93. Tesileanu CMS, et al. Survival of diffuse astrocytic glioma, IDH1/2 wildtype, with molecular features of glioblastoma, WHO grade IV: a confirmation of the cIMPACT-NOW criteria. Neuro Oncol. 2020;22(4):515–23.
94. Lee Y, et al. The frequency and prognostic effect of TERT promoter mutation in diffuse gliomas. Acta Neuropathol Commun. 2017;5(1):62.
95. Batista R, et al. The prognostic impact of TERT promoter mutations in glioblastomas is modified by the rs2853669 single nucleotide polymorphism. Int J Cancer. 2016;139(2):414–23.
96. Koelsche C, et al. Distribution of TERT promoter mutations in pediatric and adult tumors of the nervous system. Acta Neuropathol. 2013;126(6):907–15.
97. Jones C, Baker SJ. Unique genetic and epigenetic mechanisms driving paediatric diffuse high-grade glioma. Nat Rev Cancer. 2014;14(10):651–61.

98. Nicolaides TP, et al. Targeted therapy for BRAFV600E malignant astrocytoma. Clin Cancer Res. 2011;17(24):7595–604.
99. Wu G, et al. Somatic histone H3 alterations in pediatric diffuse intrinsic pontine gliomas and non-brainstem glioblastomas. Nat Genet. 2012;44(3):251–3.
100. Skene PJ, Henikoff S. Histone variants in pluripotency and disease. Development. 2013;140(12):2513–24.
101. Wan YCE, Liu J, Chan KM. Histone H3 mutations in cancer. Curr Pharmacol Rep. 2018;4(4):292–300.
102. Fontebasso AM, et al. Recurrent somatic mutations in ACVR1 in pediatric midline high-grade astrocytoma. Nat Genet. 2014;46(5):462–6.
103. Taylor KR, et al. Recurrent activating ACVR1 mutations in diffuse intrinsic pontine glioma. Nat Genet. 2014;46(5):457–61.
104. Fontebasso AM, et al. Mutations in SETD2 and genes affecting histone H3K36 methylation target hemispheric high-grade gliomas. Acta Neuropathol. 2013;125(5):659–69.
105. Temime-Smaali N, et al. The G-quadruplex ligand telomestatin impairs binding of topoisomerase IIIalpha to G-quadruplex-forming oligonucleotides and uncaps telomeres in ALT cells. PLoS One. 2009;4(9):e6919.
106. Aihara K, et al. H3F3A K27M mutations in thalamic gliomas from young adult patients. Neuro Oncol. 2014;16(1):140–6.
107. Davis RJ, Welcker M, Clurman BE. Tumor suppression by the Fbw7 ubiquitin ligase: mechanisms and opportunities. Cancer Cell. 2014;26(4):455–64.
108. Welcker M, et al. The Fbw7 tumor suppressor regulates glycogen synthase kinase 3 phosphorylation-dependent c-Myc protein degradation. Proc Natl Acad Sci U S A. 2004;101(24):9085–90.
109. Bjerke L, et al. Histone H3.3. mutations drive pediatric glioblastoma through upregulation of MYCN. Cancer Discov. 2013;3(5):512–9.
110. Li M, Liu GH, Izpisua Belmonte JC. Navigating the epigenetic landscape of pluripotent stem cells. Nat Rev Mol Cell Biol. 2012;13(8):524–35.
111. Hirabayashi Y, Gotoh Y. Epigenetic control of neural precursor cell fate during development. Nat Rev Neurosci. 2010;11(6):377–88.
112. Jenuwein T, Allis CD. Translating the histone code. Science. 2001;293(5532):1074–80.
113. Klonou A, et al. Chromatin remodeling defects in pediatric brain tumors. Ann Transl Med. 2018;6(12):248.
114. Plass C, et al. Mutations in regulators of the epigenome and their connections to global chromatin patterns in cancer. Nat Rev Genet. 2013;14(11):765–80.
115. Lewis PW, et al. Inhibition of PRC2 activity by a gain-of-function H3 mutation found in pediatric glioblastoma. Science. 2013;340(6134):857–61.
116. Chan KM, et al. The histone H3.3K27M mutation in pediatric glioma reprograms H3K27 methylation and gene expression. Genes Dev. 2013;27(9):985–90.
117. Di Lorenzo A, Bedford MT. Histone arginine methylation. FEBS Lett. 2011;585(13):2024–31.
118. Killela PJ, et al. TERT promoter mutations occur frequently in gliomas and a subset of tumors derived from cells with low rates of self-renewal. Proc Natl Acad Sci U S A. 2013;110(15):6021–6.
119. Kam KL, et al. Is next-generation sequencing alone sufficient to reliably diagnose gliomas? J Neuropathol Exp Neurol. 2020;79(7):763–6.
120. Jones C, et al. Pediatric high-grade glioma: biologically and clinically in need of new thinking. Neuro Oncol. 2017;19(2):153–61.
121. Coleman C, et al. Pediatric hemispheric high-grade glioma: targeting the future. Cancer Metastasis Rev. 2020;39(1):245–60.
122. Toll SA, et al. Sustained response of three pediatric BRAF(V600E) mutated high-grade gliomas to combined BRAF and MEK inhibitor therapy. Oncotarget. 2019;10(4):551–7.
123. Laetsch TW, et al. Larotrectinib for paediatric solid tumours harbouring NTRK gene fusions: phase 1 results from a multicentre, open-label, phase 1/2 study. Lancet Oncol. 2018;19(5):705–14.

124. Drilon A, et al. Efficacy of larotrectinib in TRK fusion–positive cancers in adults and children. N Engl J Med. 2018;378(8):731–9.
125. Ziegler DS, et al. Brief Report: Potent clinical and radiological response to larotrectinib in TRK fusion-driven high-grade glioma. Br J Cancer. 2018;119(6):693–6.
126. Grasso CS, et al. Functionally defined therapeutic targets in diffuse intrinsic pontine glioma. Nat Med. 2015;21(6):555–9.
127. Hashizume R, et al. Pharmacologic inhibition of histone demethylation as a therapy for pediatric brainstem glioma. Nat Med. 2014;20(12):1394–6.

Chapter 10
Immunohistochemical Surrogates for Molecular Pathology

Ayca Ersen Danyeli

The classification of central nervous system (CNS) tumors has undergone an evolution from the first AFIP fascicle published in 1952, until now [1]. The World Health Organization (WHO) "blue books" for CNS tumor classifications were published as four different editions in 1979, 1993, 2000, and 2007 [2–5]. The intensive knowledge regarding the molecular biology of CNS tumors that increased after 2007 and accelerated since 2010, was the driving force of publishing the update of the 4th Edition in 2016, instead of waiting for the 5th Edition for more years [6]. The 2016 classification has incorporated well-established molecular parameters into the classification of CNS tumors by "integrated diagnosis". As of 2017, cIMPACT-NOW (the Consortium to Inform Molecular and Practical Approaches to CNS Tumor Taxonomy) was established to propose changes to future CNS tumor classifications based on molecular alterations [7].

The molecular alterations playing role in classification, prognostication, and prediction of therapeutic response gain more importance especially within the diffuse glioma group. The main subject of this book is glioblastoma. However, in the light of cIMPACT updates, there are major changes in the nomenclature of glioblastoma. For this reason, this chapter will focus on the immunohistochemical surrogates of molecular alterations of Grade IV diffuse gliomas rather than the immunohistochemical counterparts of molecular alterations in GBM.

In the past, tumors with glial morphology, infiltrative pattern, increased mitotic activity, vascular endothelial proliferation (VEP) and/or necrosis findings, were reported as "Glioblastoma, WHO Grade IV". However with cIMPACT update 3; *IDH* wild type diffuse gliomas with molecular alterations of either *TERTp* mutation or *EGFR* amplification or Chromosome 7 gain/chromosome 10 loss are suggested to be classified as "Diffuse astrocytic glioma, *IDH* wild type, with molecular

A. Ersen Danyeli (✉)
Acibadem MAA University, Faculty of Medicine, Pathology Department, Istanbul, Turkey

© The Author(s), under exclusive license to Springer Nature Switzerland AG 2021
J. J. Otero, A. P. Becker (eds.), *Precision Molecular Pathology of Glioblastoma*, Molecular Pathology Library, https://doi.org/10.1007/978-3-030-69170-7_10

features of Glioblastoma" [8]. These tumors do not have to reveal high grade morphologic features such as VEP or necrosis. On the other hand, cIMPACT update 5 suggested to classify *IDH* mutant diffuse gliomas as grade 2, grade 3, grade 4 "astrocytoma, IDH mutant", by omitting glioblastoma term in this group [9].

H3K27M mutant tumors with diffuse, infiltrative pattern located in the midline structures had already been classified as "Diffuse midline glioma, H3K27M mutant, WHO Grade IV" in the WHO CNS tumors classification 2016 [6]. H3.3 G34 mutant diffuse gliomas were also suggested to be classified as Grade 4 tumors in cIMPACT update 6 [10].

These molecular alterations that have to be checked for the integrated diagnosis of high grade diffuse glial tumors are ideally detected by DNA sequencing methods. However, it is a major budget problem to create molecular pathology laboratories with enough equipment, competent staff, and validated methods especially for the developing countries. Yet even in well-developed countries, it is not always possible to perform the diagnostic molecular tests because the high expenses are not covered by the social health system or insurance companies. At this point, most of the pathologists all over the world prefer or have to use immunohistochemical technics to detect molecular alterations. It is a much more affordable and faster way. But there are important points to consider while using immunohistochemistry to detect a molecular alteration. Some of them are in means of general immunohistochemistry technics, and some are related to the features of the particular alteration. These important considerations are listed below:

- The selected antibody has to be specific for the questioned molecular alteration. You may easily find an antibody that suggests a molecular alteration with a similar name but a different target. You need to check the literature for the sensitivity and specificity of the antibody. The selection of the correct antibody is the first and the most important step to successfully identify the molecular alteration in question using immunohistochemistry. As a very simple example; anti-H3K27me3 antibody would not be the antibody to detect the H3K27M mutation, and any antibody with low sensitivity for *IDH* R132H would not help you to detect the mutation. So the selection of the correct antibody is essential.
- The optimization of the antibody should be performed with a positive control; which was proven to harbor the targeted molecular alteration by the gold standard molecular method. A positive control should then be used for each case within the same slide, each time.
- The antibody should be kept in the optimal conditions suggested by the manufacturer, and the date of expiration has to be checked routinely. The laboratories with low case volumes should pay attention to aliquote and keep the antibodies in small vials to prevent staling.
- The appropriate techniques in formalin fixation of the tissue are very important to ensure optimal antigen-antibody reaction during immunohistochemical staining. Fixation of tissues should not exceed 18–24 hours for most applications.
- It is important to avoid using previously frozen tissue. These tissues may cause false-positive or false-negative results. Decalcification procedures also negatively affect the antigen-antibody reaction.
- If possible; choose blocks of the tumor with areas of no or minimal necrosis.
- The sections from the tumor block should be obtained just before the staining process. The antibody will not work perfectly on the slides with the tumor section, kept in room temperature or even refrigerator for prolonged periods.

- If there is any positive or negative internal control for the antibody in the tissue, along with the external controls, it should be checked carefully during the interpretation.
- The interpretation should be done with the histologic details of the tumor since diffuse glioma with an infiltrative pattern consists of non-neoplastic cells along with the neoplastic cells; the pathologist should be aware of the staining pattern of the neoplastic cell itself, not the entrapped non-neoplastic components.
- You should well know the antibody's pattern of the staining (i.e. cytoplasmic, nuclear or membranous). Cytoplasmic staining may be meaningless for an antibody supposed to show a nuclear staining pattern in case of a particular mutation and visa versa. In some cases, the loss of expression may help you to detect an alteration. So the datasheet of the selected antibody should be read, the literature should be reviewed, and the correct staining patterns should be well-recognized.
- Your pathology report should include the immunohistochemical stains with the name of clones, and a short explanation of the staining pattern. Use the percent of stained cells in case of heterogeneous staining pattern and do not give scores that are not accepted universally. It is also advised to give a short explanation for the meaning of this staining (e.g suggestive for mutation). These explanations will be further discussed within each immunohistochemical stains below.
- None of these markers should be used regardless of the morphologic and radiologic findings of the tumor. And the diagnosis should always be given by a combination of the whole data. It should also be kept in mind that the gold standard for the detection of any molecular alteration is genomics. When immunohistochemical analyses cannot reliably identify a particular mutation or genetic alteration required for a particular entity (tumor type), the term "not otherwise specified (NOS)" can be used to underscore this uncertainty.

The main drivers and accompanying molecular alterations along with the predictive markers will be mentioned with the immunohistochemical surrogates in this chapter. Before that, it is suggested to check the Graphic 10.1 for the suggested algorithm of classifying high grade diffuse glial tumors based on immunohistochemical findings.

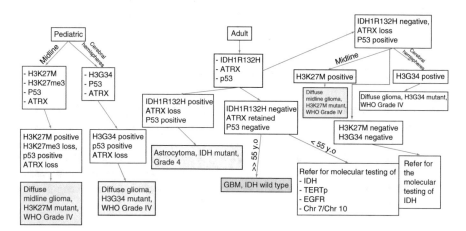

Graphic 10.1 Diagnosis of diffuse glioma with ↑ mitosis, VEP +/− necrosis by using immunohistochemistry as a tool

IDH1

IDH enzymes normally catalyze the decarboxylation of isocitrate to generate α-ketoglutarate (αKG) [11]. *IDH1* and *IDH2* play important roles in a number of cellular functions, including glucose sensing, glutamine metabolism, lipogenesis, and regulation of cellular redox status.

IDH mutation is an early event during the tumorigenesis of some of the adult diffuse gliomas [12]. For *IDH1*, the most common alteration is R132H (c.395G>A) comprising >80% of all *IDH* mutations.

The other expected *IDH1* mutations in diffuse gliomas are R132C, R132S, R132G, R132L. *IDH* mutation was first shown to be common in diffuse gliomas in 2008, and in the following year a mutation-specific IDH1 antibody for the most frequent mutation of the R132H type was developed in 2009 [13]. Although the IDH1R132H antibody is specific to IDH1R132H mutations, some tumors with IDHR132L mutations also show positive staining with this antibody.

The clones H11 and H14 had been produced. However since the clone H14 showed a more intense signal in mutated cases, it is widely used in the neuropathology practice. There are some other antibodies produced meanwhile. However, the sensitivity and the specifity of them were shown to be less reliable [14].

The mutation status of any diffuse glioma has a very strong effect on the prognosis of the tumor. It has been well-established that IDH mutant diffuse gliomas show a much better prognosis when compared with the IDH wild type diffuse gliomas [15]. Therefore it is the first stain to be ordered during the workup of an adult diffuse glioma. The pediatric cases are usually IDH wild type, although rare cases were reported especially in patients older than 14 years of age [16].

According to the WHO 2016 classification; tumors that are negative with the IDH antibody and no sequencing analysis to test for other mutations are reported as Diffuse Glioma, NOS.

However cIMPACT update 1 noted that negative IDH1R132H immunohistochemistry in a glioblastoma of patient 55 years of age and older, allows for a diagnosis of "Glioblastoma, IDH-wildtype" and that sequencing in search for other *IDH1* and for *IDH2* mutations is not necessary in this diagnostic setting [17].

The Interpretation of the Immunohistochemistry

The clone of immunohistochemical monoclonal antibody for detecting IDHR132H mutation is H09. The staining pattern is strong cytoplasmic and often weaker nuclear staining of tumor cells (Fig. 10.1). Despite of IDH1 being located in the cytoplasm, the reason behind nuclear staining is probably due to the antigen diffusion (the penetration of the soluble protein into the nucleus during tissue processing). Diffuse homogenous staining is expected in all morphologically recognizable

Fig. 10.1 A diffuse glioma, with most of the tumor cells that show positive cytoplasmic and few cells that show weak nuclear staining for mutant IDH1R132H antibody (40×). Note negative staining of non-neoplastic endothelial cells. (Primary antibody from Dianova GmbH, Hamburg)

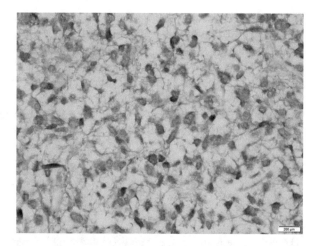

Fig. 10.2 With the mutant specific antibody, none of the cells in this glioma show the expected pattern of cellular staining. There is a faint background staining, there are few dot-like remnants of chromogen, which should be disregarded. The result should be reported as "IDH1R132H negative". (IDH1R132H (40×), (Primary antibody from Dianova GmbH, Hamburg)

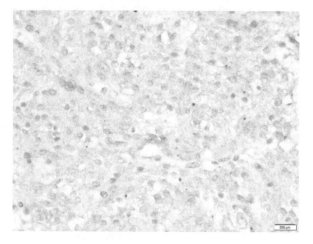

tumor cells. The background staining in the fibrillary tumor matrix with no cellular staining should require a re-evaluation of the staining procedures (Fig. 10.2).

IDH2

IDH2 mutations are much less common (<3%) in diffuse gliomas and are mutually exclusive with mutations in *IDH1* [18]. Although *IDH1* and *IDH2* are highly similar and catalyze identical reactions, *IDH1* is localized in the cytosol and *IDH2* is found in the mitochondrial matrix. The *IDH2* mutations detected in diffuse gliomas are R172K, R172M, R172W.

Since *IDH2* mutations are seen in particular lymphoma and leukemia types; routine use of immunohistochemistry for *IDH2* mutations is more common for hematopathology [19]. The immunohistochemical antibodies designed for IDH2R172K seem to have a high sensitivity and specificity. However, diffuse gliomas with *IDH2* mutations have a higher frequency of 1p/19q co-deletion. Besides, *IDH2* mutations are mutually exclusive with T*P53* and *ATRX* mutations which are frequent in IDH mutant astrocytomas. Therefore regarding the glioblastomas; it does not seem to be rational to have and routinely use the antibody for IDH2 in daily practice.

ATRX

The a-thalassemia/mental retardation syndrome X-linked (*ATRX*) gene on Xq21.1 encodes the nuclear protein ATRX. All chromosomal regions associated with *ATRX* are involved in the cell cycle. *ATRX* works together with histone chaperone death domain-associated protein (DAXX) to facilitate the incorporation of histone variant H3.3 into these regions in order to stabilize chromatin structure. Tumors maintain their telomere length either via re-activation of telomerase or through telomerase-independent mechanisms collectively called alternative lengthening of telomeres (ALT). ATRX is a repressor of ALT, which involves recombination-mediated replication of telomeric DNA. Eventually, in the telomeric region, ATRX helps to maintain telomeric integrity during DNA synthesis. ATRX deficiency triggers the alternative lengthening of telomeres (ALT) pathway. Loss of function or loss of expression of ATRX can lead to chromosomal instability such as aneuploidy. *ATRX* mutations in adult diffuse gliomas are closely associated with *IDH* and *TP53* mutations [20]. This helps in the differential diagnosis between diffuse astrocytic glioma and oligodendroglioma. In IDH wild type gliomas, ATRX loss is frequently seen in H3K27M and H3G34 mutant gliomas [21]. By itself *ATRX* mutation does not provide prognostic information for any diffuse glioma, but is helpful for the final diagnosis when combined with other immunohistochemical stains including p53, IDH and H3K27M, H3G34.

Loss of ATRX protein expression on immunohistochemistry can be used as a surrogate marker of *ATRX* mutations with high sensitivity and specificity and is almost perfectly correlates with ALT pathway activation. Missense mutations may not end up with protein loss, and genetic or epigenetic alterations other than mutations may lead to loss of protein expression. So rarely retained ATRX expression may be seen in an ATRX mutant tumor, and ATRX loss may also be seen in an ATRX wild type tumor. However, studies suggest that loss of protein expression has a better correlation with ALT status than *ATRX* mutations. So the use of ATRX immunohistochemistry is very helpful surrogate for molecular analysis of the ATRX locus.

The Interpretation of the Immunohistochemistry

The ATRX antibody commonly used in the literature (HPA001906) is polyclonal. The non-neoplastic cells are expected to show positive staining (retained expression). Nuclear positivity of non-neoplastic endothelial cells and neurons should be used as internal positive controls. Loss of nuclear expression for ATRX by immunohistochemistry supports *ATRX* mutation (Fig. 10.3). Any cytoplasmic staining should be disregarded. Since the diffuse gliomas consist of many non-neoplastic cells along with the neoplastic cells, interpretation of ATRX nuclear staining can be problematic. The morphologic evaluation of each cell within the stained slide is essential (Fig. 10.4). This may require an intense counterstaining with hematoxylin, since faint counter staining might cause you to count entrapped neurons as tumor cells with intact ATRX.

Fig. 10.3 Glioblastoma, with ATRX expression loss in tumor cells (20×). Hematoxilin counterstained nuclei of the neoplastic cells and the non-neoplastic cells with retained positivity is readily noted. (Primary antibody from Sigma Life Science, St. Louis, MO)

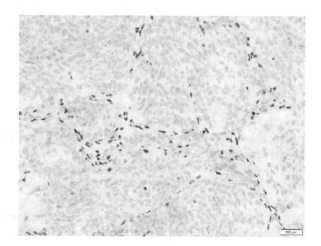

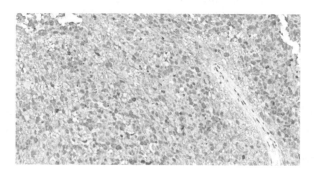

Fig. 10.4 The tumor cells do not show ATRX staining, but the endothelial cells are also negative (20×). So it is not a proper staining of the tissue with this antibody. The antibody might be staled, the staining procedure may not be correct, the tissue fixation maynot be appropriately performed or the tissue section might be old. Each step should be checked. (Primary antibody from Sigma Life Science, St. Louis, MO)

The interpretation results should be written in the report with details as "loss of nuclear expression; suggestive for ATRX mutation" or "nuclear expression is retained in the neoplastic cells; suggestive for wild type ATRX".

The loss of ATRX expression should be homogenous throughout the tumor, and if there is a patchy expression, it should be avoided to interprete the tumor as ATRX mutant. Mosaic type or patchy staining may be associated with technical issues.

In the situation of ATRX loss, if there is no staining with IDH1R132H, H3G34 or H3K27M antibody, the stains should be repeated, and if there is still discordance; the case should be referred for molecular studies.

P53

The *TP53* gene on chromosome 17p13.1 encodes the p53 protein, which plays a pivotal role in multiple cellular processes including G1 arrest, DNA repair, apoptosis, and differentiation. *TP53* mutation is the most frequent genetic alteration among human cancers [22]. Since *TP53* is a tumor-suppressor gene, its loss of function is involved in the development of tumors.

The p53 protein is inactivated directly by *TP53* mutations. *TP53* is frequently involved in the tumorigenesis of gliomas. It is almost invariably mutant in IDH mutant diffuse astrocytomas and is also detected in 30% of IDH wild type glioblastomas. H3 mutant tumors of either K27M or G34 also harbor *TP53* mutations in a high percentage.

Although it is usually a missense mutation causing loss of function, mutations in *TP53* often increase the half-life of the p53 protein product causing intense staining by immunohistochemistry. In fact the p53 antibody stains p53 protein of both wild type and mutant *TP53*, but in case of normally functioning *TP53*, the half-life of p53 protein is very short, so it is usually not detected by immunohistochemistry [23]. However, there are several conditions like cellular stress that prolong the half-life of normal p53 protein. For all of these reasons, p53 immunopositivity is not always an indicator of a *TP53* mutation [24]. There are also rare *TP53* alterations that impair p53 protein expression and cause complete p53 negativity.

The percentage of immunopositive cells for p53 staining suggestive for *TP53* mutation has always been an issue of contention. "A substantial percent of cells" was a subjective criterion. For a long time, accepted optimal cut-off value for the percentage of p53 positive neoplastic cells suggesting a *TP53* mutation was 10% of tumor cells under 40× magnification. In this case, the sensitivity and specificity of p53 immunoreactivity to predict a gene mutation were shown to be 78.8% and 96.7%, respectively [25]. The positive and negative predictive values were 94.5 and 86.3%, respectively.

Since the immunostaining is neither sensitive nor specific for a *TP53* mutation; the result must be interpreted in context with morphology and other immunohistochemical findings.

The Interpretation of the Immunohistochemistry

The most common antibody used for p53 immunohistochemistry is the clone DO-7. P53 immunohistochemistry shows a nuclear staining pattern. Any cytoplasmic staining should be disregarded. The expected intensity is very high, which would shade the chromatin details of the nucleus (Fig. 10.5). Any faint staining should not be reported as positive (Fig. 10.6). We suggest to give the percent of positive cells in the report instead of "positive" or "negative" statements.

Fig. 10.5 Glioblastoma with more than approximately 80% of the tumor cells showing strong nuclear positivity for p53 and negative staining of non-neoplastic cells. (20×) (Primary antibody from Leica Biosystems, Buffalo Grove, IL). The result can be interpreted as "suggestive for TP53 mutation"

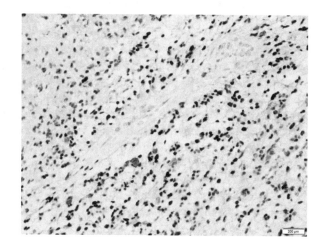

Fig. 10.6 There are few cells (<10%) that show faint nuclear p53 positivity. This pattern is not enough to accept the result as suggestive for TP53 mutation, yet it is not possible to rule out the mutation either. (Primary antibody from ScyTek Laboratories, West Logan)

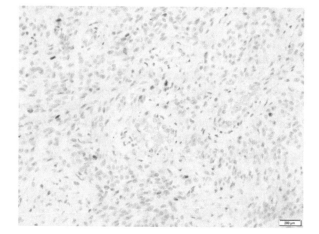

H3K27M

Mutation of the Lys 27 residue in the N-terminal tail of the H3 gene variants invokes disruption in post-translational modifications (methylation and acetylation) and alters the expression of oncogenes and tumor suppressor genes [26]. Consequently, mutation of *H3F3A* gene which results in a Lys 27-to-methionine change in the encoded protein H3.3K27M (H3.3 K27M mutation) has an important role in gliomagenesis and seen in 60% of diffuse midline gliomas [26]. H3.1 and H3.2 are more rarely mutated.

"Diffuse midline glioma, H3 K27M-mutant, WHO Grade IV" was introduced to the CNS tumor classification by WHO 2016. WHO 2016 stated that H3K27M mutation was exclusively seen in this tumor type; which is an infiltrative midline high-grade glioma with predominantly astrocytic differentiation. Yet, after the publication of WHO 2016, many cases that are not exactly diffuse midline gliomas, including ependymomas, pilocytic astrocytomas, and gangliogliomas have been reported harboring H3K27M mutation [27, 28]. Eventually cIMPACT update 2 has suggested to use the term "Difuse midline glioma, H3 K27M-mutant" just for the tumors that are diffuse gliomas, located in the midline and H3 K27M mutant, and to avoid using the term for other tumors harboring H3K27M mutation [29]. H3K27M-mutant specific immunohistochemistry is useful to identify the mutation of H3K27M with a 100% sensitivity and specificity [30]. Besides, it shows positivity for H3.3, H3.2 and H3.1 K27M mutations and therefore is more sensitive for detecting H3K27M mutant tumors than a point mutation analysis particularly for H3.3 K27M mutations.

The Interpretation of the Immunohistochemistry

The antibodies for H3K27M mutations are monoclonal RM192, and polyclonal ABE419.

The staining pattern is nuclear. The non-neoplastic cells within the tumor such as endothelial cells should be negative and it should be checked routinely during the interpretation (Fig. 10.7). The macrophages/microglial cells may show cytoplasmic staining in wild type cases, and should not be interpreted as positive for mutation. In the immunohistochemical results section of the pathology report a short explanation should be added for positive results; e.g. "suggestive for H3K27M mutation"

H3K27me3

H3K27 is trimethylated by the polycomb repressive complex 2 (PRC2). Enhancer of zest 2 (EZH2) is the main methyltransferase enzyme contained in this complex that is responsible for trimethylation of H3K27 [31]. The H3K27M mutant protein binds to EZH2 to inhibit its methyltransferase activity, resulting in a global

Fig. 10.7 Diffuse midline glioma with positive staining of tumor nuclei for mutant specific H3K27M antibody (20×). The non-neoplastic components are negative. (Primary antibody from RevMab, South San Francisco, CA)

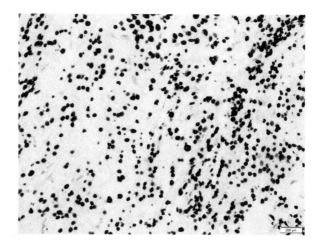

reduction of H3K27me3. As a summary, H3K27M mutation characterize a decreased genome-wide H3K27 trimethylation as a post-translational modification. The immunohistochemical studies have shown decreased H3K27me3 expression in H3K27M mutant tumors [31]. A global reduction of H3K27me3 expression is expected throughout the tumor. Therefore detecting trimethylated H3K27, started to be used to guide diagnosis of H3K27M mutant tumors. Regarding diffuse midline gliomas, H3K27me3 immunohistochemistry should only be used in conjunction with H3K27M immunohistochemistry, since the loss of H3 K27me3 expression is by itself not specific and is not always a result of H3K27M mutation [32]. H3K27me3 is enriched at unmethylated CpG islands and CpG island methylation also causes a global reduction in H3K27me3 levels. Therefore H3K27me3 reduction is also seen in posterior fossa ependymomas Group A, and oligodendrogliomas [32, 33]. Epigenetic modification on the level of histones also causes many other tumors to exhibit loss of H3K27me3 expression i.e. malignant peripheral nerve sheath tumors and high grade meningiomas [34, 35].

The Interpretation of the Immunohistochemistry

The antibody for H3K27me3 is monoclonal, clone RM175.

The staining pattern is nuclear. Non-neoplastic cells show positive staining. The decreased expression in the neoplastic cells suggests the reduction of trimethylated H3K27me3 (Fig. 10.8).

As a personal experience I have seen H3K27me3 stain mistakenly performed instead of H3K27M stain because of the similarities of the antibody names. Therefore evaluation of H3K27me3 staining requires excessive attention. On the other hand while reporting the staining results ""H3K27me3: Positive" might cause a misunderstanding of H3K27M mutation by another physician. So it would be

Fig. 10.8 The neoplastic cells show loss of nuclear H3K27me3 expression, with retained expression in the nuclei of endothelial cells cells (20×) (Primary antibody from RevMab, South San Francisco, CA)

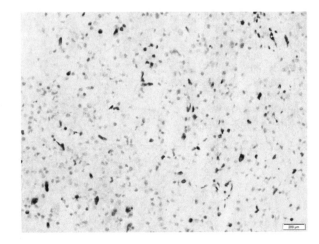

Fig. 10.9 The neoplastic cells show retained nuclear H3K27me3 expression (20×) (Primary antibody from RevMab, South San Francisco, CA)

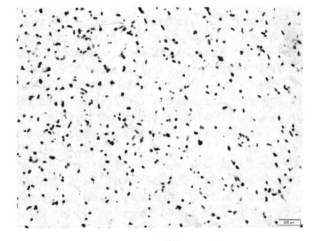

helpful to add a definition of "trimethylated H3K27 status" in paranthesis next to the name of the antibody, and in the results section note "nuclear expression is retained" either than writing "positive" (Fig. 10.9).

H3G34

The H3.3 mutations in gliomas most commonly occur in the *H3F3A* gene and is associated with one of three amino acid substitutions; K27M, G34R and G34V [26]. Unlike H3K27M mutations seen in the midline gliomas, G34 mutations are seen in supratentorial hemispheric tumors.

cIMPACT update 6 has proposed a new name; "Diffuse glioma, H3G34 mutant, WHO Grade IV" for these tumors [10]. These tumors typically show a diffusely infiltrating pattern of neoplastic cells with astrocytic differentiation and features of anaplasia (i.e. mitotic activity, microvascular proliferation and/or necrosis).

There are highly specific and sensitive antibodies against H3.3 G34R and G34V mutations [36]. Therefore; immunohistochemical detection of H3.3 G34-mutant proteins, that is, H3.3 G34R or H3.3 G34V, can serve as an alternative diagnostic method to DNA sequencing. While choosing the correct antibody, it is important not to use the commercially available antibody for H3G34W mutations; characteristically seen in giant cell tumors of bone.

The Interpretation of the Immunohistochemistry

Currently some of the commonly used clones of the antibodies for detecting Histone H3.3 G34R and G34V mutations are RM24 and RM307, respectively. The immuno-histochemical staining for G34R/V mutations are nuclear, and endothelial cells should be negative as an internal control (Fig. 10.10).

The positive immunohistochemical result requires an explanation as "suggestive for H3G34R/V mutation".

BRAFV600E

Activating mutations of the serine threonine kinase v-RAF murine sarcoma viral oncogene homolog B1 (BRAF) are frequent in benign and malignant human tumors. Over 95% of BRAF mutations are of the V600E type [37].

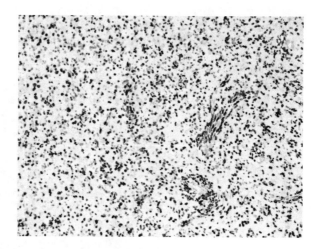

Fig. 10.10 The diffuse glioma of cerebral hemispheres revealing H3G34 mutation, as shown here with the positive nuclear expression with H3G34 R/V antibody (40×) (Primary antibodies from RevMab, South San Francisco, CA). (Courtesy of Prof Dr Tarik Tihan)

*BRAF*V600E mutation is a rare finding in glioblastoma. The epithelioid glioblastoma is the only glioblastoma variant that might harbor a *BRAF*V600E mutation [38]. Regarding pediatric cases there are low-grade diffuse gliomas showing *BRAF*V600E mutation [39]. Among pediatric cases, only the diffuse glial tumors with high-grade morphologic features would be accepted as epitheliod glioblastoma with *BRAF*V600E mutation. These cases typically show epithelioid or rhabdoid morphology. Anaplastic pleomorphic xanthoastrocytoma, another high grade tumor is a circumscribed, non-infiltrating tumor harboring *BRAF*V600E mutation, and the exclusion is based on the morphologic features. If the tumor is a high grade IDH wild type diffuse glioma, *BRAF*V600E mutation may suggest an epithelioid glioblastoma. The antibody for *BRAF*V600E mutations has been developed in 2011 and it is widely used in the routine surgical pathology practice [40].

The Interpretation of the Immunohistochemistry

BRAF immunohistochemistry using Clone VE1 is strongly concordant with *BRAF*V600E mutation. Immunostaining is diffuse, with uniform intensity throughout the cytoplasm of tumor cells, and highlights the epithelioid phenotype. The staining intensity ranges from weak to strong (Fig. 10.11).

However the intensity in glioblastoma is not strong enough as seen in extra-CNS tumors such as malignant melanoma. Importantly; staining is usually lost in the neoplastic cells adjacent to necrosis. So the interpretation should be based on the areas far from necrosis which is an important issue in GBM.

EGFR

One of the most frequent genetic alterations in glioblastoma are alterations of the epidermal growth factor (*EGFR*), reported to occur in 30–60% of cases [41]. The genomic alterations in *EGFR* include gene amplification, rearrangements, and point

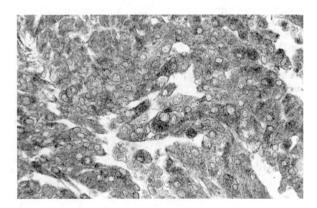

Fig. 10.11 BRAFV600E mutant epitheliod glioblastoma with neoplastic cells that show BRAF cytoplasmic positivity (40×). (Primary antibody from Spring Bioscience, Pleasanton, CA)

mutations. *EGFR* gene is located on chromosome 7q12. Deregulation of EGFR signaling contributes to tumor development and progression. Copy number alterations are the most common abnormalities in *EGFR*, with gene amplification present in >43% of glioblastoma patients [42]. However EGFR overexpression is not totally contributed to *EGFR* amplification. Therefore the routine use of EGFR immunohistochemistry for glioblastoma is not recommended. It might only be helpful in means of completely negative staining which rules out any amplification in *EGFR* since negative staining is consistent with non-amplified status.

cIMPACT 3 has proposed to classify any *IDH* wild type diffuse glioma with *EGFR* amplification as "Diffuse astrocytic glioma, *IDH* wild type with molecular features of glioblastoma" [8]. Therefore it is very important to detect the *EGFR* amplification in IDH wild type diffuse gliomas. However, the current commercially available antibodies are not helpful for detecting the amplification.

The Interpretation of the Immunohistochemistry

The anti-EGFR antibody shows a cytoplasmic and membranous staining. The expression is generally uniform throughout the tumor, and nearly all cells within the tumor express high levels of EGFR protein (>90%) by immunohistochemistry (IHC) (Fig. 10.12).

EGFRvIII

EGFR variant III which is a result of the deletion of exons 2–7, is the most common *EGFR* gene variant [42]. Both EGFR overexpression and *EGFRvIII* can enhance glioblastoma cell growth, migration and invasiveness. The variant *EGFRvIII* can be detected in 19% of glioblastomas. Diagnostically, the presence of *EGFRvIII* is

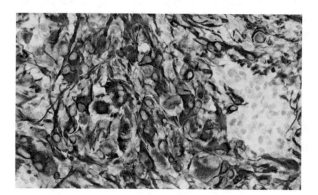

Fig. 10.12 A homogenous cytoplasmic positivity with EGFR antibody in a glioblastoma. The positivity does not confirm *EGFR* amplification, by itself. (20×). (Primary antibody from Spring Bioscience, Pleasanton, CA)

useful as a tumor-specific marker that is fairly specific to glioblastoma, as it has only rarely been identified in other cancers (eg, lung).

The Interpretation of the Immunohistochemistry

*EGFR*vIII staining is heterogeneous within the tumor. The staining pattern is expected to be cytoplasmic. The sensitivity and specificity of a non-commercial antibody were shown to be 95% and 100% respectively. Yet currently another antibody with the clone of **RM419** is available commercially which is not validated by any published glioma study.

TERT

Telomere lengthening is a fundamental hallmark of cancer, and activating telomerase promoter (*TERT*p) mutation is one of the most common regulatory mutations in cancer [43]. The telomere-lengthening process in most gliomas depends on either *TERT*p-mutations or *ATRX* mutations and these oncogenic changes are mutually exclusive.

Since *TERT*p mutation is seen in *ATRX* wild type cases, the *TERT*p mutation in case of an *IDH* mutation is highly suggestive for an oligodendroglioma, which also has to be confirmed by detecting 1p/19q codeletion [44].

However in *IDH* wild type diffuse gliomas, *TERT*p mutation is strongly correlated with an aggressive clinical course [45].

cIMPACT-NOW update 3 strictly advised to accept *IDH* wild type diffuse glial tumors as "diffuse astrocytic glioma, IDH-wildtype, with molecular features of glioblastoma, WHO grade IV" when the tumor harbors *TERT* mutation or *EGFR* amplification or Chr 7 gain/Chromosome 10 loss [8, 10]. This radical proposal means; even when a diffuse glioma does not show high grade morphologic features (e.g increased mitotic activity, VEP, necrosis) it will graded as IV based on the *TERT*p mutation.

*TERT*p status of the tumor is generally checked by molecular studies. There are commercially available antibodies for *TERT*p mutation. However studies regarding solid tumors showed that TERT protein expression did not correlate with mutation status. Also, glioma studies showed that there was an unexpected increase in TERT expression in *TERT*-wildtype as well as *TERT*-mutated gliomas and in tumor vasculature [46]. Eventually, immunohistochemical studies to detect *TERT* mutation is not recommended and molecular work-up is still needed for detecting *TERT*p mutation.

MGMT

O6-methylguanine DNA methyltransferase (MGMT) is a DNA repair protein encoded by the *MGMT* gene on 10q26. MGMT repairs DNA crosslinks and prevents cell death by removing alkyl groups from the O6-guanine position [47]. Temozolomide, a principal chemotherapeutic alkylating agent used in glioma treatment, generates DNA crosslinks that may induce apoptotic cell death in the setting of an intact mismatch repair mechanism. Silencing of MGMT protein expression because of *MGMT* gene promoter hypermethylation is considered to be associated with benefits to temozolomide therapy in glioblastoma patients [48].

Two commercial anti-MGMT antibodies (clones MT3.1 and MT23.2) are available.

Many studies have compared methylation status of *MGMT* detected by various techniques with immunohistochemistry and most of them have shown no concordance [49]. Since the studies have shown the lack of association with the *MGMT* promoter methylation status and protein expression, the use of anti-MGMT immunohistochemistry is not suggested as a clinical biomarker for routine diagnostic purposes.

CDKN2A

CDKN2A is a tumor suppressor gene located on human chromosome 9p21 and acts as a negative regulator of the cell cycle. This gene encodes for two different proteins, p16INK4a and p14ARF. *CDKN2A* is a frequent target of deletions in high-grade astrocytic tumors, with frequency ranging from 30% to 66% [50]. *CDKN2A* deletion has been reported to be more frequent in *IDH* wild type glioblastomas.

The frequencies of *CDKN2A/B* homozygous deletions reported in *IDH*-mutant astrocytic gliomas range from 0 to 12% in WHO grade II, 6–20% in WHO grade III and 16–34% in WHO grade IV tumors [51]. Multiple studies have identified homozygous deletion of *CDKN2A/B* as a marker of poor prognosis in patients with IDH-mutant diffuse astrocytic gliomas.

cIMPACT update 6 recommended discontinuing the term "Glioblastoma, *IDH*-mutant, WHO grade IV" and instead recommended referring to these tumors as "Astrocytoma, *IDH*-mutant, WHO grade 4" [10]. cIMPACT-NOW 6 also recommended that *CDKN2A/B* homozygous deletion should be a WHO grade 4 criterion for *IDH*-mutant astrocytomas. So evaluating *CDKN2A* status in *IDH* mutant astrocytoma is very important.

p16 is one of the protein products of the *CDKN2A* gene, and the expression of p16 can be detected by immunohistochemistry.

Unfortunately, studies using commercially available p16 antibody clone G175–405 did not show a satisfactory correlation between p16 immunohistochemistry and molecular detection of *CDKN2A/B* homozygous deletion [52]. The nuclear expression of p16 was too low in many samples to allow definite detection of loss of expression. Therefore, immunohistochemical stain for p16 as a surrogate for *CDKN2A/B* deletion is not suggested.

Conclusion

There are many immunohistochemical stains which are useful surrogate markers for specific molecular alterations in CNS tumors (Fig. 10.13). As the types of molecular alterations are in a broad spectrum (point mutation, deletion, amplification, translocation, hypermethylation), the meaning of the presence/absence or subcellular localization of a protein product should be explained with the knowledge of the expected molecular alteration and the associated protein expression pattern.

Every finding, during diagnostic work-up of a CNS tumor, is a piece of the puzzle. Therefore the immunohistochemical result of a particular stain must be interpreted in context with clinical, radiologic, morphologic, and other immunohistochemical findings.

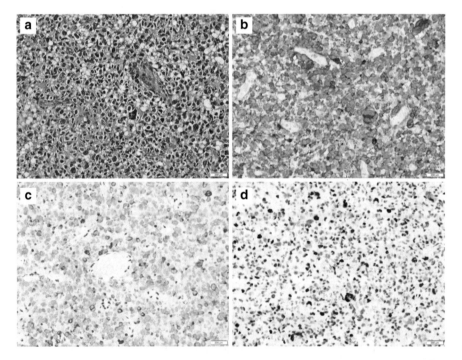

Fig. 10.13 (**a**) An IDH mutant glioblastoma (astrocytoma, *IDH* mutant, Grade 4) (**b**) IDH1R132H is diffusely positive in the cytoplasm of the neoplastic cells (20×), (**c**) nuclear ATRX expression is lost (20×). Although there is cytoplasmic staining, the loss of nuclear expression is suggestive for ATRX mutation (**d**) The neoplastic cells show diffuse and strong nuclear p53 expression (20×)

References

1. Kernohan JW, Sayre GP. Tumors of the central nervous system. Washington, DC: Armed Forces Institute of Pathology; 1952.
2. Zülch KJ. Histological typing of tumours of the central nervous system. Geneva: World Health Organization; 1979.
3. Kleihues P, Burger PC, Scheithauer BW. The new WHO classification of brain tumours. Brain Pathol. 1993;3(3):255–68.
4. Kleihues P, Cavenee WK. World Health Organization classification of tumours—pathology and genetics. 2000.
5. Louis DN, Ohgaki H, Wiestler OD, Cavenee WK, Burger PC, Jouvet A, et al. The 2007 WHO classification of tumours of the central nervous system. Acta Neuropathol. 2007;114(2):97–109.
6. Louis DN, Ohgaki H, Wiestler OD, Cavenee WK. World Health Organization histological classification of tumours of the central nervous system. 2016
7. Louis DN, Aldape K, Brat DJ, Capper D, Ellison DW, Hawkins C, et al. cIMPACT-NOW (the consortium to inform molecular and practical approaches to CNS tumor taxonomy): a new initiative in advancing nervous system tumor classification. Brain Pathol. 2017;27(6):851–2.
8. Brat DJ, Aldape K, Colman H, Holland EC, Louis DN, Jenkins RB, et al. cIMPACT-NOW update 3: recommended diagnostic criteria for "Diffuse astrocytic glioma, IDH-wildtype, with molecular features of glioblastoma, WHO grade IV". Acta Neuropathol. 2018;136(5):805–10.
9. Brat DJ, Aldape K, Colman H, Figrarella-Branger D, Fuller GN, Giannini C, et al. cIMPACT-NOW update 5: recommended grading criteria and terminologies for IDH-mutant astrocytomas. Acta Neuropathol. 2020;139(3):603–8.
10. Louis DN, Wesseling P, Aldape K, Brat DJ, Capper D, Cree IA, et al. cIMPACT-NOW update 6: new entity and diagnostic principle recommendations of the cIMPACT-Utrecht meeting on future CNS tumor classification and grading. Brain Pathol. 2020;30(4):844–56.
11. Yan H, Parsons DW, Jin G, McLendon R, Rasheed BA, Yuan W, et al. IDH1 and IDH2 mutations in gliomas. N Engl J Med. 2009;360(8):765–73.
12. Parsons DW, Jones S, Zhang X, Lin JC, Leary RJ, Angenendt P, et al. An integrated genomic analysis of human glioblastoma multiforme. Science. 2008;321(5897):1807–12.
13. Capper D, Weissert S, Balss J, Habel A, Meyer J, Jäger D, et al. Characterization of R132H mutation-specific IDH1 antibody binding in brain tumors. Brain Pathol. 2010;20(1):245–54.
14. Li J, Zhang H, Wang L, Yang C, Lai H, Zhang W, et al. Comparative study of IDH1 mutations in gliomas by high resolution melting analysis, immunohistochemistry and direct DNA sequencing. Mol Med Rep. 2015;12(3):4376–81.
15. Hartmann C, Hentschel B, Wick W, Capper D, Felsberg J, Simon M, et al. Patients with IDH1 wild type anaplastic astrocytomas exhibit worse prognosis than IDH1-mutated glioblastomas, and IDH1 mutation status accounts for the unfavorable prognostic effect of higher age: implications for classification of gliomas. Acta Neuropathol. 2010;120(6):707–18.
16. Huse JT, Rosenblum MK. The emerging molecular foundations of pediatric brain Tumors. J Child Neurol. 2015;30(13):1838–50.
17. Louis DN, Wesseling P, Paulus W, Giannini C, Batchelor TT, Cairncross JG, et al. cIMPACT-NOW update 1: not otherwise specified (NOS) and not elsewhere classified (NEC). Acta Neuropathol. 2018;135(3):481–4.
18. Wang HY, Tang K, Liang TY, Zhang WZ, Li JY, Wang W, et al. The comparison of clinical and biological characteristics between IDH1 and IDH2 mutations in gliomas. J Exp Clin Cancer Res. 2016;35:86.
19. Dupuy A, Lemonnier F, Fataccioli V, Martin-Garcia N, Robe C, Pelletier R, et al. Multiple ways to detect IDH2 mutations in angioimmunoblastic T-cell lymphoma from immunohistochemistry to next-generation sequencing. J Mol Diagn. 2018;20(5):677–85.
20. Liu XY, Gerges N, Korshunov A, Sabha N, Khuong-Quang DA, Fontebasso AM, et al. Frequent ATRX mutations and loss of expression in adult diffuse astrocytic tumors carrying IDH1/IDH2 and TP53 mutations. Acta Neuropathol. 2012;124(5):615–25.

21. Heaphy CM, de Wilde RF, Jiao Y, Klein AP, Edil BH, Shi C, et al. Altered telomeres in tumors with ATRX and DAXX mutations. Science. 2011;333(6041):425.
22. Mukhopadhyay UK, Mak AS. p53: is the guardian of the genome also a suppressor of cell invasion? Cell Cycle. 2009;8(16):2481.
23. Pardo FS, Hsu DW, Zeheb R, Efird JT, Okunieff PG, Malkin DM. Mutant, wild type, or overall p53 expression: freedom from clinical progression in tumours of astrocytic lineage. Br J Cancer. 2004;91(9):1678–86.
24. Kurtkaya-Yapicier O, Scheithauer BW, Hebrink D, James CD. p53 in nonneoplastic central nervous system lesions: an immunohistochemical and genetic sequencing study. Neurosurgery. 2002;51(5):1246–54; discussion 54–5.
25. Takami H, Yoshida A, Fukushima S, Arita H, Matsushita Y, Nakamura T, et al. Revisiting TP53 mutations and immunohistochemistry – a comparative study in 157 diffuse gliomas. Brain Pathol. 2015;25(3):256–65.
26. Schwartzentruber J, Korshunov A, Liu XY, Jones DT, Pfaff E, Jacob K, et al. Driver mutations in histone H3.3 and chromatin remodelling genes in paediatric glioblastoma. Nature. 2012;482(7384):226–31.
27. Hochart A, Escande F, Rocourt N, Grill J, Koubi-Pick V, Beaujot J, et al. Long survival in a child with a mutated K27M-H3.3 pilocytic astrocytoma. Ann Clin Transl Neurol. 2015;2(4):439–43.
28. Gessi M, Capper D, Sahm F, Huang K, von Deimling A, Tippelt S, et al. Evidence of H3 K27M mutations in posterior fossa ependymomas. Acta Neuropathol. 2016;132(4):635–7.
29. Louis DN, Giannini C, Capper D, Paulus W, Figarella-Branger D, Lopes MB, et al. cIMPACT-NOW update 2: diagnostic clarifications for diffuse midline glioma, H3 K27M-mutant and diffuse astrocytoma/anaplastic astrocytoma, IDH-mutant. Acta Neuropathol. 2018;135(4):639–42.
30. Venneti S, Santi M, Felicella MM, Yarilin D, Phillips JJ, Sullivan LM, et al. A sensitive and specific histopathologic prognostic marker for H3F3A K27M mutant pediatric glioblastomas. Acta Neuropathol. 2014;128(5):743–53.
31. Harutyunyan AS, Krug B, Chen H, Papillon-Cavanagh S, Zeinieh M, De Jay N, et al. H3K27M induces defective chromatin spread of PRC2-mediated repressive H3K27me2/me3 and is essential for glioma tumorigenesis. Nat Commun. 2019;10(1):1262.
32. Panwalkar P, Clark J, Ramaswamy V, Hawes D, Yang F, Dunham C, et al. Immunohistochemical analysis of H3K27me3 demonstrates global reduction in group-A childhood posterior fossa ependymoma and is a powerful predictor of outcome. Acta Neuropathol. 2017;134(5):705–14.
33. Pekmezci M, Phillips JJ, Dirilenoglu F, Atasever-Rezanko T, Tihan T, Solomon D, et al. Loss of H3K27 trimethylation by immunohistochemistry is frequent in oligodendroglioma, IDH-mutant and 1p/19q-codeleted, but is neither a sensitive nor a specific marker. Acta Neuropathol. 2020;139(3):597–600.
34. Pekmezci M, Cuevas-Ocampo AK, Perry A, Horvai AE. Significance of H3K27me3 loss in the diagnosis of malignant peripheral nerve sheath tumors. Mod Pathol. 2017;30(12):1710–9.
35. Katz LM, Hielscher T, Liechty B, Silverman J, Zagzag D, Sen R, et al. Loss of histone H3K27me3 identifies a subset of meningiomas with increased risk of recurrence. Acta Neuropathol. 2018;135(6):955–63.
36. Haque F, Varlet P, Puntonet J, Storer L, Bountali A, Rahman R, et al. Evaluation of a novel antibody to define histone 3.3 G34R mutant brain tumours. Acta Neuropathol Commun. 2017;5(1):45.
37. Davies H, Bignell GR, Cox C, Stephens P, Edkins S, Clegg S, et al. Mutations of the BRAF gene in human cancer. Nature. 2002;417(6892):949–54.
38. Kleinschmidt-DeMasters BK, Aisner DL, Birks DK, Foreman NK. Epithelioid GBMs show a high percentage of BRAF V600E mutation. Am J Surg Pathol. 2013;37(5):685–98.
39. Qaddoumi I, Orisme W, Wen J, Santiago T, Gupta K, Dalton JD, et al. Genetic alterations in uncommon low-grade neuroepithelial tumors: BRAF, FGFR1, and MYB mutations occur at high frequency and align with morphology. Acta Neuropathol. 2016;131(6):833–45.

40. Capper D, Preusser M, Habel A, Sahm F, Ackermann U, Schindler G, et al. Assessment of BRAF V600E mutation status by immunohistochemistry with a mutation-specific monoclonal antibody. Acta Neuropathol. 2011;122(1):11–9.
41. Ohgaki H. Genetic pathways to glioblastomas. Neuropathology. 2005;25(1):1–7.
42. An Z, Aksoy O, Zheng T, Fan QW, Weiss WA. Epidermal growth factor receptor and EGFRvIII in glioblastoma: signaling pathways and targeted therapies. Oncogene. 2018;37(12):1561–75.
43. Vinagre J, Almeida A, Pópulo H, Batista R, Lyra J, Pinto V, et al. Frequency of TERT promoter mutations in human cancers. Nat Commun. 2013;4:2185.
44. Eckel-Passow JE, Lachance DH, Molinaro AM, Walsh KM, Decker PA, Sicotte H, et al. Glioma groups based on 1p/19q, IDH, and TERT promoter mutations in tumors. N Engl J Med. 2015;372(26):2499–508.
45. Killela PJ, Reitman ZJ, Jiao Y, Bettegowda C, Agrawal N, Diaz LA, et al. TERT promoter mutations occur frequently in gliomas and a subset of tumors derived from cells with low rates of self-renewal. Proc Natl Acad Sci U S A. 2013;110(15):6021–6.
46. Masui K, Komori T, Kato Y, Masutomi K, Ichimura K, Ogasawara S, et al. Elevated TERT expression in TERT-wildtype adult diffuse gliomas: histological evaluation with a novel TERT-specific antibody. Biomed Res Int. 2018;2018:7945845.
47. Komine C, Watanabe T, Katayama Y, Yoshino A, Yokoyama T, Fukushima T. Promoter hypermethylation of the DNA repair gene O6-methylguanine-DNA methyltransferase is an independent predictor of shortened progression free survival in patients with low-grade diffuse astrocytomas. Brain Pathol. 2003;13(2):176–84.
48. Bobola MS, Tseng SH, Blank A, Berger MS, Silber JR. Role of O6-methylguanine-DNA methyltransferase in resistance of human brain tumor cell lines to the clinically relevant methylating agents temozolomide and streptozotocin. Clin Cancer Res. 1996;2(4):735–41.
49. Preusser M, Charles Janzer R, Felsberg J, Reifenberger G, Hamou MF, Diserens AC, et al. Anti-O6-methylguanine-methyltransferase (MGMT) immunohistochemistry in glioblastoma multiforme: observer variability and lack of association with patient survival impede its use as clinical biomarker. Brain Pathol. 2008;18(4):520–32.
50. Smith JS, Jenkins RB. Genetic alterations in adult diffuse glioma: occurrence, significance, and prognostic implications. Front Biosci. 2000;5:D213–31.
51. Shirahata M, Ono T, Stichel D, Schrimpf D, Reuss DE, Sahm F, et al. Novel, improved grading system(s) for IDH-mutant astrocytic gliomas. Acta Neuropathol. 2018;136(1):153–66.
52. Purkait S, Jha P, Sharma MC, Suri V, Sharma M, Kale SS, et al. CDKN2A deletion in pediatric versus adult glioblastomas and predictive value of p16 immunohistochemistry. Neuropathology. 2013;33(4):405–12.

Part III
Key Molecular Pathways in Glioblastoma Development and Progression

Chapter 11
Machine Learning-Based Automated Methods for Brain Tumor Segmentation, Subtype Classification, Tracking and Patient Survival Prediction

Linmin Pei and Khan M. Iftekharuddin

Introduction

Glioma is the most common primary brain malignancy in the central nervous system (CNS) [1, 2]. From 2011 to 2015, the annual incidence of new brain tumors has been 23 out of 100,000 in the U.S. population [3]. According to the report, among the total 392,982 new cases for this 5-year period, 30.9% are malignant tumors and 69.1% are non-malignant tumors [3]. Patients with malignant tumors have about 35% and 29.3% rates for 5- and 10- survival years, respectively [3]. Glioblastoma (GBM) is the most common and a highly aggressive type of glioma. Even though under treatment advancements, the median of the survival period for a patient with GBM still remains at 12–16 months [4]. The short survival period of patients with GBM is not only because of the rapid tumor growth, but is also due to the tumor's invasion to surrounding brain tissues [5]. Early and proper detection of the tumor grade may result in a good prognosis [6].

To achieve a proper prognosis and treatment management, accurate brain tumor detection and segmentation are very important. However, manual tumor segmentation

L. Pei
Department of Radiology, University of Pittsburgh, Pittsburgh, PA, USA

Hillman Cancer Center, University of Pittsburgh Medical Center, Pittsburgh, PA, USA

Vision Lab, Electrical & Computer Engineering, Old Dominion University, Norfolk, VA, USA
e-mail: peil@upmc.edu

K. M. Iftekharuddin (✉)
Vision Lab, Electrical & Computer Engineering, Old Dominion University, Norfolk, VA, USA
e-mail: kiftekha@odu.edu

© The Author(s), under exclusive license to Springer Nature Switzerland AG 2021
J. J. Otero, A. P. Becker (eds.), *Precision Molecular Pathology of Glioblastoma*, Molecular Pathology Library, https://doi.org/10.1007/978-3-030-69170-7_11

by radiologists is very tedious, time consuming, and prone to human error [7]. Consequently, computer-aided brain tumor analysis is desired. In the literature, many methods have been proposed to detect and segment brain tumors, such as the active contours-based [8] and atlas-based methods [9, 10]. However, performances of tumor segmentation using atlas-based methods highly depends on the quality of the tumor-bearing multimodal magnetic resonance imaging (mMRI) image registration with corresponding atlas. To overcome this issue, brain tumor segmentation may be considered as a classification problem. Traditional machine learning classifiers, including K-nearest neighbor (KNN), support vector machine (SVM), and random forest (RF), are generally used [2, 11–13] with appropriate features extraction. Due to difficulty in designing effective features extraction methods, deep learning-based classification methods for brain tumor segmentation have gained prevalence in recent years.

Tumor growth describes an abnormal growth of tissue, which usually involves cell proliferation, invasion, and mass effect to the surrounding tissues. During cell invasion, tumor cells migrate as a cohesive and multicellular group with retained cell-cell junctions and penetrate the surrounding healthy tissues. The tumor growth model may improve therapy planning (in surgery or radiotherapy) by defining the tumor invasion region based on the local estimation of the tumor cell density [14]. Many works in literature proposed cellular and microscopic models to predict tumor growth [15–17]. However, these models do not consider the interactions between cells and tissues. Macroscopic models mainly use a reaction-diffusion formalism [9, 14]. These models take both the microscopic proliferation and the macroscopic diffusion into account for tumor growth.

Even though the brain tumor segmentation and tumor growth modeling have each seen success in respective domains, these processes are studied individually. Longitudinal brain tumor prediction is not only related to the accurate segmentation of the various tumor sub-regions, but also reveals information about the tumor development over time. Monitoring longitudinal brain tumor changes is useful for follow-up of treatment-related changes, assessment of treatment response and guiding dynamically changing treatments, including surgery, radiation therapy, and chemotherapy.

In addition, brain tumor subtype classification and patient survival prediction are critical [1, 18]. An accurate tumor subtype classification results in a proper glioma grading, which benefits treatment planning and prognosis. Survival prediction estimates survival period for patients with brain tumors, which also helps the treatment management. There is a plethora of work proposed in literature about tumor subtype classification and patient survival prediction. Hou et al. proposed a convolutional neural network-based brain tumor subtype classification on whole slide image (WSI) [19]. Zeina et al. deployed an overall patient survival prediction using machine learning-based method. Even though the new tumor classification criteria released by World Health Organization (WHO) require both phenotypic and genomic information, conventional MRI is still widely used because of its non-invasive and large-scale view on brain tumor properties. It may be sufficient to use MRI only for tumor classification. In recent years, with the success of deep learning in many fields, such as computer vision [20–22], speech recognition [23], etc., deep learning-based methods have also been applied to medical imaging processing [24–26], including brain tumor detection, segmentation, tumor subtype classification, and overall patient survival prediction. There is a need to study automated learning-based automated methods for multiple tasks such as brain tumor segmentation, tracking, subtype classification, tumor growth analysis, and patient survival prediction simultaneously as each of these steps may affect multiple others.

Consequently, this chapter discusses a machine learning framework for longitudinal brain tumor volume segmentation and tracking using multimodal MRI, and combines brain tumor segmentation and tumor growth modeling. It comprises two fusion methods: feature fusion and joint label fusion (JLF). The first method fuses stochastic multi-resolution texture features with tumor cell density features to obtain tumor segmentation predictions in follow-up MRI scans. The second method utilizes JLF to combine segmentation labels obtained from (i) the stochastic texture feature-based and the Random Forest (RF)-based tumor segmentation method, and (ii) another state-of-the-art tumor growth and segmentation method, known as boosted Glioma Image Segmentation and Registration (GLISTRboost, or GB). We further discuss a context aware deep learning method (CANet) for brain tumor segmentation, tumor subtype classification, and overall survival prediction.

Background Review

The section reviews the relevant information on tumor segmentation, tumor growth modeling, longitudinal tumor tracking, the artificial neural network, and overall patient survival prediction.

Brain Tumor Segmentation

A brain tumor has highly irregular properties, including multiple cell phenotype, heterogeneous density, high intra-tumor pressure, and tortuous vasculature when comparing to normal tissues [27]. Accurate brain tumor detection and segmentation is critical for diagnosis, prognosis, and treatment planning. Brain tumors may appear with a huge variation in size, shape, heterogeneity and location on MRI, as shown in Fig. 11.1. Hence, it is very difficult to distinguish different abnormal tumor tissues such as necrosis (NC), peritumoral edema (ED), non-enhancing tumor (NE), and enhancing tumor (ET). There are many studies proposed for image-based brain tumor segmentation in the literature. Conventional machine learning-based methods, including K-nearest neighbors, support vector machine (SVM), and AdaBoost are widely used [28–30]. In recent years, deep learning-based methods outperform conventional machine learning-based methods for tumor segmentation. However, longitudinal brain tumor tracking using deep learning methods may not

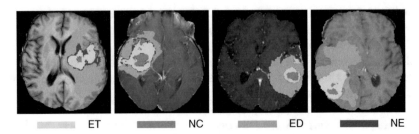

Fig. 11.1 Four cases of tumor on MRI. Note that these pre-processed images are overlaid with ground truth. All data obtained from BraTS Challenge. ET enhancing tumor, NC necrosis, ED peritumorally edema, NE non-enhancing tumor

be feasible due to a lack availability of large volume of longitudinal tumor tracking data.

Tumor Growth Modeling

Tumor growth modeling provides a trajectory of tumor changes over time. There are some works proposed for brain tumor growth modeling in the literature. According to the observation scales, it can be categorized into two groups: microscopic model and macroscopic. The microscopic models take behavior of individual cell into account for the subject, and consider the interaction between the cells and the environment as well [15–17]. For macroscopic models, they are based on local tumor cell density [9, 14]. Most of the macroscopic models employ a reaction-diffusion equation. In this work, we utilize a reaction-diffusion equation to predict brain tumor development over time as it takes both the microscopic proliferation and the macroscopic diffusion into account. There are many benefits of tumor growth simulation. First, it provides a better understanding of the physiology of the tumor growth. Second, a tumor growth model may be used to quantify a tumor's aggressiveness for a given patient. Finally, using the growth model can improve therapy planning (in surgery or radiotherapy) by better defining the tumor invasion region based on the local estimation of the tumor cell density [14]. It can help in predicting the tumor over time from a limited number of patient observations.

Longitudinal Brain Tumor Tracking

Longitudinal brain tumor segmentation prediction refers to brain tumor segmentation, and tumor growth development over time. Monitoring longitudinal brain tumor changes is useful for treatment follow-up, and assessment of different types of treatment response including surgery, radiation therapy, and chemotherapy. A reaction-diffusion equation is widely used for simulating brain tumor growth [10, 14, 31–34]. Hu et al. simulated one-dimensional tumor growth based on logistic models [35]. Sallemi et al. predicted brain tumor growth based on cellular automata and the fast marching method [36]. Clatz et al. proposed a GBM growth prediction by solving a reaction-diffusion equation [37]. In addition, we recently proposed a novel method for segmentation prediction by integrating with brain tumor segmentation [12].

Integrating with tumor segmentation, tumor growth modeling is useful in understanding the tumor development changes over time. Bauer et al. proposed a tumor growth model which is based on segmentation [38]. Boosted Glioma Image Segmentation and Registration (GLISTRboost), a state-of-the-art method, is developed for brain segmentation by incorporating a glioma growth model [39]. Brain Tumor Image Analysis (BraTumIA), another state-of-the-art tool, is used for longitudinal brain tumor segmentation [40]. However, both these tools ignore possible relationship between scans from different timepoints. Figure 11.2 illustrates a longitudinal brain tracking example. It shows the brain tumor changes at the second time scan (second row), comparing to the first-time scan (top row).

Artificial Neural Networks

Inspired by the biological neural networks of human brains, artificial neural networks (ANNs) are computing methods for estimating outputs based on the inputs. The process consists of data collection, analysis and processing, network

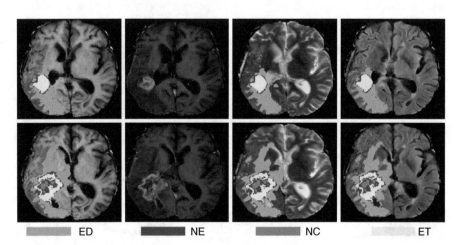

Fig. 11.2 A longitudinal brain tumor tracking example. Top row from left to right: T1, T1c, T2, T2-FLAIR, and ground truth (GT) at timepoint 1. Bottom row shows the corresponding images at timepoint 2 (89 days after timepoint 1). ED edema, NE non-enhancing tumor, NC necrosis, ET enhancing tumor

structure design, the number of hidden layers, the number of hidden units, initializing, training the network, network simulation, weights/bias adjustments, and testing the network [41]. ANNs are considered as a universal approximators that have the ability to approximate a given function distribution. Figure 11.3 illustrates a graphical representation of a perceptron.

Deep Learning Method: Convolutional Neural Network

With the availability of large dataset and the improvement of hardware, convolutional neural network (CNN) has been successfully applied in many domains, especially for visual imagery analysis. A typical CNN consists of a convolutional layer, a pooling layer, an activation function, and a fully connected layer. The convolutional layer determines the output of the neurons that are connected to the local regions of the input through convolutional operation. The pooling layer reduces the dimensionality of feature maps. The activation function is to add non-linear properties to the network. The activation functions include sigmoid, tanh, rectified linear unit (ReLU), and leaky-ReLU, among others. The fully connected layer contains neurons that are directly connected to the neurons in the two adjacent layers, without being connected to any layers within them [42]. It usually produces class scores from the activations in a classification application. A handwriting recognition application by using a CNN shown in Fig. 11.4.

Fig. 11.3 A graphical representation of a perceptron. x_i and ω_i are inputs to the neuron and the corresponding weight, respectively. $f(\bullet)$ is an active function. y is the final output

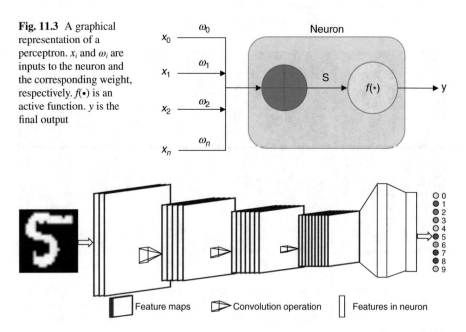

Fig. 11.4 A CNN application for handwritten digits recognition. Conv. convolutional, FC fully connected

In recent years, CNN-based methods have been successfully applied in brain tumor segmentation. According to the input data, the CNN-based methods can be generally categorized as patch-based [43], 2D slice-based [44], and 3D volume-based [45]. Each method has advantages and disadvantages. The patch-based method executes fastest in training phase, however, it may produce many misclassifications in testing phase. The 2D slice-based method has a moderate training time and generates a more accurate result than that of patch-based method in the testing phase. The 3D volume-based method takes the longest training time, yet provides the best performance in the testing phase, compared to the other two methods. All the CNN architectures for brain tumor segmentation are composed of encoding and decoding modules. The encoding module is to extract the high-dimensional dense features, and the decoding module is to reconstruct the encoded features to the corresponding segmentation. The trainable network minimizes the difference between the segmentation and ground truth.

Patient Survival Prediction

Patient survival prediction may aid in treatment management for patients. There are many studies in predicting the survivability of patients with brain tumors in the literature. These studies can be grouped as machine learning-base and deep learning-base methods. Using the machine learning-base method, handcrafted features, such as shape and texture of the brain tumor are extracted and then is followed by regression method to estimate the patient survivability. Zeina et al. propose a feature-guide deep radiomics method for glioblastoma patient survival prediction [18]. The authors extract volumetric and texture features, including piecewise triangular prism surface area (PTPSA) and multi-fractional Brownian motion (mBm) from segmented tumor tissues, and then XGBoost regression is applied on these features for the survival prediction. Due to difficulty in extracting effective handcrafted features, CNN-based deep learning method is an alternative way to predict the patient survivability [46, 47].

Methodology

In this section, we discuss a machine learning pipeline for brain tumor growth modeling, tumor segmentation and longitudinal brain tumor tracking, compromising of two methods: feature fusion and joint label fusion (JLF). Then, we describe a deep learning-based context-aware model known as CANet for brain tumor segmentation, tumor classification, and survival prediction, respectively.

Machine Learning-Based Methods: Brain Tumor Growth Modeling, Segmentation and Tracking

Biophysical Tumor Growth Model

Tumor growth refers to abnormal tissue development over time, which involves cell proliferation, invasion, and mass effect to surround tissues. We build the tumor growth model by solving a reaction-diffusion (RD) equation. The RD equation can be expressed as [34]:

$$\frac{\partial n_s}{\partial t} = D\nabla^2 n_s + \rho n_s \left(1 - n_s\right), \tag{11.1}$$

$$D\nabla n_s.\vec{n}_{\partial\Omega} = 0, \tag{11.2}$$

where n_s is the tumor cell density, D is the diffusion coefficient while infiltrating, and ρ is the proliferation rate. Equation (11.5) enforces Neumann boundary conditions on the brain domain Ω, and $\vec{n}$ is unit normal vector on the $\partial\Omega$ pointing inward to the domain.

Feature Fusion-Based Tumor Segmentation Method

The proposed method employs novel feature obtained from tumor growth pattern to improve tumor prediction in longitudinal MRI. The pipeline is shown in Fig. 11.5. Starting from the raw mMRI, we extract both non-texture and texture features. Meanwhile, based on the segmentation/ground truth at the baseline, we apply a

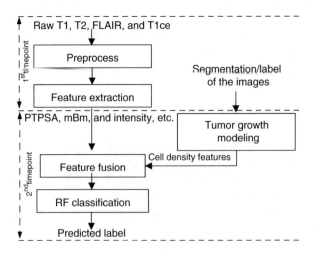

Fig. 11.5 Pipeline of the proposed method

tumor growth model by solving the reaction-diffusion equation using Lattice-Boltzmann method (more details in [2]). The cell densities of the tumors are used as novel features. Sequentially we fuse the novel features with the previous features. Finally, we perform a Random Forest (RF) classifier on the fused features to achieve prediction at the second time scan.

Joint Label Fusion-Based Tumor Segmentation

Comparing to a single-atlas based method, multi-atlas-based fusion offers a robust result. However, different atlases may generate similar label errors. To overcome the issue, a joint label fusion is proposed by Wang et al. [48]. Joint label fusion achieves consensus segmentation given as,

$$\hat{L} = \sum_{i=1}^{n} \omega_i(x) p\left(l|x,\hat{I}_n\right), \tag{11.3}$$

where $\omega_i(x)$ is individual voting weight, $\hat{I}_n$ is the n-th training image, and $p\left(l|x,\hat{I}_n\right)$ is the probability that x votes for label l. The weight is determined by:

$$\omega_x = \frac{M_x^{-1} 1_n}{1_n^t M_x^{-1} 1_n}, \tag{11.4}$$

where $1_n = [1;1;\cdots;1]$ is a vector of size n and M_x is the pairwise dependency matrix that estimates the likelihood of two atlases both producing wrong segmentations on a per-voxel basis for the target images.

The dependency matrix is computed as:

$$M_x(j,k) \sim \sum_{m=1}^{L_M} \left\langle \left| A_F^m\left(\mho\left(x(j)\right)\right) - T_F^m\left(\mho(x)\right)\right|, \left| A_F^m\left(\mho\left(x(k)\right)\right) - T_F^m\left(\mho(x)\right)\right| \right\rangle, \tag{11.5}$$

where m indices correspond to all modality channels, and $\left| A_F^m\left(\mho\left(x(j)\right)\right) - T_F^m\left(\mho(x)\right)\right|$ is the vector of absolute intensity difference between a selected atlas image and the target image over local patches $\mho$ centered at voxel $x(j)$ and x, respectively. $\langle \bullet, \bullet \rangle$ is the dot product. L_M is the total number of modalities [48].

The proposed joint label fusion-based method for tumor segmentation prediction is shown in Fig. 11.6. We utilize joint label fusion technique to fuse the label from RF and another state-of-the-art tool, known as GB.

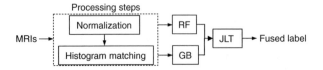

Fig. 11.6 Pipeline of joint label fusion-based tumor segmentation prediction

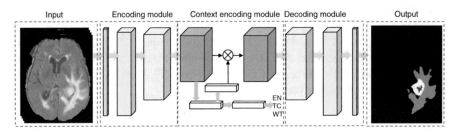

Fig. 11.7 CANet architecture for brain tumor segmentation

Deep Learning-Based Method: Brain Tumor Segmentation, Subtype Classification and Patient Survival Prediction

CANet-Based Tumor Segmentation

Even though there are many works in brain tumor segmentation, tumor subtype classification, and overall patient survival prediction in the literature, most of them are studied separately. In this section, a deep learning- based context aware network (CANet) for brain tumor analysis tasks is discussed that includes tumor segmentation, tumor subtype classification, and overall patient survival prediction [25, 49]. The CANet deep learning method for brain tumor segmentation is illustrated in Fig. 11.7. The architecture is composed of encoding, context encoding, and decoding modules. The encoding module extracts features from the input. The context encoding module generate updated features and a semantic loss to regularize the model. The decoding module reconstructs the extracted features to output prediction. Brain tumors have necrosis (NC), peritumoral edema (ED), non-enhancing tumor (NE), and enhancing tumor (ET).

CANet-Based Tumor Subtype Classification

Tumor subtype classification can be beneficial for treatment planning. The proposed pipeline for tumor classification is shown Fig. 11.8. The segmented tumor uncertainty in subregions from the above section are the inputs of tumor subtype classification. In addition, we construct a regular CNN for the classification, which includes

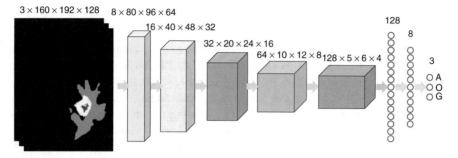

Fig. 11.8 Overview of CNN-based tumor classification. At the last convolutional layer, we apply an average pooling layer to shrink the size

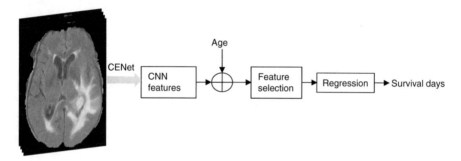

Fig. 11.9 Pipeline of proposed method for overall survival prediction

several convolutional layer, pooling layers, and fully connected layers. The output of the classification may be astrocytoma (A), oligodendroglioma (O), or glioblastoma (G).

CANet-Based Survival Prediction

The proposed pipeline for CNN-based survival prediction is shown in Fig. 11.9. We utilize the encoding module of the CANet to extract features from the input, then concatenate the age information. Subsequentially, we select features using Least Absolute Shrinkage and Selection Operator (LASSO). Finally, we perform a regression to estimate the survivability.

Experimental Setup

In this section, we describe experiment set-up, including dataset and evaluation measurement.

Dataset

As discussed, the data used for this work is taken from Multimodal Brain Tumor Segmentation Challenge (BraTS 2015 and BraTS 2019) and Computational Precision Medicine: Radiology-Pathology Challenge on Brain Tumor Classification 2019 (CPM-RadPath 2019). For longitudinal brain tumor tracking, we have nine longitudinal brain tumor data from BraTS 2015. For the tumor segmentation using CANet, we use data of BraTS 2019, including 335 cases, 125 cases, and 166 cases for training phase, validation phase, and testing phase, respectively. For the tumor subtype classification and survival prediction, there are 221, 35, and 73 cases from CPM-RadPath 2019 for training data, validation data, and testing data, respectively. Note that ground truths are only available for training data.

Brain Tumor Subregion

The evaluation in the work is based on the brain tumor subregions, including enhancing tumor (ET), tumor core (TC), and whole tumor (WT). The TC consist of enhancing tumor (ET) and necrosis (NC). The WT is the combination of all abnormal tissues, including ET, NC, and TC.

Dice Score Coefficient (DSC)

The quantality of evaluation is based on the dice score coefficient between tumor segmentation and ground truth, which can be described as $DSC = \dfrac{2 \cdot |A \cap B|}{|A| + |B|}$, where A and B represent the segmentation labels and the manually annotation (or ground truth). The DSC value ranges in $[0, 1]$, where 1 represents the regions are identical, and 0 means no overlap between these two sets.

Results and Discussions

The section reports the experimental results by using the proposed methods.

Machine Learning-Based Method

Feature Fusion

We build the biophysical brain tumor growth model by solving the RD equation using LBM. The parameters of diffusion coefficient D and proliferation rate ρ are suggested within $[0.02, 1.5]$ mm^2/day, and $\rho \epsilon [0.002, 0.2]day^{-1}$ in the literature [34]. Figure 11.10 shows examples of tumor segmentation prediction by using the proposed feature fusion-based method.

The performance comparison of tumor growth without cell density feature using the proposed method is shown in Fig. 11.11. Furthermore, we statistically analyse the significant improvement using paired t-test for all patients. The p-values for segmentation prediction obtained with and without inclusion of the cell density feature showed statistical significance for WT, TC, and ET tissues (Table 11.1).

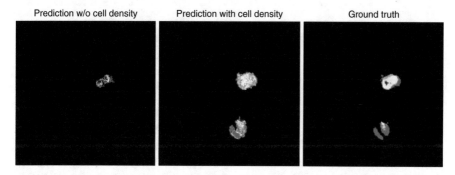

Fig. 11.10 Examples of tumor segmentation prediction by using the proposed method. (Left column) Without cell density feature, (middle column) With cell density feature, and (right column) the ground truth of second time scan

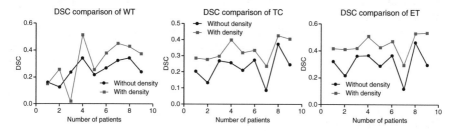

Fig. 11.11 Comparison of tumor growth prediction segmentation using proposed method [10]

Table 11.1 Paired t-test for comparison of the volume between without and with cell density by using RF only to predict the tumor segmentation labels in timepoint 2, using data from time point 1

	DSC_{WT}	DSC_{TC}	DSC_{ET}
Result w/o cell density	0.251 ± 0.08	0.229 ± 0.08	0.311 ± 0.101
Result with cell density	0.314 ± 0.16	0.332 ± 0.065	0.448 ± 0.076
p-value	0.150	0.0002	0.0002

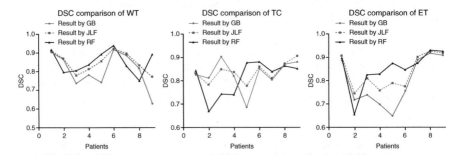

Fig. 11.12 DSC comparison results among GB, RF, and proposed method (JLF) at time 2 [10]

Label Fusion

We apply the joint label fusion-based brain tumor segmentation prediction to all nine patients at timepoint 2 (post-op scans). To evaluate the performance, we use a Leave-One-Out cross-validation schema to compute the DSC of segmentations at timepoint 2 from the proposed method and compare to the ground truth and to segmentations generated by GB. We compare the performance among the RF result, GB result, and the JLF result, as shown in Fig. 11.12. We further statistically analyse the significant importance using ANOVA, as shown in Table 11.2. The statistical analysis suggests that the joint label fusion offers significant improvement in WT and ET, comparing to the result by GB. There is an example showing the joint label fusion result in Fig. 11.13.

Furthermore, we compare the proposed work with the result using a state-of-the-art method, BraTumIA [40]. The comparison shows that our proposed method achieves much better result, as shown in Table 11.3.

Deep Learning Method

CANet-Based Tumor Segmentation

We apply the CANet for brain tumor segmentation using the validation and testing dataset of BraTS 2019, which include 125 cases and 166 cases, respectively. We then submit the segmentation for online evaluation, and performance is shown in

Table 11.2 Performance of 3D brain tumor growth prediction segmentation

	WT	TC	ET
Average DSC by GB	0.810 ± 0.095	0.829 ± 0.062	0.796 ± 0.104
Average DSC by RF	0.852 ± 0.063	0.812 ± 0.074	0.851 ± 0.083
Average DSC by JLF	0.850 ± 0.055	0.836 ± 0.041	0.837 ± 0.0074
p-value (GB and JLF)	0.047	0.579	0.023

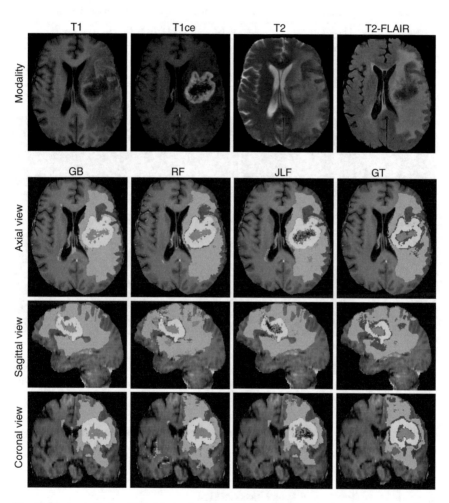

Fig. 11.13 An example of label fusion-based application. The first (top) row denotes the input brain scans. Rows 2–4 illustrate shows the axial, sagittal, and coronal views, respectively, of the T1c input can overlaid with GB, RF, JLF and GT labels

Table 11.3 Longitudinal tumor segmentation comparison of average DSC between BraTumIA [40] and JLF

	DSC_{WT}	DSC_{TC}	DSC_{ET}
BraTumIA [40]	0.761 ± 0.104	0.703 ± 0.186	0.732 ± 0.140
JLF	$.850 \pm 0.055$	0.836 ± 0.041	0.837 ± 0.075

Table 11.4 Dice coefficient results for tumor segmentation in the validation and testing datasets

Phase	Post-process	Dice_ET	Dice_WT	Dice_TC
Validation	No	0.73856	0.90496	0.81496
Validation	Yes	0.77273	0.90496	0.81496
Testing	Yes	0.8133	0.8867	0.84031

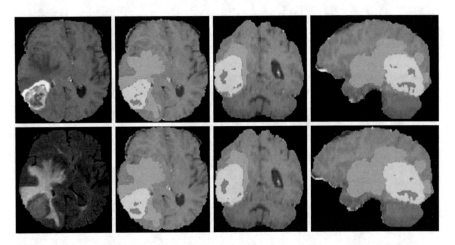

Fig. 11.14 Comparison of tumor segmentation using the proposed method and ground truth. Top row from left to right: T1ce image, segmented tumor overlaid with T1ce in axial view, in coronal view, and in sagittal view. Bottom row from left to right: FLAIR image, ground truth overlaid with T1ce in axial view, in coronal view, and in sagittal view

Table 11.4. There is an example showing the comparison between segmentation and ground truth in Fig. 11.14.

CANet-Based Tumor Subtype Classification

We apply the proposed method to the validation data and testing data of the CPM-RadPath 2019, which has 35 cases and 73 cases, respectively. In validation phase, we submit the result for online evaluation. Note that in the testing phase, we wrap the algorithm using Docker, and send to the challenge organizer. The organizer

Table 11.5 Online evaluation of tumor classification on CPM-RadPath 2019 validation and testing datasets

Phase	Dice	Average	Kappa	Balance_acc	F1_micro
Validation	0.749	0.764	0.715	0.749	0.829
Testing	0.596	NA	0.39	0.596	0.603

Table 11.6 Survival prediction performance of the validation dataset obtained from online evaluation

Phase	Accuracy	MSE	medianSE	stdSE	SpearmanR
Validation	0.586	79,146	24,362	113,801	0.502
Testing	0.439	449,009	44,604	1,234,471	0.279

executes the wrapped algorithm and rank based the performance. Our result is ranked second place in the testing phase. The tumor subtype classification performance is listed in Table 11.5.

CANet-Based Survival Prediction

We apply the proposed method to the BraTS 2019 validation and testing data for survival prediction, which contains 29 cases and 107 cases, respectively. According to the period length, the survivability can be categorized as short-term (<10 months), mid-term (between 10 and 15 months), and long-term (>15 months). The online evaluation is shown in Table 11.6.

Discussion

For longitudinal brain tumor segmentation and tracking, we discuss a novel machine learning based method comprising of feature fusion-based and joint label fusion. The feature fusion-based method shows significant prediction improvement of TC and ET abnormal tissue segmentation, while there is no significant improvement for WT tissue. On the other hand, the joint label fusion using RF and GB labels shows improvement on WT and ET abnormal tissue segmentation over that of the GB labels alone. Moreover, the performances using the method have significant improvement comparing to BraTumIA, a state-of-the-art for longitudinal brain tumor segmentation. This shows the promising application using the machine learning-based method for longitudinal tumor segmentation and tracking. However, due to availability of limited number of longitudinal tumor growth patient cases used in this study, the segmentation prediction performance is not optimal for all possible types of abnormal tissue.

For tumor classification and survival prediction using the CANet, lack of data is the main issue, which is also a limitation by using deep learning-based method. Even though we apply data augmentation to increase training sample size, 221 cases may still be insufficient number for deep learning.

Conclusion

This Chapter discusses learning-based methods for automated brain tumor growth modeling, tumor segmentation, tumor tracking, tumor subtype classification, and patient survival prediction using mMRI. Brief background is discussed for each task to introduce readers with the appropriate context. We then report a machine learning framework for brain tumor growth modeling, tumor segmentation and tracking in longitudinal mMRI scans, comprising two methods: feature fusion and joint label fusion. We further discuss a novel deep learning pipeline, known as Context-Aware Convolutional Neural Network (CANet), for tumor segmentation, tumor subtype classification and patient survival prediction. We evaluate the methods using mMRI dataset BraTS 2015, and BraTS 2019, and the Computational Precision Medicine: Radiology-Pathology Challenge on Brain Tumor Classification 2019 (CPM-RadPath), respectively. The evaluation results show the learning methods achieve state-of-the-art in longitudinal brain tumor tracking and tumor subtype classification. The performances also suggest that the methods offer promising results in tumor segmentation and overall survival prediction.

Acknowledgements This work was partially funded through NIH/NIBIB grant under award number R01EB020683.

References

1. Bakas S, et al. Identifying the best machine learning algorithms for brain tumor segmentation, progression assessment, and overall survival prediction in the BRATS challenge. arXiv preprint arXiv:1811.02629, 2018.
2. Pei L, et al. Longitudinal brain tumor segmentation prediction in MRI using feature and label fusion. Biomed Signal Process Control. 2020;55:101648.
3. Ostrom QT, et al. CBTRUS statistical report: primary brain and other central nervous system tumors diagnosed in the United States in 2011–2015. Neuro-Oncol. 2018;20(suppl_4):iv1–iv86.
4. Chen J, McKay RM, Parada LF. Malignant glioma: lessons from genomics, mouse models, and stem cells. Cell. 2012;149(1):36–47.
5. Kansal AR, et al. Simulated brain tumor growth dynamics using a three-dimensional cellular automaton. J Theor Biol. 2000;203(4):367–82.
6. Banerjee S, et al. Deep radiomics for brain tumor detection and classification from multi-sequence MRI. arXiv preprint arXiv:1903.09240, 2019.
7. Popuri K, et al. 3D variational brain tumor segmentation using Dirichlet priors on a clustered feature set. Int J Comput Assist Radiol Surg. 2012;7(4):493–506.

8. Olszewska JI. Active contour based optical character recognition for automated scene understanding. Neurocomputing. 2015;161:65–71.
9. Gooya A, Biros G, Davatzikos C. Deformable registration of glioma images using EM algorithm and diffusion reaction modeling. IEEE Trans Med Imaging. 2011;30(2):375–90.
10. Gooya A, et al. GLISTR: glioma image segmentation and registration. IEEE Trans Med Imaging. 2012;31(10):1941–54.
11. Reza SM, Mays R, Iftekharuddin KM. Multi-fractal detrended texture feature for brain tumor classification. In: Medical imaging 2015: computer-aided diagnosis: International Society for Optics and Photonics; Bellingham, USA. 2015.
12. Pei L, et al. Improved brain tumor segmentation by utilizing tumor growth model in longitudinal brain MRI. In: Medical imaging 2017: computer-aided diagnosis. International Society for Optics and Photonics; Bellingham, USA. 2017.
13. Pei L, Reza SM, Iftekharuddin KM. Improved brain tumor growth prediction and segmentation in longitudinal brain MRI. In: 2015 IEEE international conference on Bioinformatics and biomedicine (BIBM). IEEE; 2015.
14. Clatz O, et al. Realistic simulation of the 3-D growth of brain tumors in MR images coupling diffusion with biomechanical deformation. IEEE Trans Med Imaging. 2005;24(10):1334–46.
15. Retsky M, et al. Is Gompertzian or exponential kinetics a valid description of individual human cancer growth? Med Hypotheses. 1990;33(2):95–106.
16. Lazareff JA, et al. Tumor volume and growth kinetics in hypothalamic-chiasmatic pediatric low grade gliomas. Pediatr Neurosurg. 1999;30(6):312–9.
17. Bajzer Z. Gompertzian growth as a self-similar and allometric process. Growth Dev Aging. 1999;63(1–2):3–11.
18. Shboul ZA, et al. Feature-guided deep radiomics for glioblastoma patient survival prediction. Front Neurosci. 2019;13:966.
19. Hou L, et al. Patch-based convolutional neural network for whole slide tissue image classification. In: Proceedings of the IEEE conference on computer vision and pattern recognition. 2016.
20. LeCun Y, Bengio Y, Hinton G. Deep learning. Nature. 2015;521:436.
21. Goodfellow I, Bengio Y, Courville A. Deep learning. MIT Press; 2016.
22. Goodfellow I, et al. Generative adversarial nets. In: Advances in neural information processing systems; 2014.
23. Amodei D, et al. Deep speech 2: End-to-end speech recognition in english and mandarin. In: International conference on machine learning. 2016.
24. Ronneberger O, Fischer P, Brox T. U-net: Convolutional networks for biomedical image segmentation. In: International conference on Medical image computing and computer-assisted intervention. Springer; 2015.
25. Pei L, et al. Deep learning with context encoding for semantic brain tumor segmentation and patient survival prediction. In: Medical imaging 2020: computer-aided diagnosis. International Society for Optics and Photonics; 2020.
26. Akkus Z, et al. Deep learning for brain MRI segmentation: state of the art and future directions. J Digit Imaging. 2017;30(4):449–59.
27. Tang L, et al. Computational modeling of 3D tumor growth and angiogenesis for chemotherapy evaluation. PLoS One. 2014;9(1):e83962.
28. Khalid NEA, Ibrahim S, Haniff P. MRI brain abnormalities segmentation using K-nearest neighbors (k-NN). Int J Comput Sci Eng. 2011;3(2):980–90.
29. Iftekharuddin KM, et al. Brain tumor detection in MRI: technique and statistical validation. In: 2006 Fortieth Asilomar conference on signals, systems and computers. 2006.
30. Islam A, Reza SM, Iftekharuddin KM. Multifractal texture estimation for detection and segmentation of brain tumors. IEEE Trans Biomed Eng. 2013;60(11):3204–15.
31. Marušić M. Mathematical models of tumor growth. Math Commun. 1996;1(2):175–88.
32. Hogea C, Davatzikos C, Biros G. Modeling glioma growth and mass effect in 3D MR images of the brain. Med Image Comput Comput Assist Interv. 2007;10(Pt 1):642–50.

33. Konukoglu E, et al. Image guided personalization of reaction-diffusion type tumor growth models using modified anisotropic Eikonal equations. IEEE Trans Med Imaging. 2010;29(1):77–95.
34. Le M, et al. MRI based Bayesian personalization of a tumor growth model. IEEE Trans Med Imaging. 2016;35(10):2329–39.
35. RiCha H, XiaoGang R. A logistic cellular automaton for simulating tumor growth. In: Intelligent Control and Automation, 2002. Proceedings of the 4th World Congress on. 2002.
36. Sallemi L, Njeh I, Lehericy S. Towards a computer aided prognosis for brain glioblastomas tumor growth estimation. IEEE Trans Nanobioscience. 2015;14(7):727–33.
37. Clatz O, et al. Brain tumor growth simulation. INRIA; 2004.
38. Bauer S, et al. Atlas-based segmentation of brain tumor images using a Markov Random Field-based tumor growth model and non-rigid registration. In: 2010 annual international conference of the IEEE engineering in medicine and biology. 2010.
39. Bakas S, et al. GLISTRboost: Combining multimodal MRI segmentation, registration, and biophysical tumor growth modeling with gradient boosting machines for glioma segmentation. In: Brainlesion: Glioma, multiple sclerosis, stroke and traumatic brain injuries: first international workshop, Brainles 2015, Held in Conjunction with MICCAI 2015, Munich, Germany, October 5, 2015, Revised Selected Papers, Crimi A, et al., editors. Cham: Springer International Publishing; 2016. p. 144–155.
40. Meier R, et al. Clinical evaluation of a fully-automatic segmentation method for longitudinal brain tumor volumetry. Sci Rep. 2016;6:23376.
41. El-Shahat A. Advanced applications for artificial neural networks. 2018: BoD–Books on Demand.
42. O'Shea K, Nash R. An introduction to convolutional neural networks. ArXiv e-prints. 2015.
43. Havaei M, et al. Brain tumor segmentation with deep neural networks. Med Image Anal. 2017;35:18–31.
44. Zhao X, et al. A deep learning model integrating FCNNs and CRFs for brain tumor segmentation. Med Image Anal. 2018;43:98–111.
45. Myronenko A. 3D MRI brain tumor segmentation using autoencoder regularization. In: International MICCAI Brainlesion workshop: Springer; 2018.
46. Fu J, et al. An automatic deep learning-based workflow for glioblastoma survival prediction using pre-operative multimodal MR images. arXiv preprint arXiv:2001.11155. 2020.
47. Zhang Y, et al. CNN-based survival model for pancreatic ductal adenocarcinoma in medical imaging. BMC Med Imaging. 2020;20(1):1–8.
48. Wang H, et al. Multi-atlas segmentation with joint label fusion. IEEE Trans Pattern Anal Mach Intell. 2013;35(3):611–23.
49. Zhang H, et al. Context encoding for semantic segmentation. In: Proceedings of the IEEE conference on computer vision and pattern recognition. 2018.

Chapter 12
Rodent Brain Tumor Models for Neuro-Oncology Research

Yoshihiro Otani, Ryan McCormack, and Balveen Kaur

Introduction

Glioblastoma (GBM) is the most common primary malignant brain tumor with approximately 12,000 new diagnoses each year in the United States [1]. Despite advances in surgical techniques, adjuvant chemoradiation, and novel tumor treating interventions GBM prognosis continues to be grim with a median overall survival (OS) of less than 2 years [2–7]. Molecular profiling of GBM has unveiled several targets for molecular interventions, and despite the preclinical success of targeted therapies, the clinical experience has been largely disappointing. To aid in better translation of preclinical drug development to patients availability of preclinical models to evaluation of the mechanisms and interactions become critical to the development of successful therapeutics. Rodents are the choice species for these studies, for many different reasons as outlined below. Here we will discuss the utility and limitations of the different rodent models commonly utilized in neuro-oncology research.

Carcinogen Induces Rodent Brain Tumor Models

Rat GBM models were initially developed in the early 1970s and have been the mainstay of neuro-oncology for much of the last 50 years. Over time, these models have provided significant insight into the GBM progression as well as the

Y. Otani · R. McCormack · B. Kaur (✉)
The Department of Neurosurgery, McGovern Medical School, The University of Texas Health Science Center at Houston, Houston, TX, USA
e-mail: Balveen.Kaur@uth.tmc.edu

© The Author(s), under exclusive license to Springer Nature Switzerland AG 2021
J. J. Otero, A. P. Becker (eds.), *Precision Molecular Pathology of Glioblastoma*, Molecular Pathology Library, https://doi.org/10.1007/978-3-030-69170-7_12

biological mechanisms regulating GBM including chemotherapy, anti-angiogenic therapy, proteasome inhibitors, toxins, radiation therapy, photodynamic therapy, oncolytic viral therapy, and gene therapy [8–16]. Despite the limited translational success of these advances, rat brain tumor models continue to provide a wealth of information regarding the in vivo responses to GBM and different therapeutic modalities. All syngeneic rat GBM models were chemically induced by treating pregnant rats with carcinogens such as *N*-nitroso compounds [17–19]. Commonly utilized chemically induced rat brain tumor models include 9L, C6, F98, and CNS-1 (for in-depth review please see Barth and Kaur [20]). One additional caveat to these chemically induced brain tumors is that the tumor characteristics are quite different from human gliomas prompting frequent reference to "gliosarcomas" or "glioma-like tumors." This is probably a reflection of the artificial chemical-induced brain tumor development in these animals [21, 22]. Chemically induced rat glioma models have additional drawbacks when assessed histologically. Rat models do demonstrate some invasion; however, there is a lack of single-cell infiltration to the contralateral hemisphere as well as the microvascular involvement typically of human GBM. Even "invasive xenografts" in BT4C, F98, and RG-2 tumors exhibit various ranges of local invasion rather than single-cell invasion in both hemispheres [23, 24].

The major advantage of chemically induced cell lines grafted into syngeneic animals is an intact immune system permitting for studies that involve the assessment of the tumor microenvironment, microglial polarization, and interaction with the adaptive immune response [25, 26]. However, the innate and adaptive priming also has a potentially significant limitation with the inherent immunogenicity of some models resulting in a spontaneous tumor rejection. This is exemplified in studies where the C6 rat model resulted in increased rejection of tumors with reducing tumor cell inoculum such that a 30% rejection rate is observed in rats implanted with ten thousand tumor cells [27]. Later MHC allele-typing demonstrated that the C6 line was originally derived from an outbred strain and are thus not syngeneic with BDIX, Sprague-Dawley, or Wistar rats contributing towards the observed immunogenicity of this model [28].

Nevertheless, the rat GBM models have been used to provide excellent information regarding the interaction between tumor vs adaptive and innate immunity. The primary advantage of rat models lies in the significantly increased size of the rat brain when compared to that of a mouse (~1200 mg vs ~400 mg). The larger size permits a more precise tumor implantation as well as a significantly larger volume of injection. The increased brain size also provides for a larger tumor size before mortality enabling an easier opportunity for tissue analysis. While these advantages are significant, the advancements in genetic engineering have enabled the development of genetically engineered murine models that better recapitulate human disease.

Chemically Induced Murine GBM Models

Immunocompetent murine glioma models are powerful tools allowing one to investigate the therapeutic effect and interaction between tumor cells and the TME including immune cells, vasculature, neurons, and glial cells. The need for immune-competent animal models is highly significant with the increased development in immune-modulating experimental drugs being evaluated for use in brain tumor patients. Apart from the rat models described above, several chemically-induced murine glioma models have been described and are frequently utilized. GL261 was established in 1970 via chemical induction with methylcholanthrene [29]. Intracranial inoculation of GL261 cells forms reliable and reproducible tumors that have activating mutations in the Ras pathway along with loss of tumor suppressors like p53 similar to human GBM. This model has been used extensively in research to study both glioma stem cells and response to therapies.

The recent advent of biological therapies like oncolytic HSV requires a human receptor for viral entry. GL261 cells transduced with the herpes virus entry receptor nectin 1 (GL261-N4) have been created to facilitate evaluation of HSV based therapeutics. This allows the use of immune-competent GBM model to be used to evaluate the immunological benefit of HSV based therapies [30]. CT-2A was also created by chemical induction with 20-methylcholanthrene [31]. Those tumors are deficient in PTEN and have a dysregulated PI3K pathway and are thus useful to evaluate PTEN loss and/or activated PI3K signaling associated effects [32].

Genetically Induced Murine Glioma Models

During the last decade, advances in sequencing technology have increased our understanding of the genomic landscape of glioma [33, 34]. With this understanding, there have also been explorations into targeted therapeutics necessitating the development of models with specific tumor driver mutations similar to human GBM. To better recapitulate the biology of GBM, mice have been genetically engineered with specific alterations in tumor suppressors and oncogenes introduced in a tissue-specific manner using different approaches [35]. This has enabled the creation of genetically engineered mouse (GEM) models. These models have various favorable characteristics including (i) temporal and sequential induction of oncogene or depletion of tumor-suppression genes in the specific cell of origin in a specific time frame to investigate tumor development, (ii) temporal and sequential depletion of specific gene for a therapeutic feasibility proof-of-concept study, (iii) lineage-specific tracing of tumor subpopulations during tumor development and treatments, and (iv) specific induction or depletion of target genes in TME to understand the importance of such genes in TME for tumor-TME interaction.

These models dramatically changed the experimental models available for Neuro-Oncology preclinical research. The different strategies used to generate these include different recombination, transposon, and virus mediated gene transduction strategies such as: Cre/LoxP recombination, flippase/flippase recombination (Flp/FRT), avian leukosis virus (ALV)-based replication-competent ALV long terminal repeat with a splice acceptor (RCAS), transposon system (Sleeping Beauty (SB), piggyBAC, Tol2), and the CRISPR/Cas9 system. Here, we will describe some of the molecular technologies utilized to develop genetically-engineered mouse models (GEMMs) (Fig. 12.1).

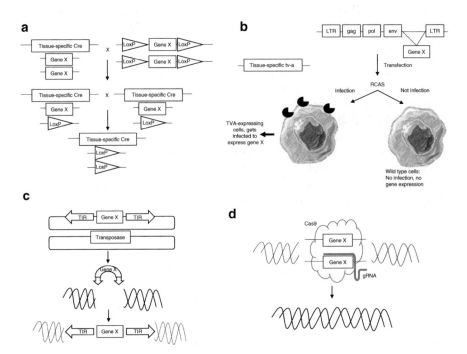

Fig. 12.1 Examples of different strategies utilized to generate genetically engineered murine glioma models. (**a**). Tissue specific Cre-expressing mice are crossed with transgenic mice engineered to have loxp sites flanking a target gene. F1 generation then generates heterozygote mice which have floxed out one allele of the gene. Subsequent mating results in homozygous mice with tissue specific loss of the target gene in both the alleles. (**b**) The RCAS-TVA system. RCAS retroviruses produced in DF1 chicken fibroblasts can enter mammalian cells expressing RCAS receptor, TVA, but not TVA-negative mammalian cells. (**c**) Transposon system. Co transfection of transposases with a genetic element that contains target gene to be inserted flanked by transposon specific terminal inverted repeats (TIRs). Transposase results in integration of the target gene into into a new target site in the mammalian genome. (**d**) CRISPR-Cas9 system. Cas9 enzyme mediated DNA incision at sequences guided by RNA (gRNA). Target genes are edited by deleting or inserting new DNA at the cut position

Cre/LoxP Site Specific Recombination Driven Murine Models

Cre-Lox is a site-specific recombinase technology derived from bacteriophage P1 [36]. This system consists of a Cre recombinase enzyme and a pair of short target sequences called Lox sequences. Lox sequence includes asymmetric 8 bp core spacer sequence and two symmetric 13 bp sequence, and Cre recombinase mediates recombination between two LoxP sites. If two LoxP sites are opposite orientation, the floxed sequence (sequence flanked by two LoxP sites) is inverted. However, if two LoxP sites are the same direction, the floxed sequence is excised.

The exact cellular origin of human GBM is still unclear; however, the best approximations of tumor initiating cells based on gene expression are utilized to generate GEM glioma models. Tissue-specific Cre transgenic mouse lines enable genomic alteration to be introduced in particular subsets of cells expressing markers of stem cell-like population. GFAP which is a specific marker for astrocytes, is also present on neural progenitor and glioma stem cells, and thus GFAP positive cells are frequently used to express tumor driving mutations [37]. A landmark study from Dr. Prada's laboratory reported the generation of mouse strains that lack p53 and harbor a conditional floxed allele of the NF1 tumor suppressor [38]. Cross-breeding of these mice with mice expressing Cre under a GFAP promotor thus generated p53 and NF1 knockout mice in GFAP+ cells. One hundred percent of these mice developed spontaneous astrocytomas that histologically resembled GBM. In another study, a pTomo-H-RasV12 plasmid that contains a human cytomegalovirus immediate-early promoter (CMV)-loxP-red fluorescent protein (RFP)-loxP-Flag-H-RasV12 and a mutant Ras, followed by internal ribosomal entry site (IRES)-GFP, was injected along with an Akt expressing lentivirus in the hippocampus or subventricular zone of adult GFAP-Cre $Tp53^{+/-}$ mice [39]. In this model, GFAP+ tumor cells express GFP which indicates GFAP-specific Cre-recombination. Isolated tumor cells (005 tumor cells) from this model are highly tumorigenic in C57Bl/6 mice and relatively non-immunogenic, lacking expression of co-stimulatory molecules (CD80 and CD86) and major histocompatibility complex I (MHCI) [40]. Thus murine 005 cells implanted in mice develop tumors with some characteristics that are similar to human GBM including tumor heterogeneity, invasion, angiogenesis, and an immunosuppressive TME [41–46]. Apart from GFAP+ cells, Nestin+ cells are also frequently exploited to be the initiating cells that harbor genetic alterations to drive GBM in mice. Nestin is a 38-kDa intermediate filament protein, initially identified in neural stem cells. Shingu et al. reported a conditional knockout of Qki, a STAR-family RNA-binding protein, using $Nes\text{-}CreER^{T2}$ line (tamoxifen-inducible Cre under $Nestin$ promoter) which increased gliomagenesis combining with $Pten^{L/L}$ and $Tp53^{L/L}$ [47]. Bardella et al. also used conditional expression of the $IDH1^{R132H}$ allele in an adult SVZ using Nes-Cre, with resultant gliomagenesis [48].

Flp/FRT

Flp/FRT is another site-directed recombination technology, analogous to Cre-Lox recombination that was derived from a yeast 2 μ plasmid [49]. Flp recombinase recognizes the gene flanked by Flp recombinase recognition target (FRT) sites with excision by homologous recombination. Although Flp/FRT and Cre/Lox are similar recombinase systems, FLP-FRT is not efficient at recombining genes in mammals since Flp has an optimal temperature of 30 degree Celsius concordant with its yeast origin [50]. Later, researchers identified an altered Flp recombinase, Flpe [51] and Flpo [52], which have an optimal temperature of 37 degrees Celsius and whose recombination efficacy is comparable to that of Cre/lox. Using the Flpo system, Hara et al. generated glioma in mice utilizing GFAP-Flpo mice to generate GFAP positive cells expressing mutant Hras^{G12V} and silenced for Tp53 using an U6-shTrp53 [53]. This mouse model enabled additional manipulation of the mouse genome by Cre/Lox, which provided for further understanding of the cellular and molecular mechanism of glioma genesis.

RCAS Avian Sarcoma Leukosis Virus Mediated GEM Model

The RCAS system is a somatic gene transfer system, derived from a family of avian sarcoma leukosis viruses (ASLVs). This virus depends on the TVA receptor for entry. Since mammalian cells do not natively express TVA, tissue specific expression of TVA is used to drive infection specificity of ASLV derived viral vectors to transport genetic cargo to a chosen cellular populations. Dr. Holland's laboratory created GEM models that developed brain tumors utilizing the RCAS system [54]. In this GBM mouse model, mice expressing the TVA receptor under the governance of a nestin promotor were used to ensure infection of only nestin positive TVA expressing cells with RCAS. Treatment of these mice with RCAS virus encoding for KrasG^{12D} a constitutively active form of Akt resulted in the development of GBM like brain tumors [54]. Further the transduction of RCAS-PDGFB in Ntv-a, Ink4a-ARF$^{-/-}$ mice spontaneously developed brainstem glioma [55]. According to the current WHO classification of tumors of the central nervous system (CNS), previously termed diffuse intrinsic pontine glioma (DIPG) is defined as midline glioma, H3 K27M-mutant which harboring K27M mutation in the histone H3 gene *H3F3A* or *HIST1H3B*. Further investigation by Hoeman et al. revealed transduction of RCAS-ACVR1 R206H with H3.1K27M in the brainstem of Ntv-a;Tp53$^{fl/fl}$ mice developed diffuse midline glioma [56]. Some of the limitations of the RCAS model is the need to prepare specific TVA-expressing mouse strains, and that the RCAS vector can only carry ~2.5 kb.

Transposon Derived GEM Models

While a majority of genes are stable entities arranged in an orderly linear pattern on definite loci on chromosomes the identification of transposons or "mobile genetic elements" facilitated the discovery of the transposon system that drives inter genomic migration. Transposon systems discovered to date include the Sleeping Beauty (SB), piggyBac (PB), Tol2, Frog Prince, Himar1, and passport. These transposon systems have not only different phylogenetic origin but also different biological properties (including cargo size and DNA sequence preference for transposition) that cause different activities. Among these transposon systems, SB and PB are widely used to develop GEMMs as well as treatment for GBM [57, 58].

SB is a two-part DNA transposon system that is used to insert tumor driver gene alteration in mouse models in several cancers including glioma. SB transposons are derived from the Tc1-mariner family that are widely encoded across all animals but silenced in vertebrates during evolution. This system is comprised of 2 components: SB transposase and a transposon containing the gene cassette that can translocate within the genome [59]. Within cells, transposase recognizes the inverted repeats of the transposon (IR/DR; inverted terminal repeat, direct repeat) and excises it from the genome, and then that transposon can be inserted at a TA dinucleotide region (~200 million potential sites in mammalian genome [60]) elsewhere in the genome. SB28 is a genetically engineered model induced by SB transposon-mediated intraventricular transfection of *NRAS*, *PDGF*, and short hairpin *Tp53* in neonatal C57Bl/6 mice [61]. This SB28 model shows less immunogenic phenotype and less number of the predicted MHC-I binding neoepitopes than the spontaneous astrocytoma model SMA-560 and the methylcholanthrene-induced GL261 models. Therefore, SB28 is resistant to ICBs [62, 63], while SMA-560 and GL261 models are responsive to checkpoint blockade immunotherapy [64–67] with unclear efficacy in human GBM [68]. Koschmann et al. investigated the role of loss of ATRX which is often concurrent with *TP53* mutation in glioma using SB system. In this model, addition of SB-mediated sh*ATRX* to sh*Tp53* and *NRAS* (NP) model significantly reduced survival of tumor-bearing mice and increased genetic instability [69]. PB is another transposon system that is isolated from the cabbage looper moth (*Trichoplusia ni*). While the original PB transposase demonstrated higher transposase activity than SB [70], subsequent efforts to improve transposon efficiency resulted in the generation of hyperactive PBase and SB100X, with better transposon efficiency [71].

Izsvak et al. found that larger elements transposed less efficiency with SB transposase, and with each kb increase in transposon length the efficiency of transposition decreased by approximately 30% [72], and cargo size limitation in SB is ~5 kb [73]. In contrast, PB elements can carry up to 9.1 kb of foreign sequence without significantly reducing integration efficiency [74]. Another advantage of PB is that

PB tolerates overproduction inhibition (OPI), permitting a tolerance to its induced expression. Thus, PB is a viable option for developing GEMMs as well as gene delivery treatment in vitro and in vivo. Chen et al. developed glioma GEMM by *in utero* electroporation of piggyBAC transposon harboring HRasV12 and AKT with GLAST-PBase into radial glial progenitors [75]. Histologically, the tumors displayed diffuse infiltration into neighboring tissues and had cells with a highly proliferative and necrotic area.

CRISPR-Cas9

As described above the goal is to create GEMMs expressing tumor drivers, however, the deletion of tumor suppressors with above techniques is a tedious time-consuming process involving homologous recombination in embryonic stem cells. Clustered regulatory interspaced short palindromic repeats (CRISPRs) were first identified in *E.coli* in 1987 [76], which play a key role in adaptive immunity as the antiviral defense. CRISPR-associated protein 9 (Cas9) is an enzyme that recognizes CRISPR sequences as a guide to cleave specific strands of DNA. This technology can be modified to cleave DNA in a sequence-specific manner leading to a very powerful technology that can result in precise gene editing without the need for cumbersome recombination strategies. This technology has revolutionized current gene editing and for this reason, Dr. Jennifer Doudna and Emmanuelle Charpentier were awarded the 2020 Nobel Prize in chemistry.

To date, several brain tumor GEMMs have been generated by CRISPR-Cas9 technology. For example, Zuckermann et al. developed sonic hedgehog (SHH) medulloblastoma, one of the childhood brain tumors with the poorest prognosis, by depleting the *Ptch1* gene [77]. Furthermore, they utilized gRNAs targeting *Nf1*, *Trp53*, and *Pten*, and were able to induce highly aggressive tumors similar to human GBM. Yu et al. developed a murine glioma model by in utero electroporation of CRISPR/Cas9 vectors targeting Nf1, Trp53, and Pten with different variants of *Pik3ca* mutations [78].

Spontaneous Tumor Derived Implantable Murine Models

Initial attempts to develop a spontaneous murine glioma model failed until 1971, despite murine, canine, and feline development of primary brain tumors [79]. In 1971, Fraser developed a spontaneous murine astrocytoma (SMA) cell line from the inbred VM/Dk strain, however, over time this model lost tumorigenicity with successive in vitro passages [80]. A decade later Dr. Bigner's laboratory established 5 cell lines (P492, P496, P497, P540, and P560) from the intracranial passaged SMA and generated five cell lines with astrocytic features that retained tumor take. Of these SMA-560 is the most highly used and has been exploited to investigate the testing of immune therapies when implanted in the VM mouse strain [81–83]. 4C8 cells also represent a non-chemically induced transplantable tumor model. These cells were originally derived from MOCH-1 glial transgenic mouse and form highly cellular tumors upon implantation into F1 generation of mice crossed between C57BL/6J (B6) female x DBA/2J (D2) male and are hence heterozygous for all strain-specific loci in their genome [84]. Lentivirus mediated transduction of H-Ras and AKT in GFAP-Cre Tp53$^{-/-}$ mice has also been used to induce spontaneous tumors in mice. As described above, primary tumor cell cultures from these tumors resulted in the isolation of 005 that formed neurosphere-like structures, and retained self-renewal and tumorigenicity upon subsequent implantation in mice. Tumors derived from the implantation of these cells are also more frequently being used [39]. Cells derived from genetic models with inactivation of NF1 and heterozygous for p53 with or without PTEN inactivation have also been used in several studies. However, it is important to note that these cells were originated from a mixed genetic background of C57/BL6, Sv129, and B6/CBA mice and will not be completely syngenic in any murine inbred strain. RNAseq analysis of end-stage tumors showed that only Mut3 tumors had an expression profile that was distinct from CT2A, GL261, or 005 murine glioma cells. Differentially expressed gene ontology pathways related to immune signaling were more enriched in the Gl261 and 005 relative to Mut3 and CT2A derived tumors [46].

Human Glioma Xenograft Models

Xenografts of human glioma derived cells implanted in immune-deficient mice are perhaps the most widely used animal model to study GBM growth and response to therapeutics. These cell lines were developed from patient-derived samples and then cultured in vitro to create a stable clonal population and engrafted orthotopically into immune-deficient mice and rats. Among these established cell line models, U87 cells derived from a glioblastoma patient is perhaps the most widely utilized model. Years of growth in vitro in tissue culture has evolved the U87 cells to undergo a clonal selection that permits rapid growth in vitro and in vivo. Stable transduction of these cells with luciferase also permits tracking of tumor growth in live animals with bioluminescence imaging [85, 86]. This cell line was developed by Dr. Ponten and Dr. McIntyre in the 1960s at the University of Uppsala, Sweden [87]. These cells were widely distributed among brain tumor researchers and were eventually deposited in the American Type Culture Collection (ATCC). Interestingly, decades later short tandem repeat sequence (STRS) profiling of these cells revealed that the U87 cells widely used and distributed by ATCC did match the profile of the patient tumor from whom these cells were originally supposed to be derived. Transcriptional profiling of the U87MG cell lines from ATCC did confirm that the cells were of CNS origin and postulated to be a human GBM cell line; however, the exact patient origin is unknown [88]. While these established human cell lines implanted into the brains of immunocompromised rodents provide a model with predictable and reliable tumor growth; they do not display histological hallmarks of GBM such as infiltrating tumor growth characteristics of invasive tumor edge, necrotic foci within tumors, and microvascular proliferation. Given the lack of histologic characteristics common to GBM, the favored xenograft models are changing to primary patient-derived stem cell-like cells maintained in vitro under conditions that do not permit differentiation or passaged in mice as xenografts [89].

Tumors derived from these traditional glioma cell lines that are maintained in serum do not fully reflect the genetic and histologic features of human GBM and the use of PDX or genetically engineered glioma models is gaining favor [90] as these models retain both the genetic and histological features of human GBM, in an immune-competent environment. The most widely used resource for GBM patient-derived cell lines is the Brain Tumor Patient-derived xenograft (PDX) National Resource at the Mayo Clinic, which has characterized and annotated a series of brain tumor PDX models with levels of multi-omic characterizations comparable to those provided for primary patient tumors by The Cancer Genome Atlas (TCGA). Unlike traditional serum grown cell lines like U87, these models more accurately mimic the histological characteristics of the human disease and express known GBM molecular alteration such as mutant *TERT*, *EGFR* amplification, *PTEN* LOH, mutant *IDH1* etc. Gene expression studies have uncovered that these models frequently also reflect different molecular subtypes identified in GBM patients. Similar to human patients these models also represent both *MGMT* methylated and un-methylated tumor types with MGMT expression mediated resistant to temozolomide observed in vitro and in vivo [6]. Integrated molecular profiling of patient-derived models has uncovered that these tumors reproduce most of the tumor driving mutations reported in patients [91]. While these models provide an excellent conduit for evaluating tumor-specific responses, these models are maintained in immuno-deficient animals and so cannot be used to evaluate immunotherapeutic responses. The additional requirement for passaging in mice, also makes these cumbersome and expensive.

Humanized Mouse Models

Development of improved xenograft models in PDX improves the reliability of tumor model characteristics; however, despite these advancements, the tumor-host interaction remains defective owing to the need for these models to be developed within immunocompromised animals. Even with immunocompetent rodent models as described above, one major drawback remains in the fact that these models rely on the rodent immune system, which does not always recapitulate the human immune response. This need has led to the development of different humanized mouse models that rely on the following pillars of an immunodeficient host mouse, populated with human immune cells, and human tumor cells.

The initial description of the possibility of engraftment of human immune cells in an immunodeficient mouse was in the nude mouse that lacks T cells (athymic nude mice) [92]. Based on this seminal characterization, it has become clear that the more immunodeficient the mice, the better the engraftment efficacy [93]. Engraftment improved with the development of scid mice deficient in T and B cell lymphocytes and crossing these animals with the nonobese diabetic (NOD) mouse background with deficiencies in NK cells, macrophage activity, and the complement system [94, 95]. Final improvements occurred through the elimination of the gamma chain of the IL-2 receptor, leading to the loss of murine NK cells and a nonfunctional IL-2, IL-4, IL-7, IL-9, IL-15, and IL-21 due to common receptor interactions [96, 97]. The final advancement in the mouse background occurred with the work of Takenaka and others with the identification of signal-regulatory protein alpha (*Sirpa*) that strongly interacts with human CD47 [98]. These advancements have created a framework allowing for a high level of engraftment following implantation of human cells.

The next major component within the humanized mouse framework is the cells used for engraftment. The first described model consisted of human PBMC reconstitution in a SCID background. This model provides for efficient T cell engraftment; however, corresponding with low levels in PBMC with lack of HSC engraftment this model has virtually no human B cells and myeloid-derived cells [99, 100]. Furthermore, utilization is limited by the development of lethal graft-versus-host-disease (GVHD) within approximately 4–6 weeks following engraftment [101, 102]. Given the robust GVHD response limiting experimental time-frames and potentially confounding results, an alternative methodology was created with engraftment of CD34+ HSC [103, 104]. In general, these models provide for the development of human T cells with the selection of human MHC molecules with limited GVHD response. CD34+ HSC models are predominantly limited by the degree of engraftment with the success of engraftment based on the recipient mouse selection (age, sex, strain), source of CD34+ cells, and route by which engraftment occurs [96, 97, 105, 106]. The CD34+ model success is also contingent on the depletion of the mouse HSC compartment with sub-lethal gamma-irradiation to facilitate human HSC engraftment. Optimization of these variables enables human engraftment to approach >90% in many immune compartments including the peripheral blood lymphocytes (PBL), spleen, thymus, and gut [103]. However due to the lack of cross reactivity between murine and human cytokines, all of these models provide a hostile environment for the maturation of the injected human PBMC or CD34+ stem cells and thus hinder an efficient repopulation into a mature immune system. This can be overcome by either repeat injections of human cytokines, or gene encoding plasmids in mice which can be cumbersome. The use of transgenic mice that also express human cytokines instead of murine cytokines ensures appropriate dosage and tissue specificity show improved maturation and population of mature human T, macrophage and NK cells.

While these models are not allogenic, they do permit the usage of defined HLA types with reconstitution allows for monitoring and tracking epitope-specific responses. These models summarized in a recent review [107] provide an advancement over currently used models however the high costs of these transgenic mice limits their wide spread usage.

Conclusion and Future Prospects

In this chapter, we have summarized the different rodent animal models frequently utilized for Neuro-oncology research. While some of the first animal models relied on carcinogen induced spontaneous tumors that were then used to generate tumorigenic cells to create implantable models these models did not frequently have the genetic alterations seen in human tumors. Current deep sequencing and single-cell technologies has uncovered the multiple genetic alterations in tumor biology to develop novel treatments. The emergence of GEMMs with fast and reliable techniques to genetically engineer cells in a tissue and cell type specific manner accelerated the utility of these models to ask key questions about molecular drivers that led to oncogenesis. Mice with these specific genetic alterations also provided a resource to evaluate targeted therapies designed to precisely treat a cell population with a specific genetic target. However these murine models do not replace the need for testing human tumors, something made highly essential for species specific biotherapies like viruses and antibodies. Drug development efforts for such biotherapies are thus for the most part limited to immune deficient models that can harbor a human tumor graft. The development of human cell lines from brain tumors started decades ago and these cells grown in serum formed reproducible homogenous tumors but lacked the heterogeneity observed with GBM. The advent of the development of primary patient derived neurosphere cultured cells or cells routinely passaged through mice as PDX models was the next improvement, although still suffered from being limited to usage in immune deficient mice. The gold standard to study human tumors in an intact tumor microenvironment is perhaps in the humanized mouse models that can accept human tumors and develop a mature human immune system. These models while cutting edge are extremely costly to use which limits their wide spread utility. More research to generate cost effective and possibly isogenic humanized murine models is needed to facilitate translation of targeted drug development efforts in the future.

References

1. Ostrom QT, Gittleman H, Truitt G, Boscia A, Kruchko C, Barnholtz-Sloan JS. CBTRUS statistical report: primary brain and other central nervous system tumors diagnosed in the United States in 2011–2015. Neuro Oncol. 2018;20(suppl_4):iv1–iv86.
2. Lacroix M, Abi-Said D, Fourney DR, Gokaslan ZL, Shi W, DeMonte F, et al. A multivariate analysis of 416 patients with glioblastoma multiforme: prognosis, extent of resection, and survival. J Neurosurg. 2001;95(2):190–8.
3. Zhu P, Du XL, Zhu JJ, Esquenazi Y. Improved survival of glioblastoma patients treated at academic and high-volume facilities: a hospital-based study from the National Cancer Database. J Neurosurg. 2019;132(2):491–502.
4. Ostrom QT, Gittleman H, Fulop J, Liu M, Blanda R, Kromer C, et al. CBTRUS statistical report: primary brain and central nervous system tumors diagnosed in the United States in 2008–2012. Neuro Oncol. 2015;17 Suppl 4:iv1–iv62.

5. Stupp R, Mason WP, van den Bent MJ, Weller M, Fisher B, Taphoorn MJ, et al. Radiotherapy plus concomitant and adjuvant temozolomide for glioblastoma. N Engl J Med. 2005;352(10):987–96.
6. Stupp R, Taillibert S, Kanner A, Read W, Steinberg D, Lhermitte B, et al. Effect of tumor-treating fields plus maintenance temozolomide vs maintenance temozolomide alone on survival in patients with glioblastoma: a randomized clinical trial. JAMA. 2017;318(23):2306–16.
7. Esquenazi Y, Friedman E, Liu Z, Zhu JJ, Hsu S, Tandon N. The survival advantage of "supra-total" resection of glioblastoma using selective cortical mapping and the subpial technique. Neurosurgery. 2017;81(2):275–88.
8. Doblas S, Tesiram Y, Saunders D, Kshirsagar P, Pye Q, Pearson J, et al. Tumor regression and angiogenesis inhibition by phenyl-tert-butyl nitrone and its main metabolite in C6 rat glioma model. AACR; 2007.
9. Solly F, Fish R, Simard B, Bolle N, Kruithof E, Polack B, et al. Tissue-type plasminogen activator has antiangiogenic properties without effect on tumor growth in a rat C6 glioma model. Cancer Gene Ther. 2008;15(10):685–92.
10. Ahmed AE, Jacob S, Nagy AA, Abdel-Naim AB. Dibromoacetonitrile-induced protein oxidation and inhibition of proteasomal activity in rat glioma cells. Toxicol Lett. 2008;179(1):29–33.
11. Sheehan J, Ionescu A, Pouratian N, Hamilton DK, Schlesinger D, Oskouian RJ, et al. Use of trans sodium crocetinate for sensitizing glioblastoma multiforme to radiation. J Neurosurg. 2008;108(5):972–8.
12. Mannino S, Molinari A, Sabatino G, Ciafrè S, Colone M, Maira G, et al. Intratumoral vs systemic administration of meta-tetrahydroxyphenylchlorin for photodynamic therapy of malignant gliomas: assessment of uptake and spatial distribution in C6 rat glioma model. Int J Immunopathol Pharmacol. 2008;21(1):227–31.
13. Yang WQ, Lun X, Palmer CA, Wilcox ME, Muzik H, Shi ZQ, et al. Efficacy and safety evaluation of human reovirus type 3 in immunocompetent animals: racine and nonhuman primates. Clin Cancer Res. 2004;10(24):8561–76.
14. Tanriover N, Ulu MO, Sanus GZ, Bilir A, Canbeyli R, Oz B, et al. The effects of systemic and intratumoral interleukin-12 treatment in C6 rat glioma model. Neurol Res. 2008;30(5):511–7.
15. Furnari FB, Fenton T, Bachoo RM, Mukasa A, Stommel JM, Stegh A, et al. Malignant astrocytic glioma: genetics, biology, and paths to treatment. Genes Dev. 2007;21(21):2683–710.
16. Krakstad C, Chekenya M. Survival signalling and apoptosis resistance in glioblastomas: opportunities for targeted therapeutics. Mol Cancer. 2010;9(1):135.
17. Dagle G, Zwicker G, Renne R. Morphology of spontaneous brain tumors in the rat. Vet Pathol. 1979;16(3):318–24.
18. Druckrey H, Ivanković S, Preussmann R. Selektive Erzeugung maligner Tumoren im Gehirn und Rückenmark von Ratten durch N-methyl-N-nitrosoharnstoff. Z Krebsforsch. 1965;66(5):389–408.
19. Schmidek HH, Nielsen SL, Schiller AL, Messer J. Morphological studies of rat brain tumors induced by N-nitrosomethylurea. J Neurosurg. 1971;34(3):335–40.
20. Barth RF, Kaur B. Rat brain tumor models in experimental neuro-oncology: the C6, 9L, T9, RG2, F98, BT4C, RT-2 and CNS-1 gliomas. J Neurooncol. 2009;94(3):299–312.
21. Samkange-Zeeb F, Schlehofer B, Schüz J, Schlaefer K, Berg-Beckhoff G, Wahrendorf J, et al. Occupation and risk of glioma, meningioma and acoustic neuroma: results from a German case–control study (Interphone study group, Germany). Cancer Epidemiol. 2010;34(1):55–61.
22. Samanic CM, De Roos AJ, Stewart PA, Rajaraman P, Waters MA, Inskip PD. Occupational exposure to pesticides and risk of adult brain tumors. Am J Epidemiol. 2008;167(8):976–85.
23. He J, Yin Y, Luster TA, Watkins L, Thorpe PE. Antiphosphatidylserine antibody combined with irradiation damages tumor blood vessels and induces tumor immunity in a rat model of glioblastoma. Clin Cancer Res. 2009;15(22):6871–80.

24. Mariani CL, Kouri JG, Streit WJ. Rejection of RG-2 gliomas is mediated by microglia and T lymphocytes. J Neurooncol. 2006;79(3):243–53.
25. Maleszewska M, Steranka A, Smiech M, Kaza B, Pilanc P, Dabrowski M, et al. Sequential changes in histone modifications shape transcriptional responses underlying microglia polarization by glioma. Glia. 2021;69:109–23.
26. Gieryng A, Pszczolkowska D, Bocian K, Dabrowski M, Rajan WD, Kloss M, et al. Immune microenvironment of experimental rat C6 gliomas resembles human glioblastomas. Sci Rep. 2017;7(1):1–14.
27. Parsa AT, Chakrabarti I, Hurley PT, Chi JH, Hall JS, Kaiser MG, et al. Limitations of the C6/Wistar rat intracerebral glioma model: implications for evaluating immunotherapy. Neurosurgery. 2000;47(4):993–1000.
28. Beutler AS, Banck MS, Wedekind D, Hedrich HJ. Tumor gene therapy made easy: allogeneic major histocompatibility complex in the C6 rat glioma model. Hum Gene Ther. 1999;10(1):95–101.
29. Ausman JI, Shapiro WR, Rall DP. Studies on the chemotherapy of experimental brain tumors: development of an experimental model. Cancer Res. 1970;30(9):2394–400.
30. Yoo JY, Swanner J, Otani Y, Nair M, Park F, Banasavadi-Siddegowda Y, et al. oHSV therapy increases trametinib access to brain tumors and sensitizes them in vivo. Neuro Oncol. 2019;21:1131–40.
31. Seyfried TN, el-Abbadi M, Roy ML. Ganglioside distribution in murine neural tumors. Mol Chem Neuropathol. 1992;17(2):147–67.
32. Marsh J, Mukherjee P, Seyfried TN. Akt-dependent proapoptotic effects of dietary restriction on late-stage management of a phosphatase and tensin homologue/tuberous sclerosis complex 2-deficient mouse astrocytoma. Clin Cancer Res. 2008;14(23):7751–62.
33. Brennan CW, Verhaak RG, McKenna A, Campos B, Noushmehr H, Salama SR, et al. The somatic genomic landscape of glioblastoma. Cell. 2013;155(2):462–77.
34. Suzuki H, Aoki K, Chiba K, Sato Y, Shiozawa Y, Shiraishi Y, et al. Mutational landscape and clonal architecture in grade II and III gliomas. Nat Genet. 2015;47(5):458–68.
35. Robertson FL, Marqués-Torrejón MA, Morrison GM, Pollard SM. Experimental models and tools to tackle glioblastoma. Dis Model Mech. 2019;12(9):dmm040386.
36. Sauer B. Functional expression of the cre-lox site-specific recombination system in the yeast Saccharomyces cerevisiae. Mol Cell Biol. 1987;7(6):2087–96.
37. Garcia AD, Doan NB, Imura T, Bush TG, Sofroniew MV. GFAP-expressing progenitors are the principal source of constitutive neurogenesis in adult mouse forebrain. Nat Neurosci. 2004;7(11):1233–41.
38. Zhu Y, Guignard F, Zhao D, Liu L, Burns DK, Mason RP, et al. Early inactivation of p53 tumor suppressor gene cooperating with NF1 loss induces malignant astrocytoma. Cancer Cell. 2005;8(2):119–30.
39. Marumoto T, Tashiro A, Friedmann-Morvinski D, Scadeng M, Soda Y, Gage FH, et al. Development of a novel mouse glioma model using lentiviral vectors. Nat Med. 2009;15(1):110–6.
40. Cheema TA, Wakimoto H, Fecci PE, Ning J, Kuroda T, Jeyaretna DS, et al. Multifaceted oncolytic virus therapy for glioblastoma in an immunocompetent cancer stem cell model. Proc Natl Acad Sci U S A. 2013;110(29):12006–11.
41. Friedmann-Morvinski D, Narasimamurthy R, Xia Y, Myskiw C, Soda Y, Verma IM. Targeting NF-κB in glioblastoma: a therapeutic approach. Sci Adv. 2016;2(1):e1501292.
42. Saha D, Martuza RL, Rabkin SD. Macrophage polarization contributes to glioblastoma eradication by combination immunovirotherapy and immune checkpoint blockade. Cancer Cell. 2017;32(2):253–67.e5.
43. Chen P, Zhao D, Li J, Liang X, Li J, Chang A, et al. Symbiotic macrophage-glioma cell interactions reveal synthetic lethality in PTEN-null glioma. Cancer Cell. 2019;35(6):868–84.e6.

44. Flores-Toro JA, Luo D, Gopinath A, Sarkisian MR, Campbell JJ, Charo IF, et al. CCR2 inhibition reduces tumor myeloid cells and unmasks a checkpoint inhibitor effect to slow progression of resistant murine gliomas. Proc Natl Acad Sci U S A. 2020;117(2):1129–38.
45. Saha D, Rabkin SD, Martuza RL. Temozolomide antagonizes oncolytic immunovirotherapy in glioblastoma. J Immunother Cancer. 2020;8(1):e000345.
46. Khalsa JK, Cheng N, Keegan J, Chaudry A, Driver J, Bi WL, et al. Immune phenotyping of diverse syngeneic murine brain tumors identifies immunologically distinct types. Nat Commun. 2020;11(1):3912.
47. Shingu T, Ho AL, Yuan L, Zhou X, Dai C, Zheng S, et al. Qki deficiency maintains stemness of glioma stem cells in suboptimal environment by downregulating endolysosomal degradation. Nat Genet. 2017;49(1):75–86.
48. Bardella C, Al-Dalahmah O, Krell D, Brazauskas P, Al-Qahtani K, Tomkova M, et al. Expression of Idh1(R132H) in the murine subventricular zone stem cell niche recapitulates features of early gliomagenesis. Cancer Cell. 2016;30(4):578–94.
49. Broach JR, Guarascio VR, Jayaram M. Recombination within the yeast plasmid 2mu circle is site-specific. Cell. 1982;29(1):227–34.
50. Buchholz F, Ringrose L, Angrand PO, Rossi F, Stewart AF. Different thermostabilities of FLP and Cre recombinases: implications for applied site-specific recombination. Nucleic Acids Res. 1996;24(21):4256–62.
51. Buchholz F, Angrand PO, Stewart AF. Improved properties of FLP recombinase evolved by cycling mutagenesis. Nat Biotechnol. 1998;16(7):657–62.
52. Raymond CS, Soriano P. High-efficiency FLP and PhiC31 site-specific recombination in mammalian cells. PLoS One. 2007;2(1):e162.
53. Hara T, Verma IM. Modeling gliomas using two recombinases. Cancer Res. 2019;79(15):3983–91.
54. Holland EC, Celestino J, Dai C, Schaefer L, Sawaya RE, Fuller GN. Combined activation of Ras and Akt in neural progenitors induces glioblastoma formation in mice. Nat Genet. 2000;25(1):55–7.
55. Becher OJ, Hambardzumyan D, Walker TR, Helmy K, Nazarian J, Albrecht S, et al. Preclinical evaluation of radiation and perifosine in a genetically and histologically accurate model of brainstem glioma. Cancer Res. 2010;70(6):2548–57.
56. Hoeman CM, Cordero FJ, Hu G, Misuraca K, Romero MM, Cardona HJ, et al. ACVR1 R206H cooperates with H3.1K27M in promoting diffuse intrinsic pontine glioma pathogenesis. Nat Commun. 2019;10(1):1023.
57. Wu A, Oh S, Ericson K, Demorest ZL, Vengco I, Gharagozlou S, et al. Transposon-based interferon gamma gene transfer overcomes limitations of episomal plasmid for immunogene therapy of glioblastoma. Cancer Gene Ther. 2007;14(6):550–60.
58. Lohe AR, Hartl DL. Autoregulation of mariner transposase activity by overproduction and dominant-negative complementation. Mol Biol Evol. 1996;13(4):549–55.
59. Ivics Z, Hackett PB, Plasterk RH, Izsvák Z. Molecular reconstruction of Sleeping Beauty, a Tc1-like transposon from fish, and its transposition in human cells. Cell. 1997;91(4):501–10.
60. Bell JB, Podetz-Pedersen KM, Aronovich EL, Belur LR, McIvor RS, Hackett PB. Preferential delivery of the Sleeping Beauty transposon system to livers of mice by hydrodynamic injection. Nat Protoc. 2007;2(12):3153–65.
61. Kosaka A, Ohkuri T, Okada H. Combination of an agonistic anti-CD40 monoclonal antibody and the COX-2 inhibitor celecoxib induces anti-glioma effects by promotion of type-1 immunity in myeloid cells and T-cells. Cancer Immunol Immunother. 2014;63(8):847–57.
62. Johanns TM, Ward JP, Miller CA, Wilson C, Kobayashi DK, Bender D, et al. Endogenous neoantigen-specific CD8 T cells identified in two glioblastoma models using a cancer immunogenomics approach. Cancer Immunol Res. 2016;4(12):1007–15.
63. Genoud V, Marinari E, Nikolaev SI, Castle JC, Bukur V, Dietrich PY, et al. Responsiveness to anti-PD-1 and anti-CTLA-4 immune checkpoint blockade in SB28 and GL261 mouse glioma models. Onco Targets Ther. 2018;7(12):e1501137.

64. Fecci PE, Ochiai H, Mitchell DA, Grossi PM, Sweeney AE, Archer GE, et al. Systemic CTLA-4 blockade ameliorates glioma-induced changes to the CD4+ T cell compartment without affecting regulatory T-cell function. Clin Cancer Res. 2007;13(7):2158–67.
65. Reardon DA, Gokhale PC, Klein SR, Ligon KL, Rodig SJ, Ramkissoon SH, et al. Glioblastoma eradication following immune checkpoint blockade in an orthotopic, immunocompetent model. Cancer Immunol Res. 2016;4(2):124–35.
66. Wainwright DA, Chang AL, Dey M, Balyasnikova IV, Kim CK, Tobias A, et al. Durable therapeutic efficacy utilizing combinatorial blockade against IDO, CTLA-4, and PD-L1 in mice with brain tumors. Clin Cancer Res. 2014;20(20):5290–301.
67. Aslan K, Turco V, Blobner J, Sonner JK, Liuzzi AR, Núñez NG, et al. Heterogeneity of response to immune checkpoint blockade in hypermutated experimental gliomas. Nat Commun. 2020;11(1):931.
68. Reardon DA, Brandes AA, Omuro A, Mulholland P, Lim M, Wick A, et al. Effect of nivolumab vs bevacizumab in patients with recurrent glioblastoma: the CheckMate 143 phase 3 randomized clinical trial. JAMA Oncol. 2020;6(7):1–8.
69. Koschmann C, Calinescu AA, Nunez FJ, Mackay A, Fazal-Salom J, Thomas D, et al. ATRX loss promotes tumor growth and impairs nonhomologous end joining DNA repair in glioma. Sci Transl Med. 2016;8(328):328ra28.
70. Wu SC, Meir YJ, Coates CJ, Handler AM, Pelczar P, Moisyadi S, et al. piggyBac is a flexible and highly active transposon as compared to sleeping beauty, Tol2, and Mos1 in mammalian cells. Proc Natl Acad Sci U S A. 2006;103(41):15008–13.
71. Balasubramanian S, Rajendra Y, Baldi L, Hacker DL, Wurm FM. Comparison of three transposons for the generation of highly productive recombinant CHO cell pools and cell lines. Biotechnol Bioeng. 2016;113(6):1234–43.
72. Izsvák Z, Ivics Z, Plasterk RH. Sleeping Beauty, a wide host-range transposon vector for genetic transformation in vertebrates. J Mol Biol. 2000;302(1):93–102.
73. Huang X, Guo H, Tammana S, Jung YC, Mellgren E, Bassi P, et al. Gene transfer efficiency and genome-wide integration profiling of Sleeping Beauty, Tol2, and piggyBac transposons in human primary T cells. Mol Ther. 2010;18(10):1803–13.
74. Ding S, Wu X, Li G, Han M, Zhuang Y, Xu T. Efficient transposition of the piggyBac (PB) transposon in mammalian cells and mice. Cell. 2005;122(3):473–83.
75. Chen F, Becker AJ, LoTurco JJ. Contribution of tumor heterogeneity in a new animal model of CNS tumors. Mol Cancer Res. 2014;12(5):742–53.
76. Ishino Y, Shinagawa H, Makino K, Amemura M, Nakata A. Nucleotide sequence of the iap gene, responsible for alkaline phosphatase isozyme conversion in Escherichia coli, and identification of the gene product. J Bacteriol. 1987;169(12):5429–33.
77. Zuckermann M, Hovestadt V, Knobbe-Thomsen CB, Zapatka M, Northcott PA, Schramm K, et al. Somatic CRISPR/Cas9-mediated tumour suppressor disruption enables versatile brain tumour modelling. Nat Commun. 2015;6:7391.
78. Yu K, Lin CJ, Hatcher A, Lozzi B, Kong K, Huang-Hobbs E, et al. PIK3CA variants selectively initiate brain hyperactivity during gliomagenesis. Nature. 2020;578(7793):166–71.
79. Berens ME, Bjotvedt G, Levesque DC, Rief MD, Shapiro JR, Coons SW. Tumorigenic, invasive, karyotypic, and immunocytochemical characteristics of clonal cell lines derived from a spontaneous canine anaplastic astrocytoma. In Vitro Cell Dev Biol Anim. 1993;29a(4):310–8.
80. Fraser H. Astrocytomas in an inbred mouse strain. J Pathol. 1971;103(4):266–70.
81. Serano RD, Pegram CN, Bigner DD. Tumorigenic cell culture lines from a spontaneous VM/Dk murine astrocytoma (SMA). Acta Neuropathol. 1980;51(1):53–64.
82. Heimberger AB, Crotty LE, Archer GE, McLendon RE, Friedman A, Dranoff G, et al. Bone marrow-derived dendritic cells pulsed with tumor homogenate induce immunity against syngeneic intracerebral glioma. J Neuroimmunol. 2000;103(1):16–25.
83. Miller J, Eisele G, Tabatabai G, Aulwurm S, von Kürthy G, Stitz L, et al. Soluble CD70: a novel immunotherapeutic agent for experimental glioblastoma. J Neurosurg. 2010;113(2):280–5.

84. Oh T, Fakurnejad S, Sayegh ET, Clark AJ, Ivan ME, Sun MZ, et al. Immunocompetent murine models for the study of glioblastoma immunotherapy. J Transl Med. 2014;12:107.
85. Russell L, Bolyard C, Banasavadi-Siddegowda Y, Weiss A, Zhang J, Shakya R, et al. Sex as a biological variable in response to temozolomide. Neuro Oncol. 2017;19(6):873–4.
86. Sun T, Patil R, Galstyan A, Klymyshyn D, Ding H, Chesnokova A, et al. Blockade of a laminin-411-notch axis with CRISPR/Cas9 or a nanobioconjugate inhibits glioblastoma growth through tumor-microenvironment cross-talk. Cancer Res. 2019;79(6):1239–51.
87. Pontén J, Macintyre EH. Long term culture of normal and neoplastic human glia. Acta Pathol Microbiol Scand. 1968;74(4):465–86.
88. Allen M, Bjerke M, Edlund H, Nelander S, Westermark B. Origin of the U87MG glioma cell line: good news and bad news. Sci Transl Med. 2016;8(354):354re3.
89. Lathia JD, Mack SC, Mulkearns-Hubert EE, Valentim CL, Rich JN. Cancer stem cells in glioblastoma. Genes Dev. 2015;29(12):1203–17.
90. Koga T, Chaim IA, Benitez JA, Markmiller S, Parisian AD, Hevner RF, et al. Longitudinal assessment of tumor development using cancer avatars derived from genetically engineered pluripotent stem cells. Nat Commun. 2020;11(1):550.
91. Vaubel RA, Tian S, Remonde D, Schroeder MA, Mladek AC, Kitange GJ, et al. Genomic and phenotypic characterization of a broad panel of patient-derived xenografts reflects the diversity of glioblastoma. Clin Cancer Res. 2020;26(5):1094–104.
92. Fogh J, Fogh JM, Orfeo T. One hundred and twenty-seven cultured human tumor cell lines producing tumors in nude mice. J Natl Cancer Inst. 1977;59(1):221–6.
93. Hudson W, Li Q, Le C, Kersey J. Xenotransplantation of human lymphoid malignancies is optimized in mice with multiple immunologic defects. Leukemia. 1998;12(12):2029–33.
94. Bosma GC, Custer RP, Bosma MJ. A severe combined immunodeficiency mutation in the mouse. Nature. 1983;301(5900):527–30.
95. Shultz LD, Ishikawa F, Greiner DL. Humanized mice in translational biomedical research. Nat Rev Immunol. 2007;7(2):118–30.
96. Ito M, Hiramatsu H, Kobayashi K, Suzue K, Kawahata M, Hioki K, et al. NOD/SCID/γ c null mouse: an excellent recipient mouse model for engraftment of human cells. Blood. 2002;100(9):3175–82.
97. Traggiai E, Chicha L, Mazzucchelli L, Bronz L, Piffaretti J-C, Lanzavecchia A, et al. Development of a human adaptive immune system in cord blood cell-transplanted mice. Science (New York, NY). 2004;304(5667):104–7.
98. Takenaka K, Prasolava TK, Wang JC, Mortin-Toth SM, Khalouei S, Gan OI, et al. Polymorphism in Sirpa modulates engraftment of human hematopoietic stem cells. Nat Immunol. 2007;8(12):1313–23.
99. Shultz LD, Pearson T, King M, Giassi L, Carney L, Gott B, et al. Humanized NOD/LtSz-scid IL2 receptor common gamma chain knockout mice in diabetes research. Ann N Y Acad Sci. 2007;1103(1):77–89.
100. Ito A, Ishida T, Yano H, Inagaki A, Suzuki S, Sato F, et al. Defucosylated anti-CCR4 mono-clonal antibody exercises potent ADCC-mediated antitumor effect in the novel tumor-bearing humanized NOD/Shi-scid, IL-2Rγ null mouse model. Cancer Immunol Immunother. 2009;58(8):1195–206.
101. Mosier DE, Gulizia RJ, Baird SM, Wilson DB. Transfer of a functional human immune sys-tem to mice with severe combined immunodeficiency. Nature. 1988;335(6187):256–9.
102. King M, Covassin L, Brehm M, Racki W, Pearson T, Leif J, et al. Human peripheral blood leucocyte non-obese diabetic-severe combined immunodeficiency interleukin-2 receptor gamma chain gene mouse model of xenogeneic graft-versus-host-like disease and the role of host major histocompatibility complex. Clin Exp Immunol. 2009;157(1):104–18.
103. Gonzalez L, Strbo N, Podack ER. Humanized mice: novel model for studying mechanisms of human immune-based therapies. Immunol Res. 2013;57(1–3):326–34.

104. Lan P, Tonomura N, Shimizu A, Wang S, Yang Y-G. Reconstitution of a functional human immune system in immunodeficient mice through combined human fetal thymus/liver and CD34+ cell transplantation. Blood. 2006;108(2):487–92.
105. Holyoake TL, Nicolini FE, Eaves CJ. Functional differences between transplantable human hematopoietic stem cells from fetal liver, cord blood, and adult marrow. Exp Hematol. 1999;27(9):1418–27.
106. Brehm MA, Bortell R, Leif J, Laning J, Cuthbert A, Yang C, et al. Human immune system development and rejection of human islet allografts in spontaneously diabetic NOD-Rag1null IL2rynull Ins2Akita mice. Diabetes. 2010;59(9):2265–70.
107. Tian H, Lyu Y, Yang YG, Hu Z. Humanized rodent models for cancer research. Front Oncol. 2020;10:1696.

Chapter 13
Stem Cell Based Modelling of Glioblastoma

Abigail A. Zalenski, Miranda M. Tallman, and Monica Venere

Introduction

Curative treatment options for glioblastoma (GBM) continue to be elusive for a myriad of reasons, including the extensive intratumoral cellular heterogeneity that exists within these tumors. Of critical clinical importance is the presence of a sub-population of cells inherently more resistant to current treatment options, referred to as cancer stem cells (CSCs) or alternatively called GBM CSCs (GSCs) [1, 2]. CSCs have been identified in many different tumor types, and were first discovered in the context of leukemia [3, 4]. This cell population harbors unique characteristics centered on the ability to initiate tumor formation, self-renew, and maintain the bulk tumor by giving rise to the non-GSCs, or more differentiated cells, within the tumor [5, 6]. Importantly, GSCs are radio-resistant and chemo-resistant [1, 2]. Additionally,

A. A. Zalenski
Department of Radiation Oncology, James Cancer Hospital and Comprehensive Cancer Center, The Ohio State University College of Medicine, Columbus, OH, USA

Neuroscience Graduate Program, The Ohio State University, Columbus, OH, USA
e-mail: Abigail.zalenski@osumc.edu

M. M. Tallman
Department of Radiation Oncology, James Cancer Hospital and Comprehensive Cancer Center, The Ohio State University College of Medicine, Columbus, OH, USA

Biomedical Graduate Program, The Ohio State University, Columbus, OH, USA
e-mail: Miranda.tallman@osumc.edu

M. Venere (✉)
Department of Radiation Oncology, James Cancer Hospital and Comprehensive Cancer Center, The Ohio State University College of Medicine, Columbus, OH, USA
e-mail: Monica.venere@osumc.edu

J. J. Otero, A. P. Becker (eds.), *Precision Molecular Pathology of Glioblastoma*,
Molecular Pathology Library, https://doi.org/10.1007/978-3-030-69170-7_13

they are highly invasive and can migrate away from the bulk tumor into the surrounding, non-neoplastic tissue. Treatment resistance, along with the invasive nature that precludes removal by surgical resection, allows for GSCs to contribute to tumor recurrence [7]. Hence, it is imperative to study this subpopulation of cells when considering new therapeutics for GBM patients. In this chapter, we will cover the many aspects and techniques that go into studying the GSC population in GBM. We will first discuss how to identify and isolate GSCs from a bulk tumor by using cell surface markers. Then we will cover how to grow and expand these cells in culture. Lastly, we will talk about the ways we can validate that a given cell actually is a GSC, as well as techniques to determine if experimental treatments can compromise the GSC phenotype.

Studying Glioblastoma Cancer Stem Cells

Isolating GSCs

The cellular heterogeneity present in tumors such as GBM is driven by the tumor microenvironment (TME). These tumors interact with their surrounding microenvironment, and this close relationship between the tumor and TME is what drives the presence of GSCs and non-GSCs. With this in mind, the ideal scenario to study GSCs would be to do so in their inherent TME to keep all microenvironmental cues and dynamics intact. However, as there are technical limitations in doing so, the GSC field has developed other methods to enrich for the GSC population in a given tumor so that it can be further evaluated experimentally. Typically, this is accomplished by using cell surface markers that have higher expression on GSCs.

CSCs in GBM were first identified using a marker called CD133, which is enriched on the cell surface of GSCs [5, 8]. CD133 is an extracellular glycosylated antigen and is most commonly identified on GSCs by a monoclonal antibody to the AC133 epitope (also known as CD133/1). It is important to note that the glycosylated surface epitope is what marks GSCs, not just the protein associated with CD133 called prominin-1 (PROM1) [9], mRNA for this gene can be found in many cell types, while the surface epitope is present on GSCs and other CSCs and some non-neoplastic stem cells [9]. One of the first publications to demonstrate the presence of GSCs sorted the cells from a patient-derived tumor based on CD133-positive and CD133-negative, and showed that the CD133-positive cells reliably formed tumors, with as few as 100 cells orthotopically injected into a mouse brain, while CD133-negative cells did not form tumors. In years since this initial publication identifying GSCs by the use of CD133, many other markers have been identified. Furthermore, some of these markers have been shown to not only mark GSCs, but may be important in maintaining the GSC-phenotype and malignant characteristics.

L1CAM is a cellular adhesion molecule that is involved in neurodevelopment, and because of this role, was investigated as a possible GSC marker. It was demonstrated that L1CAM was found on CD133-positive cells, and that depleting L1CAM had the ability to decrease tumor cell proliferation *in vitro,* as well as decrease tumor growth in an orthotopic mouse model [10]. Another marker that has been identified and verified is integrin α6. Integrin α6 was investigated as it was enriched in the perivascular niche in patient GBM specimens (a region where GSCs are thought to be preferentially located). Upon further investigation, it was shown that integrin α6 enriched for GSCs and was found on CD133-positive cells. Similar to L1CAM, depleting integrin α6 slowed tumor cell proliferation and also inhibited self-renewal [11].

The actual practice of sorting GSCs based on cell surface markers is accomplished by the use of flow cytometry or magnetic sorting. First, a patient tumor biopsy or patient-derived xenograft passaged (PDX) tumor is dissociated in tissue culture using enzymatic digestion to create a single cell suspension. PDX tumors are either grown orthotopically or in the flank of an immunocompromised mouse, but for GSC enrichment the flank model is more routinely used. The removed PDX tumor or the patient biopsy is digested into a single cell suspension, and then the cells are incubated with an antibody for one of the GSC cell surface epitopes that is either fluorescently or magnetically labeled. Then the cells are sorted by either fluorescence activated cell sorting (FACS) or magnetic activated cell sorting (MACS), respectively. The cells that do not bind to the antibody are collected as the negative, or surface receptor low, population and kept as the non-GSCs. At the end of this process, the tumor cells are effectively sorted for study of GSCs and matched non-GSCs. It should be noted that there are many stem cell genes (e.g., *NANOG, SOX2,* and others) that are specifically expressed by GSCs but these are all internal proteins [12–15]. Hence, due to the need to prospectively label these cells while keeping them alive, a cell surface marker must be used as opposed to an intracellular protein.

Despite their necessity, there are significant caveats to using these markers that must be considered. For example, fluctuation in cell surface protein expression linked to the cell cycle and receptor turnover can both create temporal challenges to efficiently capturing all of the positive cells and hence can create false positives or false negatives [16]. Additionally, some markers are not highly specific for GSCs, and can lead to false-positives as well. Careful attention must also be paid to the enzyme used for tumor dissociation to ensure it does not cleave the surface marker of choice. Despite these limitations, markers currently used for enrichment of GSCs have led to numerous insights into tumor biology that were not previously appreciated from bulk tumor evaluation.

Alternative Approaches to Isolating and Studying GSCs

While using markers to sort GSCs and studying them in culture has been standard practice for many years, scientists have begun to explore new ways to study this elusive cell population. These advances in the GSC field are beginning to address some of the short-comings in the traditional method of sorting GSCs by cell surface markers. Scientists are now considering ways to isolate GSCs without using markers, or to not isolate the GSCs at all, and study them within their microenvironment.

While sorting GSCs based on cell surface markers is an important and efficacious technique for many experiments, there are other ways to enrich for the GSC population. For example, it has been shown that GSCs and non-GSCs can be sorted based on their differential abilities to regulate iron within the cell [17]. It was recently demonstrated that GSCs have higher transferrin and ferritin levels and are able to uptake and store more iron than non-GSCs [18]. Because of this difference in iron uptake and storage, when GSCs and non-GSCs were exposed to iron and then subsequently exposed to magnets, the two cell types had different magnetic susceptibilities. In the first publication to explore this phenomenon, iron-exposed GSCs and non-GSCs were successfully separated by a quadrupole magnetic separator (QMS) which is used to separate cells based on different magnetic susceptibility [17]. While this method does not get rid of the caveat that these cells must be removed from their microenvironment to sort, it is an alternative to using the traditional cell surface markers.

In addition to finding new ways to isolate GSCs, there have also been advances which allow for study of GSCs in a pseudo-microenvironment in culture. As previously mentioned, the heterogeneity of GBM is due to the interaction of the tumor cells with their microenvironment. Further, the TME is responsible for maintaining the stem-phenotype and associated characteristics present in GSCs [19]. To study GSCs in their TME, scientists are beginning to use new culturing conditions, such as growing GSCs in microfluidic devices and 3D scaffolds. Microfluidic devices contain a network of microtubes, and can be used to study tumor cell invasion while maintaining a consistent gradient of nutrients and/or chemoattractants. They can also be coated with different ECM components such as hyaluronic acid (HA), which is highly expressed in the GBM TME [20]. Another strategy is to use a 3D scaffold system, which is composed of ECM components that mimic the TME in the brain [21]. These types of models can also incorporate co-cultures of cells found in the TME, and can contain essential TME proteins such as HA. It has even been shown that changing the coating in these 3D scaffolds can change the rates of invasion and migration for patient-derived GBM cells, as well as change gene expression in the cells [21]. This highlights the need to consider the TME when studying GSCs and GBM as a whole, and demonstrates that studying isolated GSCs may be missing crucial information in some cases.

In addition to growing tumor cells in these engineered culture systems, other groups have begun studying GSCs in an organoid culture. Organoids can be derived from a patient-tumor and are grown for months in culture to create a 3D tumor model that closely mirrors a patient tumor [22]. These tumor organoids can retain the cellular heterogeneity of GSCs and non-GSCs, as well as contain a hypoxic core. Additionally, the non-GSCs within these organoids will succumb to radiotherapy, while the GSCs will not – a hallmark of GSCs and a phenomenon that is seen in patients [22]. Another way to employ organoids in the study of GSCs is to create a cerebral organoid derived from human embryonic stem cells, and then placing patient-derived GBM cells in with the organoid. It has been demonstrated that in this model, the GBM cells will invade the cerebral organoid and create tumors that reflect patient tumors [23]. These tumors will invade and proliferate into the surrounding cerebral organoid, mimicking the actions of patient GBM tumors. Both of these approaches, microfluidic devices and organoids, allow for study of the complex and critical interactions between the GSCs and their environment, and are a welcome addition to the current repertoire of studying GSCs sorted by cell surface markers.

Expanding Isolated GSCs

After GSCs and non-GSCs are sorted, they are then ready for direct evaluation (e.g., mRNA analysis) or expansion in tissue culture for experiments that require larger cell numbers (e.g., viability studies). The culture conditions for GSCs initially stemmed from knowledge established in the normal neural stem cell/neural progenitor (NSC/NPC) field. For NSCs/ NPCs, cells are grown in suspension as neurospheres and without the addition of serum in what is known as "defined media". Serum causes NSCs/NPCs to differentiate into downstream lineages (e.g., astrocytes). GSCs can also be differentiated into a state similar to non-GSCs using serum but these non-GSCs are only a surrogate as they were not prospectively enriched from the same tumor as the GSCs. Culture conditions for GSCs as tumorspheres, or gliomaspheres, were confirmed by studies that demonstrated that cell lines grown with serum do not match the genetic abnormalities typically found in patient-derived GBM, and also often harbor mutations not found in patients [24, 25]. Furthermore, these studies showed that GSCs grown in defined media (without serum) more closely reflect the patient tumor genotype [24, 25]. Defined media maintains the cancer stem-like state of the cells and prevents the cells from differentiating as there is no serum present. However, because these are serum-independent conditions, B27 (a mix of growth supplements), basic fibroblast growth factor (bFGF), and epidermal growth factor (EGF) are added to provide growth stimuli to the cells. To keep the non-GSCs locked into the more differentiated state following FACS or MACS sorting, they are grown in media containing serum should they need to be expanded in tissue culture.

It is not always experimentally desirable to culture GSCs as floating spheres, so researchers have also determined a method to grow GSCs adherently [26]. Typically, adherent cells need serum to grow, which cannot be used in the maintenance of GSCs. However, it has been shown that GSCs can be grown on an extracellular matrix-coated plate (such as laminin), while using the same media as GSCs grown as tumorspheres [26].

Validating GSCs Functionally

Markers are obviously a crucial part in identifying and studying GSCs. As previously discussed, the CSC state is microenvironmentally driven and this state is dynamic. Therefore, functional validation is central to confirming GSCs have been isolated by any given marker. To do this, self-renewal and tumor initiation properties are evaluated by a technique called a limited dilution assay (LDA). LDAs can be done *in vitro* or *in vivo*, but it is important to note that functional validation using an *in vivo* LDA and orthotopic injection is considered by the field the gold standard for GSC confirmation. To perform an *in vivo* LDA, cells are sorted based off a GSC marker, and then both GSCs and matched non-GSCs are orthotopically injected into the brain of immunocompromised mice at lower and lower cell numbers to see if a tumor forms (e.g., 100,000 cells, 10,000 cells, 1000 cells, 100 cells, and 1 cell). In theory, one GSC should be sufficient to grow a patient-like tumor in an orthotopically-injected mouse whereas not even 100,000 non-GSCs, in this example, would form a tumor. An *in vitro* LDA is technically a surrogate for self-renewal, but is more manageable to employ in a study. It also does not necessarily recreate the tumor microenvironment or tumor heterogeneity. The premise is similar to an *in vivo* LDA, where cells are plated at lower and lower cell numbers, down to one cell per well in a 96-well plate (Fig. 13.1). After approximately 10–14 days, each well is scored for whether or not a tumorsphere formed and then a stem-cell frequency can be calculated using a freely available webtool called ELDA (extreme limiting dilution analysis) [27]. These methods allow the determination if a given marker or other sorting method can reliably mark cells that will behave with GSC-characteristics when placed into the tumor microenvironment.

Another way to confirm that a given marker does reliably enrich for GSCs is to evaluate if cells sorted by this marker consistently form tumors over the non-GSCs. The ideal way to demonstrate consistent tumor formation would be to take the sorted GSCs and perform an *in vivo* serial transplantation. This refers to a method where the GSCs would be orthotopically injected in a mouse model, and once the tumor forms, remove it, sort for the GSCs, and then reinject in a new mouse (Fig. 13.2). In theory, this serial transplantation could go on infinitely, with the GSCs forming tumors in every new mouse, and non-GSCs never forming tumors. This is not necessarily done in practice, but is a way to confirm that a marker has reliably marked a continually self-renewing population of GSCs. Additionally, this assay could be performed in an *in vitro* setting, where sorted GSCs should repeatedly form tumorspheres, whereas non-GSCs will not.

Evaluating Changes in the Stem Cell State

Enriching, expanding, and validating GSCs are critical to be able to study this cell type. After these steps, experiments can be designed to understand unique characteristics of GSCs, as well as test potential therapeutics. This includes understanding

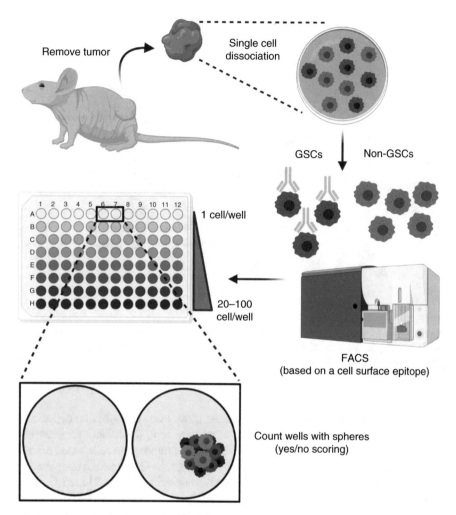

Fig. 13.1 Protocol for enriching for GSCs from a bulk tumor. The tumor is removed and dissociated into a single cell suspension. The cells are exposed to a GSC-specific cell surface antibody which will fluorescently label GSCs. Fluorescence-activated cell sorting (FACS) is then used to sort the GSCs at lower and lower numbers into a 96 well plate, from 20–100 cells per well down to 1 cell per well. After approximately 10 days, wells are scored based on the presence of a sphere so that a stem-cell frequency can be calculated. Created with BioRender.com

when GSCs have lost the stem cell phenotype, colloquially known as a "loss or a shift in stemness". There are several strategies to evaluate changes in the stem cell state, starting with an *in vitro* LDA on GSCs that have been exposed to a given drug or other treatment either in tissue culture or exposed while growing as a flank xenograft.

To use an *in vitro* LDA to investigate how a therapy impacts the GSC population when exposed while growing within an *in vivo* xenograft, the first step is to inject GBM cells into mice. The flank is chosen over orthotopic for technical feasibility of

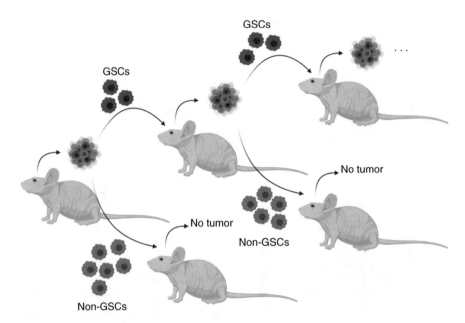

Fig. 13.2 Model of *in vivo* serial transplantation. A bulk tumor is sorted into GSCs and non-GSCs, and these two separate populations are each orthotopically injected into a mouse model. No tumor will form from the non-GSCs, but a tumor will form in the GSC-injected mouse. This new tumor is removed, sorted, and reinjected to another mouse model. The GSCs will again form a tumor, while non-GSCs do not. In theory, this process could go on indefinitely. Created with BioRender.com

harvesting just tumor tissue. Once the tumors form, mice are either treated with a vehicle or the experimental therapeutic. After treatment, the tumors are removed and dissociated, and then each tumor is sorted into stem/nonstem cells based off one of the GSC markers. Then, cells that are positive for the GSC marker are plated at decreasing dilutions, down to one cell per well, as described above. These LDAs are scored for both vehicle and experimental conditions, and the stem cell frequencies of different conditions can be compared. In other words, if results indicate that the stem cell frequency decreased following a given treatment it would indicate that that treatment is able to target the GSC subpopulation by either directly killing the GSCs or by shifting them to a more differentiated, non-GSC phenotype.

In addition to the *in vitro* LDA, flank or orthotopic tumors can be removed from vehicle control and experimental mice and processed for immunofluorescence to evaluate for a shift in stemness by immunolabeling the tumors with antibodies to stem cell genes followed by quantification. For example, tumors can be immunola-beled and quantified for the number of Sox2 positive cells, a known stem cell gene that is also used to identify GSCs [12]. This method allows for the visualization of the presence or absence of GSCs and also allows for the evaluation of where within the tumor GSCs are located.

While the previous two methods are examples that allow for *in vivo* administration of a therapy, there are also ways to evaluate changes in the stem cell fate entirely in an *in vitro* system. One such way is to use a GBM cell line where a fluorescent reporter is driven by the promoter of a cancer stem cell gene. For example, a cell line that has a GFP reporter driven by the *Sox2* promoter could be used [28, 29]. If there is one cohort of cells that are treated with vehicle, and another cohort treated with a drug, as stemness shifts, so should the levels of stem cell gene expression, and therefore GFP expression. Cells can be treated and then immunolabeled for GFP and imaged to quantify the percentage of GFP-positive cells, or cells could be quantified through FACS. Similar to this approach, it is also possible to take populations of treated versus non-treated cells, and examine mRNA or protein levels of GSC genes, such as Sox2, NANOG, and OCT4.

Conclusions and Future Directions

The cancer stem cell field has rapidly expanded over the past few decades, and the ways in which GSCs are evaluated continues to evolve. Despite these changes in how GSC are studied, the underlying motive for investigating this population remains the same. These cells are resistant to current therapies, and to make substantial progress in the way that GBM patients are treated, therapies that target this elusive population of cells must be identified.

References

1. Bao S, et al. Glioma stem cells promote radioresistance by preferential activation of the DNA damage response. Nature. 2006;444(7120):756–60.
2. Chen J, et al. A restricted cell population propagates glioblastoma growth after chemotherapy. Nature. 2012;488(7412):522–6.
3. Lapidot T, et al. A cell initiating human acute myeloid leukaemia after transplantation into SCID mice. Nature. 1994;367(6464):645–8.
4. Bonnet D, Dick JE. Human acute myeloid leukemia is organized as a hierarchy that originates from a primitive hematopoietic cell. Nat Med. 1997;3(7):730–7.
5. Singh SK, et al. Identification of a cancer stem cell in human brain tumors. Cancer Res. 2003;63(18):5821–8.
6. Singh SK, et al. Identification of human brain tumour initiating cells. Nature. 2004;432(7015):396–401.
7. Wakimoto H, et al. Human glioblastoma-derived cancer stem cells: establishment of invasive glioma models and treatment with oncolytic herpes simplex virus vectors. Cancer Res. 2009;69(8):3472–81.
8. Beier D, et al. CD133(+) and CD133(−) glioblastoma-derived cancer stem cells show differential growth characteristics and molecular profiles. Cancer Res. 2007;67(9):4010–5.
9. Kemper K, et al. The AC133 epitope, but not the CD133 protein, is lost upon cancer stem cell differentiation. Cancer Res. 2010;70(2):719–29.
10. Bao S, et al. Targeting cancer stem cells through L1CAM suppresses glioma growth. Cancer Res. 2008;68(15):6043–8.

11. Lathia JD, et al. Integrin alpha 6 regulates glioblastoma stem cells. Cell Stem Cell. 2010;6(5):421–32.
12. Hemmati HD, et al. Cancerous stem cells can arise from pediatric brain tumors. Proc Natl Acad Sci U S A. 2003;100(25):15178–83.
13. Tunici P, et al. Genetic alterations and in vivo tumorigenicity of neurospheres derived from an adult glioblastoma. Mol Cancer. 2004;3:25.
14. Ligon KL, et al. Olig2-regulated lineage-restricted pathway controls replication competence in neural stem cells and malignant glioma. Neuron. 2007;53(4):503–17.
15. Suva ML, et al. Reconstructing and reprogramming the tumor-propagating potential of glioblastoma stem-like cells. Cell. 2014;157(3):580–94.
16. Sun Y, et al. CD133 (Prominin) negative human neural stem cells are clonogenic and tripotent. PLoS One. 2009;4(5):e5498.
17. Park KJ, et al. Quantitative characterization of the regulation of iron metabolism in glioblastoma stem-like cells using magnetophoresis. Biotechnol Bioeng. 2019;116(7):1644–55.
18. Schonberg DL, et al. Preferential iron trafficking characterizes glioblastoma stem-like cells. Cancer Cell. 2015;28(4):441–55.
19. Dirkse A, et al. Stem cell-associated heterogeneity in Glioblastoma results from intrinsic tumor plasticity shaped by the microenvironment. Nat Commun. 2019;10(1):1787.
20. Logun M, et al. Microfluidics in malignant glioma research and precision medicine. Adv Biosyst. 2018;2(5):1700221.
21. Sood D, et al. 3D extracellular matrix microenvironment in bioengineered tissue models of primary pediatric and adult brain tumors. Nat Commun. 2019;10(1):4529.
22. Hubert CG, et al. A three-dimensional organoid culture system derived from human glioblastomas recapitulates the hypoxic gradients and cancer stem cell heterogeneity of tumors found in vivo. Cancer Res. 2016;76(8):2465–77.
23. Linkous A, et al. Modeling patient-derived glioblastoma with cerebral organoids. Cell Rep. 2019;26(12):3203–3211 e5.
24. Lee J, et al. Tumor stem cells derived from glioblastomas cultured in bFGF and EGF more closely mirror the phenotype and genotype of primary tumors than do serum-cultured cell lines. Cancer Cell. 2006;9(5):391–403.
25. Li A, et al. Genomic changes and gene expression profiles reveal that established glioma cell lines are poorly representative of primary human gliomas. Mol Cancer Res. 2008;6(1):21–30.
26. Pollard SM, et al. Glioma stem cell lines expanded in adherent culture have tumor-specific phenotypes and are suitable for chemical and genetic screens. Cell Stem Cell. 2009;4(6):568–80.
27. Hu Y, Smyth GK. ELDA: extreme limiting dilution analysis for comparing depleted and enriched populations in stem cell and other assays. J Immunol Methods. 2009;347(1–2):70–8.
28. Thiagarajan PS, et al. Development of a fluorescent reporter system to delineate cancer stem cells in triple-negative breast cancer. Stem Cells. 2015;33(7):2114–25.
29. Tang B, et al. A flexible reporter system for direct observation and isolation of cancer stem cells. Stem Cell Reports. 2015;4(1):155–69.

Chapter 14
The Neuroscience of Glioblastoma

Kwanha Yu

Introduction

Unrelenting cell growth is a hallmark of all cancers [1], and some of the major drivers of this growth are mitogenic pathways which govern cell proliferation and survival in the non-disease state. Over the past several decades we have observed that synaptic activity and neurotransmitter signaling can exhibit a trophic effect, suggesting that synaptic activity may be important in the regulation of cell proliferation and survival, expanding their role beyond cell-cell communication [2]. This proposes an interesting question of whether cancers can hijack the neurotrophic properties of synapse biology to drive the aforementioned, unrelenting cell growth. The compartmentalization of the central nervous system (CNS) and specificity of synaptic structures to neuronal cells has necessitated and facilitated the development of specialized tools to answer neuroscience-related questions [3]. Using these tools to probe the relationship between synapse biology and cancer cell growth has ushered in a new area of research where the concepts and techniques of neuroscience are applied to the topics and models of brain cancer. This nuanced approach also provides a molecular perspective on how cancers in the brain are associated with common comorbidities, specifically neurological disorders. With this in mind, in this chapter we will focus two major themes: (1) the interaction of the synaptic microenvironment and glioma and (2) the molecular connection between glioma and epilepsy. While synapses are present elsewhere, their abundance in the brain make CNS tumors the prime system to study this phenomenon. Additionally, glioma constitutes about 80% of malignant brain tumors, glioblastoma is among the

K. Yu (✉)
Center for Cell and Gene Therapy, Department of Neurosurgery, Baylor College of Medicine, Houston, TX, USA
e-mail: kyu@bcm.edu

J. J. Otero, A. P. Becker (eds.), *Precision Molecular Pathology of Glioblastoma*, Molecular Pathology Library, https://doi.org/10.1007/978-3-030-69170-7_14

deadliest of cancers, and there have been no significant improvements in patient outcomes; thus, there are critical knowledge gaps in molecular pathology for future therapeutic development. Lastly, while there are other potential comorbidities (depression, motor coordination deficits, cognitive changes), the molecular and pathological connections between synapses and epilepsy have been more clearly defined.

Synapses Drive Glioma

As introduced earlier, cancers will repurpose existing non-disease pathways for their growth, and we propose synapse biology as one such path. In this section, we will categorize the evidence for the neurotrophic and mitogenic effect of synapses, focusing primarily on the subventricular zone (SVZ) and dentate gyrus (DG), two stem cells pools that persist into adulthood [4]. We will focus on these pools because gliomas are thought to be derived from them, and cancers as a whole can be described as a dedifferentiation into a more stem-like state [5]. We will then present the evidence for potential correlative mechanisms in glioma, concluding with an exploration of evidence that gliomas may be increasing synaptic activity in or around the tumors to promote their growth.

During embryogenesis and postnatal development, neurotransmitters play a critical role in the cellular proliferation, growth, survival, differentiation, and migration of neural precursor/progenitor cells (NPCs) into mature neurons/glia [2]. In the mature adult brain, there are two distinct pools of NPCs: one in the SVZ along the lateral ventricle and another in DG of the hippocampus [4]. NPCs in the SVZ differentiate into neuroblasts which migrate to the olfactory bulb along the rostral migratory stream and integrate into olfactory synaptic networks. The subgranular zone cells of the DG generate granule cells, which are DG specific neurons critical for many aspects of learning and memory. Research for over 20 years demonstrates that synaptic activity and neurotransmitter release can influence the proliferation, growth, migration, and survival of these NPCs into neurons and glia in the mature brain.

Glutamate functions as the principle excitatory neurotransmitter in the CNS, interacting with ionotropic receptors NMDA and AMPA/kainate, or with metabotropic glutamate receptors (mGluRs). While mGluR binding results in secondary messaging cascades, glutamate binding to NMDAR and/or AMPAR results in membrane voltage change by increasing intracellular Na+ and Ca^{2+} [6]. When cultured with glutamate, NPCs from the DG [7] and SVZ [8] both demonstrated increased survival, proliferation, and differentiation. *In vivo* pharmacological treatments that increase intracellular Ca^{2+}, result in similar increases in neurogenesis in the hippocampus [7]. Additionally, increasing the excitability of olfactory bulb neurons improved the integration and survivability of newborn neurons from the SVZ [9]. These studies reveal that excitatory glutamate signaling is sufficient for NPC proliferation. But they beg the questions: to what range can other neurotransmitter activities elicit a similar effect? Is there a necessary dependence on these activities? What are the molecular mechanisms driving these cellular behaviors?

To this end, many studies have demonstrated both common and individual modes by which specific neurotransmitters affect NPC proliferation. Gamma aminobutyric acid (GABA) functions as the major inhibitory neurotransmitter in the CNS. The majority of adult neurons derived from the SVZ are inhibitory. As such, if any brain region required GABA for cell viability, one would suspect it be between the SVZ and olfactory bulb. However, in adulthood GABA, secreted from the migrating neuroblasts, appears to suppress this proliferation of NPCs through nonsynaptic signaling [10]. Additionally, genetic manipulation of *DBI* (Diazepam Binding Inhibitor), which reduces GABA activity, revealed that DBI is necessary and sufficient for neuroblast proliferation from the SVZ [11]. These studies reveal a suppressive mechanism of inhibitory neurotransmitter signaling towards NPC proliferation.

While GABA appears to suppress adult NPC proliferation, most other neurotransmitters demonstrate a positive effect similar to glutamate. This includes dopamine (associated with the brain's pleasure pathways), where direct brain infusion of dopamine receptor agonists promotes NPC proliferation and differentiation into neurons [12]; and depletion of dopaminergic fibers, which mimics dopamine depletion, reduces SVZ proliferation. Additionally, this same study reveals that EGF acts downstream of dopamine signaling [13]. The mood modulating neurotransmitter serotonin also promotes NPC proliferation. Treatment with serotonin agonist and antagonist generally increases and decreases, respectively, NPC proliferation in the SVZ [14] and DG [15]; however, the specific effects may be nuanced as different serotonin receptors may elicit different effects. Acetylcholine [16] and its agonist nicotine also appear to promote proliferation; however, the neurotrophic effects of nicotine appear to be prominent in the SVZ over the DG, acting in part through FGF2 and FGFR1 [17]. Collectively, these studies highlight a mitogenic effect of various neurotransmitters and interestingly reveal that some of the downstream pathways include receptor tyrosine kinase (RTK) components.

The extended evidence that neurotransmitters are necessary and sufficient for some degree of NPC proliferation leads to the question whether it is the action of the synapses that contributes to NPC behavior. We already mentioned it is a nonsynaptic function of GABA that suppresses NPC proliferation [10], and nonsynaptic roles for other neurotransmitters have been reviewed [18]. Over the last two decades, a specialized set of genetically encoded optic tools have been developed in neuroscience. Among these optogenetic tools are channelrhodopsins, a family of light-gated ion channels which are transgenically expressed at the presynaptic terminal. These channels can be activated by light signals (photostimulation) sent through fiberoptic cables implanted into rodent brains. The photostimulation opens these channels, forcing ionic exchange and synaptic communication. Genetic or stereotaxic control can restrict which cell populations are forcefully activated upon photostimulation. Use of these approaches has demonstrated an increase in NPC proliferation from the SVZ [16] to the olfactory bulb, as well as an increase in glia (specifically oligodendrocytes) within activated regions [19]. Given the extensive evidence that neurotransmitters and synaptic activity have mitogenic roles in the CNS, we now ask if gliomas could utilize these mechanisms for their own growth, and if so, where and how does this mechanism begin?

To this end, a series of studies over the past decade have revealed a parallel phenomenon and molecular mechanisms governing this process. Similar to normal, healthy glia [19], channelrhodopsin stimulation of neurons increases the proliferation of surrounding glioma cells in patient derived xenograft (PDX) models [20]. This observation suggests that gliomas may utilize similar trophic mechanisms from enhanced neuronal communication. To identify candidate molecules, the same study combined optogenetic activation with *ex vivo* and *in vitro* culture systems. Culture media from photostimulated *ex vivo* brain slices expressing channelrhodopsin increased the proliferation of primary glioma cells *in vitro*. Of note, the channelrhodopsin is restricted to neurons, thus it is a consequence of the neuronal activity that drives this tumor growth. Proteomics analysis revealed the neuronal protein Neuroligin3 (NLGN3) as a secreted mitogen for glioma. Along with a subsequent study, it was found that the absence of NLGN3 greatly reduced PDX growth, NLGN3 activated a number of known glioma driver pathways including PI3K-AKT-mTOR and Ras-Raf (among others), and glioma cells will upregulate their own NLGN3 production in a positive feedback loop [21].

Clearly gliomas respond to microenvironmental synaptic activity to potentiate their growth, but could tumors bypass these cell-extrinsic mechanisms and intrinsically form synapses? Recent studies suggest this may be the case [22, 23]. In these studies, primary patient derived samples were found to express neurotransmitter receptors. Electron microscopy imaging reveals synapse like structures between PDX and surrounding neurons. Electrophysiological recordings demonstrate that these synapses are functionally active. All these data support the notion that gliomas can form functional synapses. But to address whether these synapses can promote glioma growth, PDX expressing channelrhodopsin were activated and changes in tumor growth were assayed. These differ from the previously mentioned studies in that channelrhodopsin in expressed in glioma cells instead of microenvironmental neurons [20]. Photostimulation of PDX results in increased glioma growth, and overexpression of a dominant negative glutamate receptor (thereby decreasing a cells glutamate sensitivity) on PDX decreased glioma growth and slowed tumor associated death [22, 23]. In sum, these data begin to paint a picture where gliomas will not only hijack the neurotrophic effects of surrounding synaptic activity but will also reprogram themselves to mimic some neuronal behavior for their own growth.

The complexities of healthy synapse biology is further complicated by glial contributions. While synapses are neuronal structural, they are supported by astrocytes in a structure known as the tripartite synapse [24]. Astrocytes are the support glial cells of the CNS, and their progenitors are thought to be a potential lineage for the glioma cell of origin [5, 25]. Among their multiple functions, astrocytes are critical for proper synaptogenesis. Given this inherent trait of astrocytes and the advantages it could convey towards their malignant cancerous analogous, could gliomas also directly influence the synaptic microenvironment to promote their own growth? Several key studies suggest this is a likely scenario.

Recent studies have validated that a subpopulation of astrocytes that can specifically promote the formation of synapses [26, 27]. One mechanism they do so, is through secreted proteins including Glypicans (GPCs), Thrombospondins (THBSs), SPARC, and SPARCL1 [28]. Interestingly, these same secreted factors appear to promote different aspects of glioma growth. GPC3 is present in human tumors, *GPC3* overexpression accelerates tumor-associated death, and *GPC3* loss can slow it [29]. Members of the *THBS* family are highly expressed in human gliomas [30]. Lastly, SPARC and SPARCL1 have been found to complex with Pleiotrophin and HSP90 to promote glioma growth and invasion [31]. While these pro-synaptogenic astrocyte factors function for gliomagenesis, is it through modulating synapses? As this is a relatively new topic, it has not been heavily explored, but work with GPC3 appears to indicate that this is the case. *GPC3* overexpression in mouse gliomas increases the number of excitatory and inhibitory synapses at the peritumoral margins. Additionally, the disruption of proper synapse number may also contribute to seizures (discussed later), and the overexpression or knockout of *GPC3* in a mouse glioma model increases or decreases seizure activity, respectively [29].

Together, these recent studies provide an interesting perspective into cancer biology that are ideally addressed by neuroscience approaches and in the brain. Research in other cancers reveals a similar phenomenon in other tissue types, where cancers will preferentially undergo growth at innervation of the peripheral nervous system [32]. Yet the abundance of synapses and decades of tool development and expertise make the brain the ideal place to study this phenomenon. Recent work has also demonstrated that metastases of other primary cancers into the brain may be governed by similar mechanisms [33]. These topics were avoided for this chapter but further highlight the contributions of these mechanisms towards tumorigenesis.

How Gliomas and Seizures Interact

Among cancer comorbidities, epilepsy is particularly associated with cancers in the brain. One of the more apparent mechanism brain tumors induce epilepsy is through the destruction of a stable neural network. While smaller or shorter-lived tumors may have a reduced effect, as tumors persist longer and grow larger, they do so at the expense of non-tumorous, healthy tissue. This would view seizures as a consequence of a destabilized neural network from tumor growth. However, we described previously that enhanced synaptic activity can promote glioma growth and how gliomas will modulate the neuronal milieu to this end. Therefore, is it possible that the same mechanisms that promote seizures can drive glioma? We will first describe the resting state of a healthy brain and then propose how tumors alter these systems to promote a hyperexcited brain state. We will also summarize evidence of what effects seizures may have on the glioma. Lastly, we will explore what pathways and mechanisms may preferentially promote a more hyperexcited brain state in glioma brains.

The connection between seizures and glioma is complex. Many glioma patients will experience seizures as the presenting symptom drawing them into clinic for their dreadful diagnosis. While headaches are the most common symptom, they are too ubiquitous, and brain cancer is not primarily assumed as the cause. However, unless a patient has a history of epilepsy, a sudden seizure will cause most to seek out a neurological consultation. In general, patients with lower grade gliomas more frequently present with seizures, and presenting with seizures associates with more favorable prognosis for both low and high grades patients [34–37]. Despite the stronger association with lower grades, seizures do affect a significant amount of high grade patients (ranging from 30% to 80%) [35, 38]. However, these clinical trends do not describe the underlying biology of this phenomenon. Work in the last decade using preclinical research models has provided greater illumination to the molecular changes which may be driving this comorbidity, particularly in the higher grades.

One rudimentary way to view seizures or network hyperexcitability, is through the lens of synaptic imbalance, as a net increase in excitatory and/or decrease in inhibitory brain profile. While oversimplified (as excitatory and inhibitory neurons can synapse onto others like themselves and each other), there is still some value to this perspective. In the non-disease state astrocytes play a critical role in maintaining excitatory-inhibitory homeostasis. As mentioned previously, glutamate is the principal excitatory neurotransmitter of the CNS, and after release into the synaptic cleft, astrocytes will uptake extracellular glutamate through excitatory amino acid transporters (EAATs). Through a glutamine intermediate, glutamate will be recycled and repackaged into synaptic vesicles in the presynaptic terminal [24]. This process is critical for maintaining homeostasis, as high extracellular glutamate levels are toxic for neurons in a phenomenon called excitotoxicity. Continuous binding to ionotropic receptors lead to deadly intracellular Ca^{2+} levels [6]. Thus healthy astrocytes are contributing to, if not maintaining, synaptic balance and cellular survival in the neuronal network. In fact, models of chronically reactive astrocytes (which are associated with disease or injury) can lead to hyperexcitability [39].

Given the importance of astrocytes towards extracellular glutamate and the contributions of glutamate towards NPC proliferation, could glioma cells directly modulate extracellular glutamate levels to potentiate their own growth? More simply, are there astrocytic mechanisms that increase extracellular glutamate independent of neurons, and is there evidence that gliomas utilize these systems? One system is the cystine/glutamate exchanger xCT, encoded by *SLC7A11*, is the transporter subunit which catalyzes the 1:1 exchange of cystine intracellularly and glutamate extracellularly [40]. Cystine can then be reduced to cysteine for glutathione synthesis, an intracellular antioxidant [41]. In a study comparing nearly a dozen primary human glioblastoma samples, tumors with the highest xCT level demonstrated higher glutamate release, a decrease in peritumoral neurons (suggestive of excitotoxicity), increased brain hyperexcitability, and poorer survival based on PDX and human genomics data [42]. Treating mice bearing PDX tumors [43] and an endogenous mouse model of glioblastoma [44] with sulfasalazine, an xCT antagonist, significantly reduced hyperexcitability by reducing extracellular glutamate. Moreover,

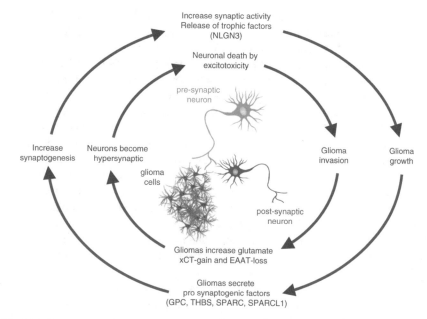

Fig. 14.1 The vicious cycle within the tumor microenvironment. The synaptic activity of neurons promotes glioma growth while the glioma will increase the synaptic activity of microenvironment neurons. This cyclic pathway contributes to peritumoral neuronal death by excitotoxicity, making room for glioma invasion, which further extends this poisonous behavior in the brain

higher grade gliomas demonstrate decreased *EAAT1* and *EAAT2* expression compared to lower grade [45], together suggesting that more pathogenic tumors not only lose the ability to clear, but actively contribute to extracellular glutamate levels. Unsurprisingly, as dysregulation of glutamatergic mechanisms are associated with epilepsy [46], glioma patients that suffered seizures also demonstrated tumors with high glutamate, decrease EAAT2, and increased xCT [47].

Collectively, this poses an interesting model (Fig. 14.1) where microenvironmental increased extracellular glutamate increases synaptic activity. In response to this enhanced activity, glioma cells proliferate (in response to molecules such as NLGN3). This phenomenon is further exacerbated (or possibly initiated) by molecules secreted from gliomas such as GPCs and THBSs which increase peritumoral synaptic activity, feeding back into this vicious cycle. As the extracellular glutamate level increases and crosses the threshold from hyperexcitable to excitotoxic, neurons die thereby making space for glioma to invade into. As the tumor grows, more of the neuronal network is destabilized by its destruction in combination with the excessive glutamate levels which increase the excitatory profile of the peritumoral microenvironment. These insults compound to levels detectable by electroencephalograms, manifesting in interictal spikes and seizures.

This proposed model suggests seizures are largely a consequence of molecular, cellular, and physiological activities driven by tumors. However, is it possible that seizures feed back into the system to promote growth? Analysis of seizures induced in rodent brains through pilocarpine administration (which activates cholinergic receptors) or perforant path induction reveal an increase in NPC proliferation and differentiation into neurons and glia [48–50]. Kainic acid (an AMPAR agonist) induced seizures also increases NPC proliferation from the DG [51]. These studies could suggest an indirect effect of seizures towards glioma growth (likely through similar pathways governing synapse-associated proliferation mentioned prior), and this may be further hinted at by conserved molecular pathway between glioma and epilepsy (discussed later). Inversely, a study longitudinally tracked an endogenous mouse glioblastomas model generated in a seizure-protective genetic background, which could be viewed as a "seizure knockdown" model. Along with decreased hyperexcitability, there was a modest (non-significant) increase in the survival of these "seizure knockdown" glioma mice [44]. While these studies might suggest that seizure-suppressive mechanisms may slow glioma growth, they contend against clinical trends where patients that present with seizures have better prognosis [34, 35, 38]. Perhaps it is simply serendipitous, that in those individuals, the tumor grew in a more network-sensitive brain region, thus seizures revealed the disease at an earlier, more treatable state.

As the sensitivity of specific brains regions has not been heavily investigated, what is known about the factors driving glioma-associated epilepsy? One possibility is that seizures are inherent to glioma progression. As the tumor grows, it alters the environment to better supports its growth, molding it into a more hyperexcitable state. Eventually, all glioma brains would eventually develop seizures without intervention, thus different patients are simply at different points along the same disease trajectory. There may be some evidence to support this view of glioma-epilepsy pathogenesis. PDX studies comparing low and high xCT lines reveal that even low xCT models eventually demonstrate seizures but at later time points [42]. Studies in an endogenous mouse glioblastoma model reveal that tumor brain hyperexcitability increases over time [26, 44]. Additionally, there is a concomitant increase in the constituency of a pro-synaptic subpopulation in these mouse tumors, and there is an increase of xCT levels in the whole brain (tumoral, peritumoral, and distally away from the tumor). This supports the notion that seizures are a pathological consequence of gliomas. However, with the birth of cancer genomics, we have demonstrated there is great inter-tumoral heterogeneity across patients. Are there differences across patient genomics that could also address the heterogeneity of this pathophysiology?

The advent of cancer genomics has revealed an enormous amount of information concerning glioma, as glioblastoma was among the first solid tumors to be systematically characterized [52]. A subsequent question that followed was whether the annotated information were of functional drivers for tumorigenesis or non-functional passengers. This theme lies at the heart of cancer functional genomics. In a recent functional genomics study utilizing both endogenous mouse and PDX glioblastoma models, a group characterized different mutations in *PIK3CA* [29], a known driver gene mutated in 11% of glioblastomas. Mutations in the *RTK-PI3K-ATK* pathway are found in 90% of glioblastoma patients. Researchers found that different mutations demonstrated different effects on gliomagenesis. One means by which variants exerted different effects on tumor growth was altering the synaptic milieu of the microenvironment. More precisely, transcriptomic analysis of tumors driven by 2 mutations, those encoding for the C420R and H1047R variants, demonstrated dysregulated synapses. Electroencephalogram analyses revealed that these two tumors brains demonstrated enhanced hyperexcitability. There was also a concomitant increase in excitatory and decrease in inhibitory synapses at the peritumoral margins. Additionally, C420R driven tumors, which demonstrated even more pronounced synapse dysregulation compared to H1047R, exhibited a greater abundance of GPC3. This suggests that differences in tumor genetics can differentially alter the tumor-synaptic microenvironment to promote glioma growth. More broadly, it implicates that unique genetics may contribute to more excitable tumor brains.

This study hints at the immense complexity and value of functional genomics, that even single residue differences can have drastically different effects on tumorigenesis with immense implications towards patient specific therapies. Interestingly, the same study revealed that outside the context of tumors, H1047R can induced epileptiform activity more potently than C420R, further emphasizing differential mechanism across these variants. Genomics approaches have been applied to other diseases such as PI3K Related Overgrowth Spectrum (PROS) disorders, a pediatric disorder driven by mutations in the *PI3K-AKT-mTOR* pathway. Patients demonstrate segmental overgrowth phenotypes in body regions that mosaically carry mutations. Many *PIK3CA* mutations that drive PROS are also found in cancer [53–55]. When restricted to the brain, patients present megalencephaly, cortical dysplasia (both which correspond with cancer's unrelenting cell growth), and epilepsy [56–58]. It is difficult to distinguish in each patient whether the epileptiform activity is a consequence of the megalencephaly/dysplasia-mediated network disruption or if the hyperexcitability is independent of these morphological changes. However, work in genetic mouse models reveals that the $PIK3CA^{H1047R}$ mutation can induce hyperexcitability independent of tissue morphology defects [29, 59]. Given that the same mutations can induce seizures with and without tumorigenesis, this supports the notion of glioma-independent mechanisms towards hyperexcitability. These mechanisms may work in parallel with glioma-specific mechanism to increase the excitability of the tumor microenvironment and brain, potentiating tumor growth. Collectively, it further supports the possibility that specific tumors genetics may promote hyperexcitability microenvironmentally and network-globally.

Concluding Thoughts

Collectively we stand in the early days, wading in the shallow waters of cancer neuroscience [60], emerging from the collaboration between cancer biology and neuroscience research. In compiling this chapter, we aimed to highlight how pathways familiar to neuroscience are utilized by glioma for its own growth. Due to the scope of the chapter and space considerations, many topics were not addressed but are critically important in considering, moving forward in, and growing this hybrid field. How conserved are these molecular mechanisms in other cancer systems with respect to the peripheral nervous systems? What are the contributions of neuro-immunology as it is involved in the tumor microenvironment, synaptic pruning, and epilepsy? What other technologies can collaborate just as optogenetics and electro-encephalograms have? Can therapeutics be repurposed between neurological disorders and glioma?

As we continue to fill the knowledge gaps of the molecular pathology of glioblastoma, we hope this advances therapeutics for this incurable disease. The questions and answers that lie ahead are countless. The ocean before us is vast.

Acknowledgements We would like to acknowledge the efforts of Drs Benjamin Deneen, Jeffrey L Noebels, and Asante Hatcher for their efforts in reviewing and proofreading this manuscript. We would like to acknowledge the contributions of Rachel N Curry towards generating Fig. 14.1. Work for compiling this manuscript was supported by the following grants: NIH R01-CA223388, U01-CA217842, and R50-CA252125.

Suggested Readings We suggest these additional references for the following topics: additional reviews on the glioma neuroscience [61, 62], including clinical perspectives between glioma and seizures [34, 63], the peripheral nervous system's influence of non-CNS tumors [32], comprehensive view of glutamate in glioma [6], healthy astrocyte biology [24], and glia in epilepsy [64].

References

1. Hanahan D, Weinberg RA. Hallmarks of cancer: the next generation. Cell. 2011;144:646–74.
2. Nguyen L, et al. Neurotransmitters as early signals for central nervous system development. Cell Tissue Res. 2001;305:187–202.
3. Kim CK, Adhikari A, Deisseroth K. Integration of optogenetics with complementary methodologies in systems neuroscience. Nat Rev Neurosci. 2017;18:222–35.
4. Obernier K, Alvarez-Buylla A. Neural stem cells: origin, heterogeneity and regulation in the adult mammalian brain. Dev Camb Engl. 2019;146:dev156059.
5. Zong H, Parada LF, Baker SJ. Cell of origin for malignant gliomas and its implication in therapeutic development. Cold Spring Harb Perspect Biol. 2015;7:a020610.
6. Robert SM, Sontheimer H. Glutamate transporters in the biology of malignant gliomas. Cell Mol Life Sci. 2014;71:1839–54.
7. Deisseroth K, et al. Excitation-neurogenesis coupling in adult neural stem/progenitor cells. Neuron. 2004;42:535–52.
8. Brazel CY, Nuñez JL, Yang Z, Levison SW. Glutamate enhances survival and proliferation of neural progenitors derived from the subventricular zone. Neuroscience. 2005;131:55–65.
9. Lin C-W, et al. Genetically increased cell-intrinsic excitability enhances neuronal integration into adult brain circuits. Neuron. 2010;65:32–9.
10. Liu X, Wang Q, Haydar TF, Bordey A. Nonsynaptic GABA signaling in postnatal subventricular zone controls proliferation of GFAP-expressing progenitors. Nat Neurosci. 2005;8:1179–87.
11. Alfonso J, Le Magueresse C, Zuccotti A, Khodosevich K, Monyer H. Diazepam binding inhibitor promotes progenitor proliferation in the postnatal SVZ by reducing GABA signaling. Cell Stem Cell. 2012;10:76–87.

12. Van Kampen JM, Hagg T, Robertson HA. Induction of neurogenesis in the adult rat subventricular zone and neostriatum following dopamine D3 receptor stimulation. Eur J Neurosci. 2004;19:2377–87.

13. O'Keeffe GC, et al. Dopamine-induced proliferation of adult neural precursor cells in the mammalian subventricular zone is mediated through EGF. Proc Natl Acad Sci U S A. 2009;106:8754–9.

14. Tong CK, et al. Axonal control of the adult neural stem cell niche. Cell Stem Cell. 2014;14:500–11.

15. Banasr M, Hery M, Printemps R, Daszuta A. Serotonin-induced increases in adult cell proliferation and neurogenesis are mediated through different and common 5-HT receptor subtypes in the dentate gyrus and the subventricular zone. Neuropsychopharmacol Off Publ Am Coll Neuropsychopharmacol. 2004;29:450–60.

16. Paez-Gonzalez P, Asrican B, Rodriguez E, Kuo CT. Identification of distinct ChAT+ neurons and activity-dependent control of postnatal SVZ neurogenesis. Nat Neurosci. 2014;17:934–42.

17. Mudò G, Belluardo N, Mauro A, Fuxe K. Acute intermittent nicotine treatment induces fibroblast growth factor-2 in the subventricular zone of the adult rat brain and enhances neuronal precursor cell proliferation. Neuroscience. 2007;145:470–83.

18. Vizi ES, Fekete A, Karoly R, Mike A. Non-synaptic receptors and transporters involved in brain functions and targets of drug treatment. Br J Pharmacol. 2010;160:785–809.

19. Gibson EM, et al. Neuronal activity promotes oligodendrogenesis and adaptive myelination in the mammalian brain. Science. 2014;344:1252304.

20. Venkatesh HS, et al. Neuronal activity promotes glioma growth through neuroligin-3 secretion. Cell. 2015;161:803–16.

21. Venkatesh HS, et al. Targeting neuronal activity-regulated neuroligin-3 dependency in high-grade glioma. Nature. 2017;549:533–7.

22. Venkatesh HS, et al. Electrical and synaptic integration of glioma into neural circuits. Nature. 2019;573:539–45.

23. Venkataramani V, et al. Glutamatergic synaptic input to glioma cells drives brain tumour progression. Nature. 2019;573:532–8.

24. Khakh BS, Deneen B. The emerging nature of astrocyte diversity. Annu Rev Neurosci. 2019;42:187–207.

25. Laug D, Glasgow SM, Deneen B. A glial blueprint for gliomagenesis. Nat Rev Neurosci. 2018;19:393–403.

26. John Lin C-C, et al. Identification of diverse astrocyte populations and their malignant analogs. Nat Neurosci. 2017;20:396–405.

27. Morel L, et al. Molecular and functional properties of regional astrocytes in the adult brain. J Neurosci. 2017;37:8706–17.

28. Allen NJ, Eroglu C. Cell biology of astrocyte-synapse interactions. Neuron. 2017;96:697–708.

29. Yu K, et al. PIK3CA variants selectively initiate brain hyperactivity during gliomagenesis. Nature. 2020;578:166–71.

30. Rege TA, Fears CY, Gladson CL. Endogenous inhibitors of angiogenesis in malignant gliomas: nature's antiangiogenic therapy. Neuro Oncol. 2005;7:106–21.

31. Qin EY, et al. Neural precursor-derived pleiotrophin mediates subventricular zone invasion by glioma. Cell. 2017;170:845–859.e19.

32. Faulkner S, Jobling P, March B, Jiang CC, Hondermarck H. Tumor neurobiology and the war of nerves in cancer. Cancer Discov. 2019;9:702–10.

33. Zeng Q, et al. Synaptic proximity enables NMDAR signalling to promote brain metastasis. Nature. 2019;573:526–31.

34. Samudra N, Zacharias T, Plitt A, Lega B, Pan E. Seizures in glioma patients: an overview of incidence, etiology, and therapies. J Neurol Sci. 2019;404:80–5.

35. van Breemen MSM, Wilms EB, Vecht CJ. Epilepsy in patients with brain tumours: epidemiology, mechanisms, and management. Lancet Neurol. 2007;6:421–30.

36. Kerkhof M, Benit C, Duran-Pena A, Vecht CJ. Seizures in oligodendroglial tumors. CNS Oncol. 2015;4:347–56.
37. Vecht CJ, Kerkhof M, Duran-Pena A. Seizure prognosis in brain tumors: new insights and evidence-based management. Oncologist. 2014;19:751–9.
38. van Breemen MSM, et al. Efficacy of anti-epileptic drugs in patients with gliomas and seizures. J Neurol. 2009;256:1519–26.
39. Robel S, et al. Reactive astrogliosis causes the development of spontaneous seizures. J Neurosci. 2015;35:3330–45.
40. Sato H, Tamba M, Ishii T, Bannai S. Cloning and expression of a plasma membrane cystine/glutamate exchange transporter composed of two distinct proteins. J Biol Chem. 1999;274:11455–8.
41. Deneke SM, Fanburg BL. Regulation of cellular glutathione. Am J Phys. 1989;257:L163–73.
42. Robert SM, et al. SLC7A11 expression is associated with seizures and predicts poor survival in patients with malignant glioma. Sci Transl Med. 2015;7:289ra86.
43. Buckingham SC, et al. Glutamate release by primary brain tumors induces epileptic activity. Nat Med. 2011;17:1269–74.
44. Hatcher A, et al. Pathogenesis of peritumoral hyperexcitability in an immunocompetent CRISPR-based glioblastoma model. J Clin Invest. 2020;130:2286–300.
45. de Groot JF, Liu TJ, Fuller G, Yung WKA. The excitatory amino acid transporter-2 induces apoptosis and decreases glioma growth in vitro and in vivo. Cancer Res. 2005;65:1934–40.
46. Barker-Haliski M, White HS. Glutamatergic mechanisms associated with seizures and epilepsy. Cold Spring Harb Perspect Med. 2015;5:a022863.
47. Yuen TI, et al. Glutamate is associated with a higher risk of seizures in patients with gliomas. Neurology. 2012;79:883–9.
48. Parent JM, et al. Dentate granule cell neurogenesis is increased by seizures and contributes to aberrant network reorganization in the adult rat hippocampus. J Neurosci. 1997;17:3727–38.
49. Parent JM, Valentin VV, Lowenstein DH. Prolonged seizures increase proliferating neuroblasts in the adult rat subventricular zone-olfactory bulb pathway. J Neurosci. 2002;22:3174–88.
50. Parent JM, von dem Bussche N, Lowenstein DH. Prolonged seizures recruit caudal subventricular zone glial progenitors into the injured hippocampus. Hippocampus. 2006;16:321–8.
51. Shtaya A, et al. AMPA receptors and seizures mediate hippocampal radial glia-like stem cell proliferation. Glia. 2018;66:2397–413.
52. Cancer Genome Atlas Research Network. Comprehensive genomic characterization defines human glioblastoma genes and core pathways. Nature. 2008;455:1061–8.
53. Keppler-Noreuil KM, Parker VER, Darling TN, Martinez-Agosto JA. Somatic overgrowth disorders of the PI3K/AKT/mTOR pathway & therapeutic strategies. Am J Med Genet C Semin Med Genet. 2016;172:402–21.
54. Keppler-Noreuil KM, et al. PIK3CA-related overgrowth spectrum (PROS): diagnostic and testing eligibility criteria, differential diagnosis, and evaluation. Am J Med Genet A. 2015;167A:287–95.
55. Mirzaa G, et al. PIK3CA-associated developmental disorders exhibit distinct classes of mutations with variable expression and tissue distribution. JCI Insight. 2016;1:e87623.
56. Marin-Valencia I, Guerrini R, Gleeson JG. Pathogenetic mechanisms of focal cortical dysplasia. Epilepsia. 2014;55:970–8.
57. Jansen LA, et al. PI3K/AKT pathway mutations cause a spectrum of brain malformations from megalencephaly to focal cortical dysplasia. Brain J Neurol. 2015;138:1613–28.
58. D'Gama AM, et al. Mammalian target of rapamycin pathway mutations cause hemimegalencephaly and focal cortical dysplasia. Ann Neurol. 2015;77:720–5.
59. Roy A, et al. Mouse models of human PIK3CA-related brain overgrowth have acutely treatable epilepsy. elife. 2015;4:e12703.
60. Monje M, et al. Roadmap for the emerging field of cancer neuroscience. Cell. 2020;181:219–22.
61. Johung T, Monje M. Neuronal activity in the glioma microenvironment. Curr Opin Neurobiol. 2017;47:156–61.

62. Jung E, et al. Emerging intersections between neuroscience and glioma biology. Nat Neurosci. 2019;22:1951–60.
63. Venkataramani V, Tanev DI, Kuner T, Wick W, Winkler F. Synaptic input to brain tumors: clinical implications. Neuro Oncol. 2020. https://doi.org/10.1093/neuonc/noaa158.
64. Patel DC, Tewari BP, Chaunsali L, Sontheimer H. Neuron-glia interactions in the pathophysiology of epilepsy. Nat Rev Neurosci. 2019;20:282–97.

Index

Printed in the United States
by Baker & Taylor Publisher Services